Glass-Ionomers in Dentistry

Sharanbir K. Sidhu
Editor

Glass-Ionomers in Dentistry

Springer

Editor
Sharanbir K. Sidhu
Adult Oral Health
Institute of Dentistry
Barts and The London School of Medicine and Dentistry
Queen Mary University of London
London
UK

ISBN 978-3-319-37134-4 ISBN 978-3-319-22626-2 (eBook)
DOI 10.1007/978-3-319-22626-2

Springer Cham Heidelberg New York Dordrecht London

Softcover re-print of the Hardcover 1st edition 2016

Printed on acid-free paper

Springer International Publishing AG Switzerland is part of Springer Science+Business Media (www.springer.com)

Foreword

I welcome the publication of a book which sets out to establish the current status and future prospects for the development of an important group of materials. Dr Alan Wilson, who is considered the father of glass-ionomer chemistry, would have been delighted that a group of materials based on his original ideas back in the 1970s had come to such prominence. Acknowledgement of the work of Dr Denis Smith in identifying the potential of polycarboxylate-based materials in dentistry also needs to be made. The initial limitations of glass-ionomers which restricted their clinical use have been addressed by various additions and modifications over many years. This has led to some confusion amongst dentists and researchers who have quite rightly asked the question – 'when is a glass-ionomer not a glass-ionomer?' Even ISO standards which set out to define composition and minimum performance requirements for materials remain somewhat equivocal on this subject.

The group of authors, brought together from the UK and Australia/New Zealand, not forgetting a key contribution from Malta, have tried to address the confusion in a logical way. They represent all stakeholders, including manufacturers, materials scientists, academic clinicians and general practitioners. Overall, it is a useful addition to the bookshelves of all interested parties.

John McCabe
Emeritus Professor
Newcastle-upon-Tyne
UK

Preface

As editor of this monograph, I am grateful to the distinguished colleagues who so willingly gave up their time to contribute to it with their expertise. It would not have been possible without their passion and hard work in sharing their knowledge. I am also grateful to several individuals notably Professors Timothy F Watson, John F McCabe and Martin J Tyas, as well as Dr Graham J Mount, who have been so inspirational and provided me with much-valued mentorship in glass-ionomer cements over the years. I would also like to thank my family for the forbearance and support in my endeavours.

This monograph was inspired by the continuing and new roles of glass-ionomer cement materials in restorative dentistry. The indications for their use have extended over the years and now cover a wide range from lining, bonding, sealing, luting or restoring a tooth, as well as assisting in healing and hypersensitivity. Of particular interest, these materials have paved the way to new and modified approaches to dealing with established and early caries. Modern-day glass-ionomers are considered as bioactive adhesive restorative materials that release ions that can play a part in remineralization or healing of tooth structure. They now have specific or niche roles in clinical techniques such as minimally invasive approaches.

The monograph is somewhat deliberately structured to commence with the first chapter providing a rare historical perspective regarding the discoveries in the laboratory in London that led to the invention of glass-ionomer cements. This forms the basis for an introduction to the subject matter and is followed by chapters dealing mainly with clinical aspects. The next chapters focus on the nature of these materials, how they perform clinically as well as the benefits and limitations of their use. The shift in emphasis from a purely restorative to a therapeutic role, in terms of the anticaries and remineralizing potential of glass-ionomer cements, is highlighted in the chapter on minimum intervention which also reflects their impact on the minimally invasive era. The next section continues with contemporary views on their use in endodontics and in paediatric dentistry. The final chapter discusses future avenues and developing technologies for further improvement of glass-ionomers. While it is impossible to cover every aspect of these materials, it is hoped that the contents are of interest to undergraduate and postgraduate students, a wide range of dental clinical professionals as well as researchers and scientists.

Although there is little doubt that more needs to be done before they reach their full potential, the future for this group of materials would appear relatively promising.

Sharanbir K. Sidhu
London, UK

Contents

Contributors

Katie Bach, BDS, DCD Oral Health Unit, Auckland District Health Board, Auckland, New Zealand

Avijit Banerjee, BDS, MSc, PhD Conservative & MI Dentistry, King's College London Dental Institute at Guy's Hospital, King's Health Partners, Guy's Dental Hospital, London, UK

Michael F. Burrow, BDS, MDS, PhD, DDSc, MEd Restorative Dentistry, Melbourne Dental School, The University of Melbourne, Carlton, VIC, Australia

Josette Camilleri, BChD, MPhil, PhD Department of Restorative Dentistry, Faculty of Dental Surgery, Medical School, Mater Dei Hospital, University of Malta, Msida, Malta

Joshua J. Cheetham, BE, MBA, PhD Department of Research and Development, SDI Limited, Bayswater, VIC, Australia

Geoffrey M. Knight, BDSc, MSc, MBA, PhD Private Practice, Brighton, VIC, Australia

David John Manton, BDSc, MDSc, PhD Department of Growth and Development, University of Melbourne, Melbourne Dental School, Carlton, VIC, Australia

John W. Nicholson, BSc, PhD, DSc Bluefield Centre for Biomaterials, London, UK

1 The History and Background to Glass-Ionomer Dental Cements

John W. Nicholson

Abstract

This chapter provides a historical perspective and an insight into how the glass-ionomer cement was invented following a long series of studies on dental cements, beginning with the now obsolete dental silicate cement. It reviews the experiments on the predecessor materials and also the early studies of the glass-ionomer dental cement. Glass-ionomer cements emerged from research on the former dental silicate cement and the zinc polycarboxylate cement. Dental silicates were poorly understood materials in the early 1960s when studies were started at the Laboratory of the Government Chemist in the UK. These studies showed for the first time that dental silicates were acid–base materials that set to form a matrix of metal phosphates containing unreacted glass filler. From this, the role of the glass was understood for the first time and, in particular, the importance of its alumina/silica ratio in controlling basicity. Following this discovery, the means of producing a practical glass-polyacrylate dental cement was clear and was achieved by altering the alumina/silica ratio of the glass to increase its basicity and balance the reduced acidity of the poly(acrylic acid). The original glass capable of forming a practical cement, known as G200, was high in fluoride and hence fairly opaque compared with modern ionomer glasses. Consideration of the role of fluoride led to the concept of chelating additives to control the setting reaction which led to the discovery of the effect of tartaric acid. This allowed glass-ionomer cements of good translucency for clinical use to be developed. These inventions led on to the pioneering work described in this chapter in which the setting reactions were elucidated, the role of water established, the release of fluoride studied and the factors affecting strength determined. This knowledge informed early ideas of how these materials might be used in dentistry, and the chapter concludes with a review of these early clinical applications.

J.W. Nicholson, BSc, PhD, DSc
Director, Bluefield Centre for Biomaterials, London, UK
e-mail: john.nicholson@bluefieldcentre.co.uk

S.K. Sidhu (ed.), *Glass-Ionomers in Dentistry*, DOI 10.1007/978-3-319-22626-2_1

1.1 Introduction

A substantial part of modern dentistry is concerned with the restoration of function and increasingly the appearance of the teeth following damage by caries, non-carious tooth surface loss or occasionally through trauma.

The topic of dental materials is a critical aspect of restorative dentistry (Wilson 1978). It is a complicated subject, as it is not only concerned with mechanical and chemical function, i.e. strength and toxicity/biocompatibility. It also includes considerations of aesthetics, as increasingly good matches for the appearance of the natural tooth are required as patients are concerned about the cosmetic aspects of tooth repair at least as much as function (Mount and Hume 2005).

For much of the history of restorative dentistry, functional repair was considered paramount, and aesthetic considerations simply did not feature in the process of selection of materials. Repairs were made using either silver amalgam or gold foil (Skinner and Phillips 1960). The former was more economical, and silver amalgam has remained until now a widely used material within restorative dentistry throughout the world, particularly in certain geographical locations (Kovarick 2009).

However, for well over a hundred years, dental cements have been available to the profession which, if not fully matching the appearance of the natural tooth, were at least white and less obtrusive than either gold foil or silver amalgam. The first of these cements was the zinc oxychloride cement invented by Sorel in 1855 (Sorel 1855). It was prepared by reaction of zinc oxide powder with aqueous solutions of zinc chloride. The concentration of zinc chloride was quite high, typically of the order of 40–50 % by mass, so that reaction with zinc oxide powder was rapid and quickly led to the formation of a solid ceramic-like mass of reasonable strength and insolubility in oral fluids. This cement was pioneered in dentistry in 1858, but proved unsuccessful (Wilson 1978). It was difficult to manipulate and subject to erosion within the mouth; hence, its overall clinical performance was poor.

Next came the zinc phosphate cement, which was invented around 1878 (Pierce 1879). It was not particularly successful as first formulated, but was refined by Fleck in 1902 (Fleck 1902), as a result of which it was much easier to use and capable of satisfactory service in clinical dentistry. The refinements introduced by Fleck were necessary in order to reduce the excessively vigorous setting reaction between the components, zinc oxide and aqueous phosphoric acid. The modifications involved changes to both components to slow down the setting reaction and to reduce the exotherm. The zinc oxide powder was deactivated by heat treatment in the range 1100–1200 °C. This causes a degree of sintering between the particles of the powder and also a slight loss of the oxygen to form a nonstoichiometric compound $Zn_{(1+x)}O$, where x is up to 70 ppm (Dollimore and Spooner 1971). The resulting solid is pale yellow in colour and reacts much more slowly with the phosphoric acid solution than untreated zinc oxide, so that a satisfactory paste can be mixed and placed prior to setting.

The phosphoric acid solution was also deactivated to prevent the reaction with zinc oxide occurring too quickly. This was achieved by incorporation of controlled amounts of aluminium and zinc salts. They have the effect of pre-reacting with a small portion of the acid to form salts of the type which make up the matrix of the set cement and hence can be readily incorporated as the cement solidifies. The overall effect of these additives is to reduce reactivity and contribute to the ease of mixing of the final cement formulation.

The resulting cement has excellent properties and is still widely used in clinical dentistry, notably for luting crowns (Hill and Lott 2011). The cement is easy to mix, forms a smooth off-white paste and hardens at an appropriate rate to give a strong solid with good dimensional stability.

The third cement in this group is the now obsolete dental silicate cement. Of the three cements, it attained the highest degree of clinical importance and was also critical to the development of the glass-ionomer cement. Although successful, it was a material with deficiencies in clinical service, and it was because of these deficiencies that the Laboratory of the Government Chemist in the UK was called upon to investigate these materials

(Wilson 1996a). A small group was established under the leadership of Dr. Alan Wilson, whose pioneering work in understanding the setting and structure of the dental silicate cement paved the way for the invention of the far superior glass-ionomer cement (Wilson and Kent 1971).

The early history of the dental silicate cement is obscure (Wilson 1978) though there is evidence that it may date back as far as the zinc phosphate cement. However, it was not until 1908 that a successful version appeared (Schoenbeck 1980). This cement, like the others already described, is a two-component material. The powder was a glass based on calcium aluminosilicate with added fluoride flux, and the liquid was a concentrated solution of phosphoric acid. Like the zinc phosphate cement, the dental silicate cement was improved considerably by the inclusion of salts in the aqueous phosphoric acid component, as this reduced the vigour of the setting reaction and allowed workable pastes to be mixed and placed. The paste that was formed was off-white and set rapidly to form a solid, strong material with a degree of translucency. This translucency gave an appearance that was superior to that of the zinc phosphate cement, and this made the cement suitable for the aesthetic repair of the anterior teeth (Wilson 1978). Another advantage of the dental silicate cement was that the strength was high, of the order of 250–300 MPa in compression at 24 h. This was also a superior property of these cements compared with the zinc phosphate cement.

Development of a proper understanding of the setting and structure of dental silicate cements was slow. Due to its importance in the genesis of the glass-ionomer cement, this topic is considered in detail in the next section of this chapter.

1.2 Dental Silicate Cement

Until the 1960s, dental silicate cement was the most widely used filling material for the anterior teeth. In fact, until the first simple acrylic-based composite materials appeared in the mid-1950s, it was the only aesthetic (tooth-coloured) dental material available to dental clinicians (Kakaboura and Vougiouklakis 2001; Wilson and Nicholson 1993). In the mid-1960s, 40 brands were available (Wilson 1969), but with the advent of the first bis-GMA composite resins in 1962, and then the glass-ionomer in 1971, its use has dwindled and it is now almost completely obsolete.

The name dental silicate is incorrect and was applied early in its history in the erroneous belief that the setting involved the formation of a silicate structure (Voelker 1916). It was the early work of Wilson and his co-workers in the 1960s that established that the cement is, in fact, phosphate-bonded (Wilson and Nicholson 1993).

The earliest successful dental silicate cement was developed by Steenbock in the early years of the twentieth century (Steenbock 1904). This cement used glasses based on blends of calcium alumina-silicates and beryllium silicates (Steenbock 1904), compositions which almost certainly gave cements of poor translucency (Wilson and Nicholson 1993). An early development was the inclusion of fluoride, initially as a flux to lower the melting temperature of the glass-forming mixture. The presence of fluoride not only lowered the melting temperature of the glass; it also improved both the strength and the translucency of the set cement (Wilson and Nicholson 1993). By 1938, all dental silicate glasses were fluoride-containing and also were no longer formulated with beryllium silicates (Paffenbarger et al. 1938). In other words, they were calcium fluoro-aluminosilicates of the same general type as modern glasses for glass-ionomer cements (Wilson and Nicholson 1993).

Although dental silicate cements were strong and aesthetic, and also offered the therapeutic benefit of sustained fluoride release, they had several drawbacks. These were noted by early workers in the field (Wilson and Nicholson 1993) and included porosity, a tendency to stain, a susceptibility to acid attack in the mouth, dimensional instability and the absence of adhesion to the tooth. In certain patients, the acid attack could be so severe that the restoration eroded significantly and even disappeared completely in extreme cases (Wilson and Nicholson 1993)

These problems were tolerated for many years, but in the early 1960s, it was no longer considered acceptable within the UK. At this time, the UK Department of Scientific and Industrial Research (DSIR) set up a committee to stimulate and co-ordinate research in universities and government research establishments on the subject of dental materials and equipment (Wilson 1996a). It was through this committee that the Laboratory of the Government Chemist became involved. This organisation is now a private company, operating as LGC and based in Teddington but was originally established as a public sector laboratory in 1842, based in central London (Hammond and Egan 1992). It has a wide-ranging brief to apply chemical analysis in the service of government, mainly where issues of revenue are at stake. Improving the reliability of dental silicate cements fell within this remit because of the cost of this failure to the tax payer-funded National Health Service in the UK. The original commission to the Laboratory of the Government Chemist from the DSIR was to examine the structure and properties of silicate cements with the aim of determining whether or not they had any potential for improvement (Wilson 1996a).

1.2.1 Composition of Dental Silicates

As we have seen, dental silicate glasses were based on the SiO_2–Al_2O_3–CaF_2 system, with a relatively high aluminium to silicon (Al/Si) ratio. This composition is necessary in order to make the glass basic, a requirement for reaction with aqueous phosphoric acid in the setting process. The Al/Si ratio controls the basicity of the glass and hence the ability of the glass to react with acid solutions (Wilson 1996b). The Al/Si ratio is lower in dental silicate glasses than that in glasses for glass-ionomer cements because of the different strengths of the acids involved in the setting reaction. The acid in glass-ionomers is a weak organic acid based on a water-soluble polymer such as poly(acrylic acid), whereas the acid in dental silicates is strong. However, the discovery of the rate-modifying effects of (+)-tartaric acid in glass-ionomer cements has somewhat obscured these differences. A wider range of glasses, including those with Al/Si ratios approaching those in dental silicate glasses, are capable of forming glass-ionomer cements when (+)-tartaric acid is present in the acid liquid (Wilson 1996a).

Table 1.1 Composition of typical dental silicate liquid

Species	Mass (%)
H_3PO_4	48.8
Al	1.6
Zn	6.1
H_2O	43.3

Based on data from Wilson and Nicholson (1993)

The liquids in dental silicate cements were concentrated solutions of orthophosphoric acid H_3PO_4, generally with additions of aluminium and zinc (Wilson et al. 1968), as shown in Table 1.1. The optimum acid concentration was 48–55 % by mass (Wilson et al. 1970a), although higher concentrations were used in certain brands. Important properties of dental silicate cements relate to the concentration of the phosphoric acid in the liquid component, including strength and resistance to acid attack (Wilson et al. 1970a, 1979).

The sensitivity of these properties to acid concentration led to practical difficulties in the deployment of dental silicate cements. The optimum concentration of phosphoric acid is stable only in an atmosphere of 70 % relative humidity. In more humid atmospheres, the solution takes up water, reducing the acid concentration and leading to inferior cements (Paffenbarger et al. 1938; Wilson et al. 1970a; Worner and Docking 1958). Similarly, in less humid atmospheres, the acid liquid loses water and increases the concentration of the acid. Cements made from such solutions are also inferior. This sensitivity to the prevailing humidity was a further disadvantage of these cements as practical dental materials.

1.2.2 The Setting Reaction of Dental Silicate Cements

A critical step in the development of the glass-ionomer cement was the understanding of the setting reaction of the dental silicate cement, which was achieved by Wilson et al. from 1968. The earliest view had been that the cement was formed by gelation of silicic acid in the solid state (Ray 1934). This was shown to be incorrect in a study of the effect of acid storage environments on dental silicates, from which Wilson and Batchelor concluded that the matrix could not be silica gel (Wilson and Batchelor 1968). They suggested initially that the matrix might be a silico-phosphate material instead, but it was then found that infrared spectroscopy could not detect the presence of any P–O–Si bonds (Wilson and Mesley 1968). The nature of the setting reaction was finally established in 1970 in a paper by Wilson et al. (1970b) which, while primarily concerned with the role of water in these cements, showed that the main products of setting were amorphous aluminium phosphates. Some siliceous material was formed, but it remained as a coating around the partly reacted glass filler particles. The set cement was thus shown to consist of partly reacted glass particles embedded in a matrix of calcium phosphate.

Careful examination of the results obtained led Wilson to conclude that the setting of the dental silicate cement took place as follows. As the powder and liquid are mixed, the reaction begins with the attack on the basic glass particles by hydrogen ions from the phosphoric acid solution (Wilson and Mesley 1968; Wilson and Batchelor 1967a). This causes migration of aluminium, calcium and sodium ions into the matrix (Wilson and Kent 1968) and leaves behind what is essentially silicic acid. Fluoride ions are also released into the matrix at this stage (Wilson and Kent 1968), possibly as complexes of the type AlF^{2+} and AlF_2^+, both of which are known from other studies (Connick and Poulsen 1957; O'Reilly 1960; Akitt 1989).

As the metal ions migrate into the matrix phase, the ionised acid forms metal salts based on the anionic species $H_2PO_4^-$ (Kent and Wilson 1969). As this happens, the pH of the matrix rises towards neutral and the reaction gradually ceases. The products formed are substantially insoluble and also rigid, and their formation thus causes the cement to set to a hard non-deformable body. Wilson et al. referred to this process as "precipitation", a term that is not wholly satisfactory as precipitation strictly refers to the formation of an insoluble solid that separates from the solution in which it is formed. Dental silicate cements, like other materials of this type, show no phase separation. Instead, all of the water originally present in the acid solution becomes incorporated into the final cement. In fact, one of the defining features of cements is that they consist of pastes which set hard in their entirety, without expelling water (Wilson and Nicholson 1993).

Despite this infelicity in terminology, the studies by Wilson et al. offered a brilliant explanation of the setting of dental silicate cements. Their results showed that hardening reached 65 % of its final value within 30 min and ceased after about 72 h (Wilson et al. 1972). The pH was shown to reach 5.2 after 48 h. However, electrical conductivity studies showed that some form of reaction continued slowly for at least 7 weeks (Wilson and Kent 1968), though hardness did not change. Strength had been known for some years to continue rising in these materials for at least 12 months after fabrication (Paffenbarger et al. 1938), and hence, the discovery of a slow long-term reaction in the solid state was not particularly surprising. The final matrix, as shown by electron probe microanalysis (Kent et al. 1970), is predominantly amorphous aluminium phosphate that also contains fluorite (CaF_2) and sodium acid phosphates.

As previously mentioned, silicic acid is also formed in the early stages of the setting process. This substance polymerises readily to form silica, SiO_2 (Kent et al. 1970; Tarutani 1989). This result is consistent with the known aqueous chemistry of silica (Iler 1979), in particular that low pH favours the occurrence of silicic acid, $Si(OH)_4$, but this changes rapidly in the pH range 5–6, and gelation to silica becomes favoured (Iler 1979).

Water also plays an important role in the setting and post-hardening reactions of these cements. Its initial function is as the medium for the reaction, but as the setting proceeds, it hydrates the products of reaction and becomes incorporated into the solidifying mass. Studies have shown that water exists in fully hardened cements in two states, namely, bound and unbound water. These have been named alternatively as non-evaporable and evaporable, respectively (Wilson et al. 1979). These two states differ in that bound water is retained by the cement when stored in a strongly desiccating atmosphere for 24 h, whereas the unbound water is lost under these conditions, causing a reduction in mass (Wilson et al. 1979). The precise location of the bound water is not clear, though the possibility of hydrating the components of the aluminium phosphate, particularly the Al^{3+} ions, is likely (Enderby and Nielson 1989).

In their studies of the set cement, Kent et al. 1970 (Tarutani 1989) used glass powders that had been sieved to remove the finest particles. Electron probe microanalysis showed that the matrix of the dental silicate cement contained Al, P, Na and F only, with the Si restricted to layers around the partly reacted glass filler particles. This was important in establishing how these materials set, but it is not a true picture of the elemental distribution in clinical dental silicates. In a later study, Brune and Smith (1982) showed that silicon was distributed throughout the matrix. It seems probable that this was caused by the reaction of very fine glass particles that were so small that they degraded completely as the reaction proceeded. Hence, this later observation does not invalidate the conclusions of Wilson et al. (1970b) that the setting of dental silicates does not consist of the formation of silicates but of phosphates.

1.2.3 Physical Properties of Dental Silicate Cements

Physical properties of dental silicates vary with the powder/liquid ratio and the best cements are mixed at high ratios, up to 4 g/cm^3 (Wilson et al. 1972). Mixing was done by gradually incorporating the powder, so as to minimise the effect of the reaction exotherm between the components of the cement (Brune and Smith 1982). Properties of the resulting cements are shown in Table 1.2.

The values of strength are all quoted at 24 h, but they all continue to rise for at least a year after fabrication (Paffenbarger et al. 1933). The overall strength of the dental silicate is generally considered to be higher than that of any other acid–base cement, though glass-ionomers with strengths exceeding 300 MPa in compression have been reported (Guggenberger et al. 1998).

Table 1.2 Properties of clinical dental silicate cements

Property	Value
Powder/liquid ratio	2.70–4.02
Working time (23 °C), min	3.6
Setting time (37 °C), min	3.25–7.0
Compressive strength (24 h), MPa	68.5–255
Flexural strength (24 h), MPa	24.5
Tensile strength (24 h), MPa	13.6
Solubility/disintegration strength (24 h), %	0.34–0.38
Opacity, $C_{0.7}$	0.42–0.71

Based on data from Wilson and Nicholson (1993)

1.2.4 Solubility and Ion Release

The properties of dissolution and ion release from dental silicate cements were widely investigated, as they were of such importance in the clinical performance of these materials. Erosion and dissolution limited the acceptability of dental silicates, but fluoride release was beneficial in view of the therapeutic effect of fluoride for teeth damaged by caries (ten Cate et al. 2008).

When fully set, dental silicate cements were resistant to attack in neutral solutions. The main species eluted were sodium, fluoride and silica, all in very small amounts (Wilson and Batchelor 1967a). However, before hardening was complete, the cements were vulnerable to attack even in neutral conditions because of the presence of a variety of water-soluble intermediates, including sodium salts, acid phosphates and fluorides.

The removal of such matrix-forming ionic species was found to cause significant changes to the cement surface. To prevent this, clinicians adopted the practice of covering the surface of a freshly placed dental silicate with a layer of varnish. Once a properly formulated dental silicate had hardened fully, it was safe from attack by neutral solutions. It should be noted, though, that poorly formulated cements, including those prepared from incorrect powder/liquid ratios, could contain relatively large amounts of soluble reaction products and consequently disintegrate when immersed in neutral solutions. Studies showed that the main species eluted into neutral solutions were soluble salts of sodium and phosphate and also fluoride (Wilson and Batchelor 1967a, b). As time passed, the rate of elution dropped rapidly, and acid phosphate species ($H_2PO_4^-$ and HPO_4^{2-}) ceased to be released.

By contrast, in acidic conditions, erosion of these cements was shown to be much more rapid (Wilson and Batchelor 1968). This susceptibility to acid attack was suspected as being the cause of the variable performance of these materials from the beginning (Voelker 1916), a view that was confirmed during the 1950s (Norman et al. 1957) and 1960s (Jorgensen 1963). The extent of erosion by acids was found to vary not just with pH but also with their complexing ability. Citric acid, in particular, was found to be especially erosive (Wilson and Batchelor 1968; Stralfors and Eriksson 1969), a concern given the extent to which citric acid drinks are consumed. Studies of erosion of dental silicate cements in service showed that they tended to develop a pattern of grooving at the margin of the restoration and the tooth (Tay et al. 1974, 1979) and, when left unchecked, led to eventual failure of the restoration.

Although dental silicate cements failed under acid attack, their resistance was compared favourably with all other dental cements except the glass-ionomer (Norman et al. 1959; Kuhn et al. 1984). This lack of acid resistance was not considered a particular problem; in fact, when properly prepared and placed, dental silicate cements gave very good results in patients (Robinson 1971). The problem was that the range of optimum performance was relatively narrow. Poor handling and preparation, allowing the acid concentration to change by exposure to the atmosphere at varying humidities and preparing the cement at less than the recommended powder/liquid ratio were all factors that would lead to a cement containing too much water-soluble material and result in clinical failure. It was this unreliability that gave the dental silicate cement its reputation as an unsatisfactory material and left the door open for the development of a much less sensitive material: the glass-ionomer cement.

1.3 Zinc Polycarboxylate Cements

The development of the zinc polycarboxylate cement was also an important step in the invention of the glass-ionomer cement. First reported by Smith in 1968 (Smith 1968), this cement was prepared from the reaction of zinc oxide with aqueous poly(acrylic acid). The setting process involved gelation of the poly(acrylic acid) solution with zinc ions released from the powder as a result of attack by the acid. Setting involved incorporation of all of the water in the original acid solution and the formation of a rigid mass from the initial viscous paste.

The zinc polycarboxylate cement was invented as a result of a rational exploration by Smith of factors that can cause adhesion to the tooth surface, and the work was carried out with the aim of producing a material that could act as a luting cement yet show true adhesion to the tooth (Smith 1968). It was the first inherently adhesive dental material and, as such, represented an important advance in restorative dentistry.

The zinc polycarboxylate cement remains a useful material for clinical dentistry, with applications as liners and bases, luting cements and periodontal packs (Wilson and Nicholson 1993). It can be used in all applications of zinc phosphate cements, with the possible exception of post crowns and cantilever bridges (Smith 1982). This does not mean that zinc phosphate has become obsolete or completely superseded in these applications. The choice of material varies between clinicians, and individual clinical technique may favour one material over the other. Consequently, zinc phosphate is still employed in the restorative dentist's armamentarium.

The critical aspect of the invention of the zinc polycarboxylate was the use of aqueous solutions of poly(acrylic acid) as the cement-forming liquid. Concentrations were relatively high, typically 30–43 % by mass (Wilson and Nicholson 1993), which means that the liquid had a reasonably high viscosity. Although poly(acrylic acid) is the principal acid polymer used in these cements, other polymers were quickly proposed, including copolymers of itaconic or maleic acid (Bertenshaw and Combe 1972).

The molar mass of the polymers used varies between about 22,000 and 49,000 (Bertenshaw and Combe 1976) and needs to be carefully controlled in order to obtain satisfactory cements. High molar mass polymers lead to cements of high strength; however, the consequently high viscosity of the polymer solution makes mixing the cement difficult. As a result, molar mass tends to represent a balance between these conflicting requirements and is chosen as a compromise between being low enough to allow satisfactory mixing and high enough for useful strength. Similar issues arise with the glass-ionomer cement, and molar mass of the constituent polymer for these materials also represents a compromise between the need for ease of mixing and high final strength.

The powders for zinc polycarboxylate cements are also complex and do not consist simply of pure zinc oxide (see Table 1.3). As is the case for zinc phosphate cements, the zinc oxide for zinc polycarboxylates has to be deactivated for use in practical cements. Pure powdered zinc oxide reacts too quickly with aqueous poly(acrylic acid) solution to form a smooth paste. Instead, it forms clumps of powder agglomerated by prematurely formed zinc polyacrylate, and this lumpy mixture cannot be mixed further to form a smooth usable paste.

Zinc oxide is deactivated partly by sintering, as mentioned previously for zinc phosphate, a process which results in a pale yellow powder that is very slightly oxygen-deficient (Dollimore and Spooner 1971). In addition, the zinc oxide is mixed with up to 10 % by mass of magnesium oxide powder. Powders may, in addition, contain silica, alumina or bismuth salts, the latter to impart radiopacity. Another key additive is stannous fluoride, which is added at 4–5 % by mass, and was originally added as a source of fluoride (Foster et al. 1974). In fact, stannous fluoride itself probably dissolves out of these cements, rather than free fluoride, as SnF_2 is soluble in water and exists in aqueous solution at very low levels of dissociation (Turner et al. 2013). In addition to providing a source of fluoride, stannous fluoride was found to increase the strength of zinc polycarboxylate cements (Foster et al. 1974), a phenomenon that has yet to be explained.

The majority of brands of zinc polycarboxylate cement consist of two components, an appropriately formulated deactivated zinc oxide powder and an aqueous solution of polymeric acid, typically poly(acrylic acid). Quite early on, it was found that this cement could be formulated as a dry powder consisting of the zinc oxide powder plus dried polymer, with reaction initiated by mixing this powder with the correct volume of pure water (Bertenshaw and Combe 1972). Setting of these water-activated cements proceeds satisfactorily, and there appear to be no important differences in setting, ultimate strength or clinical performance between these materials and cements formulated more conventionally from aqueous acid solutions.

The way in which zinc polycarboxylate cements are formulated has been shown to influence cement properties, including working and setting times, and strength when set. Factors affecting these include powder/liquid ratio, composition of the powder, molar mass and type of the polymeric acid and also its concentration in the cement-forming liquid (Smith 1971). Typical properties of these cements are shown in Table 1.4.

Setting and hardening of zinc polycarboxylates occur reasonably quickly. A typical formulation

Table 1.3 Composition of zinc polycarboxylate cements

Component	% by mass
Zinc oxide powder: ZnO	85.2–96.8
MgO	4.73–10.06
Poly(acrylic acid), concentration in solution	32.4–42.9

Based on data from Bertenshaw and Combe (1972, 1976)

Table 1.4 Properties of zinc polycarboxylate cements

Property	Value
Working time (23 °C)/min	2–5
Setting time (37 °C)/min	3–12
Compressive strength (24 h)/MPa	48–80
Tensile strength (24 h)/MPa	4.8–15.5
Adhesion to enamel (tensile, 24 h)/MPa	4.1–6.9
Adhesion to dentine (tensile, 24 h)/MPa	2.2–5.1

Based on data from Wilson and Nicholson (1993)

reaches its maximum strength at 24 h, after which it shows little or no change over subsequent time periods (Watts et al. 1979; Osborne et al. 1978; Paddon and Wilson 1976). The cement shows some viscoelastic properties, and measured strength is influenced by the crosshead speed of the testing machine, particularly at low speeds (Wilson and Lewis 1980). This viscoelasticity remains as zinc polycarboxylate cements age, and distinct creep has been detected under static loading conditions in samples aged for 24 h (Wilson and Lewis 1980). Significant stress relaxation was also found in specimens aged for 4 weeks (Paddon and Wilson 1976).

Zinc polycarboxylates were the first adhesive dental restorative materials and have been shown to bond to untreated dentine and enamel (Mizrahi and Smith 1969). Bond strength to enamel is higher than to dentine, as shown in Table 1.4. In general, zinc polycarboxylate appears to be mild in clinical use, having minimal effects on the dental pulp (Plant 1970; Beagrie et al. 1972; Wilson 1968). They are also nonirritating when used in implants in soft tissue and bone (Wilson 1968).

1.4 Invention of the Glass-Ionomer Cement

It is important to understand the nature of the invention of the glass-ionomer cement. It did not consist of simply mixing the glass powder of the dental silicate cement with the poly(acrylic acid) solution of the zinc polycarboxylate and finding that an excellent cement was the result (Wilson 1996a). It is true that early attempts to improve the dental silicate cement did involve experiments with aqueous solutions of organic acids, though these acids were monomeric and the results, while interesting, were not successful in producing cements with significantly improved properties (Wilson 1968).

Poly(acrylic acid) was considered in those early experiments, but the results were so disappointing that they were not reported at the time (Wilson 1968). Instead, they were hinted at some years later (Wilson and McLean 1988) and not described in detail until Wilson published his personal account of the invention of glass-ionomers (Wilson 1996a). It turned out that these early glass-polyacrylate cements were disappointing in the extreme. They formed an intractable paste which underwent a sluggish reaction, as observed by an increase in the viscosity of the paste; hardening was very slow and the product was hydrolytically unstable. This cement was clearly of no use as a potential dental material (Wilson 1996a).

The invention of the glass-ionomer cement was, in fact, not a single act but rather a series of innovative steps. One key step was the finding that the alumina/silica ratio of the glass controlled the resulting basicity and hence the readiness with which a glass powder would react with an acid solution. This pointed the way towards the first successful glass for a glass-ionomer cement, one with sufficient basicity to react with aqueous poly(acrylic acid). Controlling the alumina/silica ratio allowed the glasses to set much more rapidly than the original glass-poly(acrylic acid) mixture, where the glass was of relatively low basicity. These improved mixtures not only set more rapidly; they were also hydrolytically stable when placed in water (Wilson and Kent 1971; Kent et al. 1973).

The first glass to give at least moderately satisfactory cements was designated G200 and contained alumina and silica in the appropriate ratio to give a high basicity; it was also high in fluoride. Its composition is given in Table 1.5. The resulting cement was known as ASPA 1, the term ASPA being an acronym for aluminosilicate poly(acrylic acid). ASPA was also the brand name of the very first commercial glass-ionomer cement, launched in 1975 (Wilson and McLean 1988).

Table 1.5 Composition of the glass G200

Component	% by mass
SiO_2	30.1
Al_2O_3	19.9
AlF_3	2.6
CaF_2	34.5
NaF	3.7
$AlPO_4$	10.0

Based on data from Wilson and McLean (1988)

The first glass-ionomer, based on G200, was far from the finished article, in that it set relatively slowly and retained a high degree of water sensitivity for a considerable time after setting, which was a distinct drawback. In addition, the glass itself was not particularly translucent, and therefore, the resulting cement had poor aesthetics.

The next inventive step along the path to creating a satisfactory glass-ionomer cement was the discovery of the effect of (+)-tartaric acid on the setting reaction. This discovery came about from a consideration of the nature of the G200 glass. It was exceptionally high in fluoride, a factor that seemed to be important as G200 was the only glass capable of forming a usable cement with poly(acrylic acid) solution (Wilson 1996a). Wilson and his team inferred that fluoride ions must play an important part in controlling the setting reaction, suggesting in particular that they interacted with aluminium ions released from the glass and prevented them from prematurely cross-linking the poly(acrylate) polymer chains. This, they postulated, was because of the high affinity of aluminium for fluoride ions and the formation of complex ions of the type AlF^{2+} and AlF_2^+, which had been proposed to occur during the setting of dental silicate cements (Wilson and Kent 1968).

Slowing the reaction of aluminium via chelation seemed to be a way forward. In the gravimetric analysis of rocks, the established method to prevent premature precipitation of aluminium as the phosphate was to include either citric acid or (+)-tartaric acid, both of which were known to form water-soluble complex ions with Al^{3+} (Lundall and Hoffman 1938). These two acids were therefore examined as potential additives in the glass-ionomer cement.

The results were striking, especially with (+)-tartaric acid. The resulting cements had longer working times and sharper setting, seemingly contradictory properties, both of which made the cement mixture easier to mix and to manipulate (Crisp et al. 1975; Wilson et al. 1976). The cements also had improved compressive strength and were more resistant to acid attack. Wilson considered this to be the most important discovery made in the whole process of inventing and developing the glass-ionomer cement (Wilson 1996a). The new formulation was named ASPA II, and it can be considered to be the first really practical glass-ionomer cement.

1.5 Pioneering Studies of Glass-Ionomer Cements

Following the preliminary reports announcing the development of the glass-ionomer cement (Wilson and Kent 1971; Kent et al. 1973), detailed scientific publications on these cements began to appear in 1974. As well as scientific studies, the first clinical report appeared that year (McLean and Wilson 1974). It covered fissure sealing and restoration with glass-ionomers and was the report of a 2-year clinical study undertaken with the original ASPA formulation of glass-ionomer.

The initial scientific studies were concerned with the setting reaction of these materials (Crisp and Wilson 1974a, b; Crisp et al. 1974). They broke the reaction down into two stages: the decomposition of the glass powder (Crisp and Wilson 1974a) and the reaction of the ions released to cross-link the polyacid, which was incorrectly termed "precipitation" (Crisp and Wilson 1974b). Gelation would have been a better term for this part of the setting process.

The remaining paper in this important series describes the application of infrared spectroscopy to the study of the setting reaction (Crisp et al. 1974) and was important in showing that the main products are calcium and aluminium polyacrylates. These two possible products can be distinguished on the basis of their infrared spectra. Calcium polyacrylate shows a carboxylate band at 1540 cm^{-1}, indicating a highly ionic structure, whereas aluminium polyacrylate shows an equivalent band at about 1600 cm^{-1}, indicating a degree of covalent character with distinct chelation of the central Al^{3+} ions by the surrounding carboxylate groups (Crisp et al. 1974). This paper also showed that the fully set cement contained some residual unreacted carboxylic acid groups, trapped within the cement as it hardened and unable to react for steric reasons (Crisp et al. 1974).

1.6 Early Research on Glass-Ionomers

1.6.1 The Composition and Structure of the Glasses

The first practical glasses for use in glass-ionomer cements were calcium aluminosilicates with added fluoride (Wilson and Kent 1971; Kent et al. 1979; Wilson et al. 1980). Their alumina/silica ratio was adjusted to make them sufficiently basic to set on reaction with aqueous poly(acrylic acid). Although numerous other glass systems have been investigated since these early studies, the glasses developed by Wilson and Kent remain the basis of all practical glass-ionomer cements used clinically. The one substantial change has been the development of strontium-containing ionomer glasses (Guida et al. 2003), where the element strontium is used in place of calcium in the formulation.

Fluoride is an essential component of the glasses (Wilson and McLean 1988). This element has several functions within the glass. It lowers the fusion temperature, it improves the working behaviour of the freshly mixed cement paste by preventing premature gelation and it improves the strength of the set cement. Fluoride-containing glasses are much less opaque than pure oxide ones, and this in turn means that cements prepared from them have improved translucency.

The essential property of glasses for use in glass-ionomer cements is that they are basic and can react with aqueous solutions of acid (Hill and Wilson 1988). This property arises from the ratio of alumina to silica in the glass. Right from the start of research into workable glasses for these cements, this need for basicity and how it could be achieved were well understood. The theoretical framework for this understanding was the random network model of glass as advanced by Zachariasen in 1932 (Zachariasen 1932).

This model considers the glass structure to be a random assembly of oxygen polyhedral, each comprising a small central cation surrounded by a number of negatively charged oxygen ions. A typical polyhedron is (SiO_4). These structures are linked at the corners via the oxygen ions to form an array of chains and interconnected units. The overall concept thus views a glass as consisting essentially of a polymer based on (SiO_4) tetrahedra joined at the corners and exhibiting varying degrees of cross-linking.

The reactivity of such glass structures towards aqueous acids can be increased by including cations such as calcium that can break up the continuous Si–O–Si structural units to form non-bridging oxygen. These ions are described as "network modifying":

$$-Si-O-Si- + CaO \rightarrow -Si-O^{-}Ca^{2+}\,{}^{-}O-Si-$$

The inclusion of aluminium has more complex effects than the inclusion of simpler chemical species such as calcium or sodium. Aluminium can act as a network modifier in an analogous way to calcium, but it can also be a network former. In the latter case, the presence of reasonable amounts of silica as tetrahedral building blocks of (SiO_4) forces the aluminium to adopt a similar tetrahedral geometry and to form species equivalent to (AlO_4). Although these tetrahedra are the same size as the (SiO_4) ones, they carry more formal charge. This is because the central cation is a 3+ ion, compared to the formal 4+ charge on the central silicon in (SiO_4). The presence of the (AlO_4) tetrahedra therefore has to be balanced by additional cations (e.g. Na^+, Ca^{2+}) in the structure close to the main oxide network (Lowenstein 1954).

These ideas show that the aluminosilicate glass structure of ionomer glasses can be regarded as consisting of linked (SiO_4) and (AlO_4) tetrahedral, with additional cations to balance the charge deficiency due to aluminium. It is the alumina units and their associated cations that serve as the point of reaction with aqueous acid solution, and reaction of the acid involves removal of the charge-balancing cations, followed by rupture of the aluminosilicate network (Wilson and McLean 1988). The Al/Si ratio cannot apparently be greater than 1:1; otherwise there are insufficient (SiO_4) tetrahedral to force the aluminium into fourfold co-ordination, and high basicity does not develop (Lowenstein 1954). Glasses for ionomer cements must have a minimum Al/Si ratio of 1:2, with practical glasses having ratios above this limit (Kent et al. 1979; Wilson et al. 1980). The upper limit in this ratio was found to be 0.75:1 by mass early in these studies (Wilson and McLean 1988), this limit being the point at which the mineral phase corundum (Al_2O_3) crystallises out within the glass structure. Glasses containing two distinct phases are inherently opaque, and resulting cements lack the aesthetics for clinical use.

The three essential components of the early glasses for ionomer cements were silica, alumina and fluorite, i.e. SiO_2, Al_2O_3 and CaF_2. In practice, additional components were added in order to improve properties such as the setting rate, translucency and final strength (Wilson and McLean 1988). Practical glasses typically belonged to complex systems such as:

$$SiO_2 - Al_2O_3 - CaF_2 - AlPO_4 - Na_3AlF_2$$

Table 1.6 Relationship between composition and cement properties for early ionomer glasses

Code	G241	G278	G279	G282
Composition				
SiO_2	120	120	120	120
Al_2O_3	102	102	102	102
CaO	112	101	84	11.2
CaF_2	0	15.6	39	140
Appearance below T_g	Clear	Clear	Clear	Opaque
Powder/liquid ratio/g cm^{-3}	2.5	2.5	2.0	2.5
Setting time (37 °C)/min	2.25	2.25	[a]	3.0
Compressive strength (24 h)/MPa	74	125	[a]	165

Based on data from Kent et al. (1979)

[a]Cement unworkable (set too quickly), hence no setting time recorded, and no specimens could be made for determination of compressive strength

The glasses were prepared by fusion of these components, typically in a ceramic crucible, with fusion temperatures varying between 1100 °C and 1500 °C, depending on the precise chemical composition of the fusion mixture (Wilson and McLean 1988; Hill and Wilson 1988). After melting and allowing the mixture to become thoroughly homogeneous at an elevated temperature, the melt was cooled rapidly by pouring it either onto a metal plate or directly into water. This resulted in the formation of a glass frit consisting of large pieces of glass. It was then ground to a fine powder, typically of 20–50 μm, depending on the clinical application of the cement (Wilson and McLean 1988).

The preparation results in glasses of varying structures. Some show a degree of phase separation that leads to an opaque appearance (Hill and Wilson 1988), whereas others have no visible phase separation and are clear in appearance. Phase-separated glasses were found to give rise to stronger cements than clear glasses (Wilson and Nicholson 1993; Kent et al. 1979), as shown by the results in Table 1.6.

The structure of G200, the first successful ionomer glass, was reported in 1979 (Barry et al. 1979). Although differing somewhat from modern ionomer glasses in that it is low in sodium and very high in fluoride, G200 was found to show some distinctive features that appear to be typical of glasses capable of forming satisfactory glass-ionomer cements. It was shown by scanning electron microscopy to contain phase-separated droplets of complex structure as well as substantial deposits of crystalline fluorite (Barry et al. 1979). The phase-separated droplets had an average diameter of 1.7 μm and represented about 20 % of the volume fraction of the glass. They had a different chemical composition from the rest of the glass and in particular were found to be richer in calcium than the surroundings. These phases were found to vary in basicity, meaning that acid attack occurred preferentially at the most basic of them, causing relatively high levels of calcium to be released from the glass compared with its overall calcium content. This has also been found for the more modern ionomer glass G338 (Wasson and Nicholson 1991). This is a glass that is widely used in clinical glass-ionomer cements and whose composition is given in Table 1.7.

The fact that glasses containing a droplet phase gave stronger cements led to some early work in which the amount of the disperse phase

Table 1.7 Composition of the glass G338

Component	% by mass
SiO_2	24.9
Al_2O_3	14.2
AlF_3	4.6
CaF_2	12.8
$NaAlF_6$	19.2
$AlPO_4$	24.2

Based on data from Wasson and Nicholson (1991)

Table 1.8 Effect of phase-separated crystallites on strength of cements

Glass	Crystalline phase	Flexural strength/MPa
G228	None	21
G309	Fluorite (CaF_2), corundum (Al_2O_3)	33
G381	Baddeleyite (ZrO_2)	28
G385	Rutile (TiO_2), tieilite (Al_2TiO_5)	30

Based on data from Prosser et al. (1986)

was deliberately increased in certain experimental glasses (Prosser et al. 1986). In this study, the mechanical property studied was flexural strength rather than compressive strength, but it was found that where identifiable disperse phases could be introduced, there was indeed a rise in strength. These results are shown in Table 1.8.

1.6.2 The Acidic Polymer Component

The original polymeric acid used in glass-ionomer cements was poly(acrylic acid) (Wilson and Kent 1971). It is still the most widely used acid, though a variety of other polymers have been studied since this acid was first reported. It was, of course, the polymer used in zinc polycarboxylates (Smith 1968) and, hence, was the natural choice when the glass-ionomers were being developed (Wilson 1996a).

Poly(acrylic acid) is an example of the class of substances called polyelectrolytes (Hara 1993). These are substances which combine the features of being both polymers and electrolytes. They derive the latter feature from the presence along the polymer chain of a substantial number of functional groups that are capable of carrying an electrical charge. In the case of most of the polyelectrolytes used to prepare glass-ionomer cements, these functional groups are carboxylic acids, $-CO_2H$. The physical chemistry of polyelectrolytes is complicated (Hara 1993) but can largely be neglected in considering the use of these substances for forming glass-ionomer cements. However, the presence of the polar functional groups able to carry charge does confer one very important property, namely, that polyelectrolytes are generally soluble in water (Hara 1993).

The polyelectrolytes used to prepare glass-ionomer cements are poly(alkenoic acid)s. This was recognised many years ago in the nomenclature agreed by the International Organization for Standardization (ISO) for these materials, where the formal name is glass polyalkenoate cement (Wilson and McLean 1988). In addition to the homopolymer of acrylic acid, copolymers were also studied in the early years of research on glass-ionomers (Crisp et al. 1980a; Schmidt et al. 1981), the main ones being acrylic/itaconic acid (Crisp et al. 1980a) and acrylic/maleic acid (Schmidt et al. 1981). The latter has become commercially important (Nicholson 2000), though the majority of commercial glass-ionomer cements are still formulated with poly(acrylic acid) homopolymer.

The solution of the polymeric acid is used at relatively high concentrations, typically in the range 40–50 % by mass (Wilson and McLean 1988). An early publication demonstrated the importance of the acid concentration in a study involving cements made from the glass G200 (Crisp et al. 1977). The cements in this study were also formulated to include tartaric acid, since the effect of this substance had been discovered by this stage. However, the ratio of tartaric acid to poly(acrylic acid) was maintained constant in all experiments, in order to avoid complicating the results. Unfortunately, the study involved cements formulated at varying powder/liquid ratios, as the aim was to keep the consistency of the freshly mixed cement pastes constant. This part of the study showed, not surprisingly, that as the polymer concentration

Table 1.9 Variation in properties of glass-ionomer cements with varying polymer concentrations

Concentration property	28.6 %	42.9 %	52.0 %
Compressive strength (24 h)/MPa	35	110	152
Diametral tensile strength (24 h)/MPa	4	9	12

Based on data from Crisp et al. (1977)

Table 1.10 Variation in properties of glass-ionomer cements with varying molar masses

Molar mass property	27,000	76,000	230,000
Working time (23 °C)/min	9.25	4.75	2.75
Setting time (37 °C)/min	6.50	5.00	3.25
Compressive strength (24 h)/MPa	17.0	31.0	113.0
Diametral tensile strength (24 h)/MPa	2.9	3.4	5.8

Based on data from Wilson et al. (1977a)

was reduced, more powder was needed to produce a cement of equivalent consistency. This did make results difficult to interpret. However, there were useful findings specifically that as polymer concentrations were lowered, the strengths of the resulting cements were reduced. Selected results from this study are shown in Table 1.9.

Another feature of the polymer which is important in controlling the properties of glass-ionomer cements is the molar mass (molecular weight) (Wilson et al. 1977a). This was first shown in a study which reported the properties of cements prepared from commercial poly(acrylic acid) samples of widely differing molar masses. The polymers were all used at a concentration in water of 25 % by mass, and cements were prepared from them at several different powder/liquid ratios. Some highlights from the data obtained are shown in Table 1.10, and these results show clearly that both the speed of the setting reaction and the eventual strength of the set cement vary with the molar mass of the polymer used.

These results also showed that, as with concentration, there was a balance to be struck between the speed of setting (and also ease of mixing which this implies) and compressive strength. High molar mass polymers give strong cements but set quicker than cements made from low molar mass polymers.

1.6.3 Tartaric Acid and Its Role

An early observation was that available fluoride present in the glass had considerable influence on the working time of glass-ionomer cements (Crisp et al. 1974). This was attributed to the ready formation of aluminium fluoride complexes, with the argument being that complexed aluminium fluoride complex ions were not immediately available for interacting with polyanion chains in the cement and cross-linking them. As a result, the working time was prolonged.

This led to the search for chelating agents that could be added to the cement and extend the working time by combining with ions leached from the glass, preventing them from interacting with the polyanion chains. In this way, premature gelation would be avoided and the working time extended. It was recognised that acidic chelating agents would be advantageous, as they could aid the removal of the cations from the glass and also suppress the ionisation and uncoiling of the polymer chains, thus further prolonging working time (Wilson et al. 1976).

The initial search for a successful chelating additive included a wide range of substances (see Table 1.11). These included hydroxyacids, such as tartaric acid and citric acid, hydroxybenzoic acids, diketones, ethanolamine and urea. The study involved the use of the oscillating rheometer to monitor setting profiles, from which the working time could be determined. Working times were also confirmed using a modified Gillmore needle, where resistance to indentation by a weighted needle is taken as the criterion of workability. Two methods were used because working time is not an exact property. Defining it by laboratory tests is not straightforward, though these early papers by Wilson et al. (1976) clarified a method that has since been widely used and which replaces much of the subjectivity that otherwise surrounds the concept. In fact, the two experimental methods used gave results that were in good agreement (Wilson et al. 1976).

As well as working time, the gel time was recorded (Wilson et al. 1976). This effectively corresponded to the setting time, but at a temperature of 23 °C. It was taken to be the time at

Table 1.11 Effect of chelating agents on the setting of ASPA glass-ionomer cement

Additive	P/L ratio (g/cm^3)	Working time (min)	Gel time (min)
None	3.5	1.8	9
None	4.0	2.4	8
5 % tartaric acid	3.5	2.0	6
5 % tartaric acid	4.0	1.9	5
5 % citric acid	4.0	1.9	6
2 % 2,6-dihydroxy benzoic acid	4.0	2.1	9
2 % acetylacetone	4.0	2.3	8
5 % urea	3.5	2.2	15
5 % ethanolamine	3.5	3.5	19

Based on data from Wilson et al. (1976)

Table 1.12 Infrared absorption band (C=O asymmetric stretch) for species present in cements formulated with tartaric acid

Species	Band (cm^{-1})
Ca-tartrate	1595
Al-tartrate	1670
Ca-polyacrylate	1550
Al-polyacrylate	1559

Based on data from Nicholson et al. (1988)

which the cement was shown to be set on the oscillating rheometer, as characterised by the rheometer showing only small but constant amplitude.

Additives were found to have a variety of effects, but the best of them were tartaric acid and citric acid, with the former being superior overall. In both cases, they sharpened the setting rate, and this generally meant increasing the working time and reducing the gel time. The effects were greater with tartaric acid, and there was also some evidence that the resulting cements were less soluble in water than those containing citric acid (Wilson et al. 1976).

The effects of including tartaric acid in the cement formulation were studied in detail, mainly by infrared spectroscopy (Crisp and Wilson 1976). Samples were examined using the attenuated total reflectance (ATR) technique in which they were pressed against the face of a crystal and the spectrum recorded in reflectance mode. Also, ionic extracts were obtained from the cements at various time intervals and analysed. The results of the two approaches were combined in order to obtain a detailed account of the cement-forming reactions in the presence of tartaric acid. This study used G200 glass and a liquid comprising 47.5 % by mass poly(acrylic acid) and 5 % by mass tartaric acid. A powder/liquid ratio of 1.5 g/cm^3 was used, which is lower than that of practical cements. However, it reacted more slowly than a properly formulated cement, and this gave time to collect the spectra, which allowed the reaction to be studied in reasonable detail.

The results of the ATR infrared part of the study were not particularly informative, partly because the absorption bands were broad and ill-defined. Attempts were made to monitor the reduction in the carboxylic acid bands, whose asymmetric stretch occurs at about 1700 cm^{-1}, and to monitor the increase in carboxylate salt bands, at 1540 cm^{-1} and 1600 cm^{-1} for calcium and aluminium, respectively. It was not until FTIR was first used in 1988 (Nicholson et al. 1988) that the differences between the positions of the bands due to the metal salts of poly(acrylic acid) and tartaric acid could be identified (Table 1.12). Consequently, the early studies by Crisp and Wilson (1976) were not able to confirm the early appearance of calcium and aluminium tartrates, nor the corresponding delay in the appearance of the respective polyacrylate salts. Nonetheless, they were able to confirm the essential similarity of the setting reaction with and without tartaric acid and that the presence of tartaric acid acts in part by increasing the rate at which ions are liberated from the glass powder in the first step of the process (Crisp and Wilson 1976).

Another early study applied ^{13}C NMR spectroscopy to the setting of glass-ionomer cements (Prosser et al. 1982). This showed quite clearly that the initial reaction is between the glass powder and the tartaric acid, forming complex tartrate cations. As neutralisation proceeds and pH reaches about 3, the poly(acrylic acid) starts to be neutralised by metal ions from the glass. The cement sets to a hard mass at pH 5.0–5.5 (Wilson and McLean 1988). Prosser et al. (1982) also noted that the presence of tartaric acid suppressed the ionisation of the poly(acrylic acid) with the result that its uncoiling was delayed. This reduced the viscosity of the cement paste and slowed the onset of gelation.

Glass-ionomer cements containing tartaric acid were found to be stronger than those without any additive (Wilson and McLean 1988; Wilson et al. 1976). This led to the suggestion that these cements contain specific bridging complexes that add strength to the set matrix (Wilson et al. 1976). However, this neglects the likely effect of the lower cement viscosity on mixing. A lower viscosity paste would be easier to manipulate, would wet the glass powder better and be less likely to entrap air during mixing, thus reducing the development of pores within the set material. All of these effects would improve the homogeneity of the mixed cement, reduce flaws and consequently enhance strength.

1.6.4 Maturation and the Role of Water

The main steps in the initial setting reaction were identified and described in the earliest papers on these materials (Crisp and Wilson 1974a, b; Crisp et al. 1974). However, it was also discovered early in the development of glass-ionomers that there were slow changes in the cements that continued for a considerable time, up to at least a year after preparation. For example, compressive strength increased during this time, with the strength being proportional to the logarithm of time (Crisp et al. 1976a).

The mechanical properties as a whole were shown to change with time. A newly hardened cement was shown to behave somewhat like a zinc polycarboxylate cement in that it had a degree of plastic character. Later, as the various slow maturation processes took place, it became much less plastic and increasingly rigid (Paddon and Wilson 1976). No other cements behave in this way. Zinc polycarboxylates, for example, retain their plastic character for considerable periods of time (Paddon and Wilson 1976), and indeed, there is no evidence that they ever lose it.

The changes in mechanical properties were found to correlate with increases in the proportion of bound water within the cement (Wilson et al. 1979, 1981). It was suggested that processes analogous to the hydration reactions in Portland cement took place in glass-ionomers, possibly due to increasing hydration of the metal carboxylate units within the cement (Wilson et al. 1979, 1981).

Due to its correlation with the physical changes on maturation, the role of water in glass-ionomers attracted considerable attention in the early research on these materials. Glass-ionomers are based on water-soluble polymers, yet there is no phase separation on setting, so it was apparent from the start that water played an important part in the structure and setting of these cements (Wilson and McLean 1988). As for dental silicates, water within the set cements was classified into "loosely bound" and "tightly bound", this somewhat arbitrary division being based on whether or not the water can be removed by simple desiccation, by either storage in a desiccator over anhydrous silica gel or by heating at 105 °C for an hour (Wilson et al. 1979, 1981; Wilson and Crisp 1975; Elliot et al. 1975; Crisp et al. 1976b). It was shown that not only did glass-ionomers contain water in these two distinguishable states but also that their ratio changed on ageing. In particular, the proportion of bound water was shown to increase as maturation occurred. This change was accompanied by an increase in the compressive strength and a decrease in the plasticity (Wilson et al. 1979, 1981).

Water was found to be readily exchanged by freshly prepared cements, with water being gained under conditions of high humidity and lost at low humidity. Indeed, glass-ionomers were found to be stable to gain or loss of water only in an atmosphere of 80 % relative humidity (Hornsby 1980). As the cements aged and the proportion of bound water increased, the susceptibility to water loss in low humidity conditions was found to decrease (Hornsby 1980; Saito 1978). The period of time for which the earliest cements were at risk of losing water was found to vary with the brand and ranged between 1 and 30 days (Phillips and Bishop 1985).

Early contact with moisture was also shown to be damaging to freshly prepared glass-ionomer cements (Mount and Makinson 1982; Crisp et al. 1980b; Causton 1981; Earl and Ibbetson 1986). Such contact was shown to cause disruption to the surface, with swelling and loss of ions into the saliva. This led to roughened surfaces and reduced aesthetics (Phillips and Bishop 1985). Research around this time showed that these problems could be prevented by application of an appropriate varnish immediately after placement of the cement (Earl et al. 1985).

1.6.5 Fluoride Release

The ability of glass-ionomer cements to release fluoride is considered clinically beneficial, and it was first observed in the pioneering studies of Wilson and his co-workers (Crisp et al. 1976b). The initial report was concerned with the chemistry of erosion, and fluoride was seen to be part of that. It was soon studied as an independent phenomenon (Forsten 1977; Maldonado et al. 1978), even though the early work showed it to be accompanied by the release of other metal ions, such as sodium and calcium (Crisp et al. 1976b). Release was also shown to be sustained for considerable periods of time, initially for many months, and later for at least 5 years following fabrication of the cement (Forsten 1991).

Quite early on, the observation was made that fluoride release from glass-ionomers obeyed kinetic laws where release was proportional to the square root of time, a relationship that is consistent with release being a diffusion process, at least in part (Wilson et al. 1985; Tay and Braden 1988). The first equation proposed by Wilson et al. (1985) to describe the release process was:

$$\text{Total release} = C + At^{1/2} + Bt$$

Unfortunately, the best fit with the experimental data for this equation was found where the terms B and C were negative. This made assigning any physical meaning to the equation difficult.

The alternative form of the equation, based on just two terms, was proposed a little later by Tay and Braden in 1988 (Tay and Braden 1988). Their equation took the form

$$\text{Total release} = Bt + At^{1/2}$$

This study involved determining the release of fluoride for glass-ionomer cements for a period of two-and-a-half years. However, despite the duration of their experiments, Tay and Braden found that equilibrium was not reached by these materials, and because of this, they were not able to determine the diffusion coefficient for the release. However, they were able to confirm that fluoride release involved two processes, one short term and rapid and the other prolonged and gradual (Tay and Braden 1988). The latter followed a linear relationship with the square root of time and could thus be shown to be diffusion based. These two essential steps have been confirmed in later studies (De Witte et al. 2000), where the short-term process has been called "early wash-out" and shown to be directly proportional to time. The latter process has been confirmed as being diffusion based, on the basis of its directly proportional relationship with $t^{1/2}$.

1.6.6 Physical Properties

Glass-ionomer cements are materials that set rapidly when placed in the mouth, typically in 3–8 min. They are relatively brittle materials, an observation made for the earliest cements (Crisp et al. 1976a; Elliot et al. 1975; Prosser et al. 1984), and one that is still applicable to currently available formulations.

Typical values of physical properties of the early commercial cements are shown in Table 1.13. By the time these data were collected, both conventional and water-activated glass-ionomers were available to the profession. However, physical properties were not found to be influenced by which of these types a particular material belonged to. Other aspects of the composition were found to be much more influential, including the exact composition of the glass powder and the molar mass as well as the type of polymer and also its concentration in the overall cement formulation.

Table 1.13 Physical properties of early commercial glass-ionomer cements

Property	Range of values
Working time, 23 °C/min	1.3–3.8
Setting time, 37 °C/min	2.75–4.7
Compressive strength, 24 h/MPa	140–195
Diametral tensile strength, 24 h/MPa	9.0–19.3
Flexural strength, 24 h/MPa	8.9–30.0
Creep, 24 h/%	0.17–0.33
Water leachable material, 1 h/%	0.13–0.70
Opacity, $C_{0.7}$	0.44–0.85

Based on data from Prosser et al. (1984)

Early on in their evolution, brands of glass-ionomer were developed specifically as restorative cements and as luting cements (Wilson and McLean 1988). The latter were prepared initially from small-particle-sized glass powders in order to achieve the required consistency and flow characteristics (Wilson et al. 1977b). Such small glass particles were increasingly part of the glass blend in restorative grade materials, added to improve their overall physical properties (Wilson and McLean 1988).

Generally, glass-ionomers prepared for use as luting cements had lower strengths than those designed for use as restorative materials. The specification for them was published by the International Organization for Standardization (ISO) as early as 1986 (International Organization for Standardization 1986) and included the requirement of a minimum compressive strength of 65 MPa for luting grade glass-ionomers, compared with a minimum of 130 MPa for restorative grade cements. This is a consequence of the lower powder/liquid ratio used for luting cements (Wilson and McLean 1988). This lower powder/liquid ratio also slows down the setting and maturation reactions, so that the onset of resistance to moisture is delayed. Consequently, luting grade glass-ionomers were found to be more susceptible to early contamination by water than restorative grades (Wilson and McLean 1988).

Glass-ionomer cements are generally considered to have reasonable aesthetics (i.e. to match the appearance of the natural tooth). They are relatively inferior in this regard to composite resins, but superior to all cements available for use in clinical dentistry, including the former dental silicate cement. This derives mainly from the use of clear or opalescent glass powders in their formulation (Wilson and McLean 1988).

The earliest glass-ionomers were of poor translucency compared with materials that became available later, and because of this, they could not be made to match the appearance of the natural tooth (Crisp et al. 1979). However, quite early on, an experimental type of glass-ionomer cement called ASPA X was produced, and it had a translucency which was an excellent match for the tooth (Crisp et al. 1979).

One problem for the determination of appearance with these materials generally was its relationship to maturation. The slow hydration and other reactions that bring about increases in strength and reductions in plasticity also improve appearance, so that full translucency was not reached in the early commercial cements until at least 24 h had elapsed from placement (Wilson and McLean 1988).

A feature that adversely affected the aesthetics of glass-ionomers from the earliest days was that the darker shades were less translucent than the lighter shades (Asmussen 1983). Hence, they look less like natural tooth than the corresponding material in lighter shades. Also, if the freshly placed cement was allowed to come into contact with moisture, the surface was damaged, and this adversely affects the translucency. Overall, these problems meant that glass-ionomers need careful handling in order to optimise their appearance in vivo, and this contributed to their reputation as demanding materials to use.

1.6.7 Adhesion

The ability of glass-ionomers to form adhesive bonds to the surface of the natural tooth was recognised at the earliest point in their development. Indeed, by analogy with the zinc polycarboxylate, the use of poly(acrylic acid) in glass-ionomers was expected to make them naturally adhesive (McLean and Wilson 1974). Right from the start, the advantage of adhesion of these materials was apparent in allowing the repair of cervical erosion lesions in adult teeth and in sealing pits and fissures in children's teeth (McLean and Wilson 1977a, b).

Early studies were carried out to determine the tensile bond strengths on untreated enamel and dentine (Hotz et al. 1977; Prodger and Symonds 1977; Levine et al. 1977; Powis et al. 1982; Aboush and Jenkins 1986). Results varied with the brand used, but all types showed acceptable bond strengths to both substrates (Powis et al. 1982; Aboush and Jenkins 1986). Values on enamel varied from 2.6 to 9.6 MPa and on dentine from 1.1 to 4.1 MPa. Although these ranges overlap to an extent, all studies found higher bond strengths to enamel than to dentine (Wilson and McLean 1988). It was also found that adhesion developed rapidly, with about 80 % of the eventual bond strength being achieved by 15 min (Aboush and Jenkins 1986). Thereafter, it continued to increase for several days after attachment (Powis et al. 1982).

The mechanism of this adhesion was studied in early papers on this topic. Initially, when freshly mixed cement paste is applied to the tooth, wetting has to take place and the adhesion that develops rapidly was attributed to the formation of hydrogen bonds originating from the free carboxyl groups in the cement (Wilson 1974). It was suggested that these hydrogen bonds were later replaced by ionic bonds involving cations obtained from either the cement or the tooth mineral (Wilson 1974). Such a view is consistent with the subsequent findings of the slow formation of an ion-exchange layer between the tooth and the cement (Ngo et al. 1997; Hien-Chi et al. 2006). The concept of the formation of relatively strong bonds involving in part carboxylate groups from the poly(acrylic acid) component was also suggested by early results using infrared spectroscopy to study the bonded surface (Beech 1973).

The role of collagen in the tooth structure on the adhesion of glass-ionomers was unclear from these early studies, and indeed, there still seems to be doubt about how important it is. The finding that tensile bond strengths were greater to enamel than to dentine suggested that the most important bonds are formed with the mineral phase of the tooth. Based on this finding and the results of infrared spectroscopy, Beech stated that bonding involved the hydroxyapatite phase of the tooth only and that collagen had no role at all (Beech 1973). This was challenged by Wilson (1974), who argued that as collagen contains both amino and carboxylic acid groups, the possibility of strong interaction with both poly(acrylic acid) and polyacrylate is high, so that some degree of adhesion would be envisaged. However, he later conceded that, on balance, the evidence pointed towards the conclusion that glass-ionomers probably do not form any adhesive bonds to collagen (Wilson and McLean 1988).

In practical situations, bonding can be improved by surface conditioning. For glass-ionomers, originally this meant treating the tooth surface with a solution of 50 % aqueous citric acid (McLean and Wilson 1977a, b). This technique was found generally to increase the bond strength, though in certain cases, it had no measurable effect (Wilson and McLean 1988). However, citric acid is somewhat aggressive towards the tooth surface and was found to attack both the dentine and the enamel, and not only the smear layer as desired. The resulting loss of mineralizing ions caused substantial damage to the structural integrity of the substrate (Powis et al. 1982) and led to the recommendation that citric acid treatment should be limited to 5 s (Brannstrom 1981). Modern surface conditioning follows the procedure established by Powis et al. (1982) of using dilute solutions of poly(acrylic acid) to remove the smear layer only. They originally employed a 25 % solution, but later studies suggested that slightly higher concentrations, i.e. between 30 and 35 %, were preferred as these gave higher bond strengths (Long et al. 1986).

Adhesion by glass-ionomers is not only desirable because it aids retention of the cement within the tooth but also because it considerably reduces the problem of marginal leakage. Such leakage is a clinical problem, as gaps at the margin of restorations through which it occurs can result in the entry of harmful microorganisms, which then give rise to secondary caries beneath the restorations. In early studies of this problem, using a variety of in vitro methods, the expectation that adhesion would reduce the occurrence of leakage was confirmed (Maldonado et al. 1978; Hembree and Andrews 1978; Kidd 1978). A few years later, it was shown that glass-ionomer cements were able to provide a seal against the diffusion of radiolabelled sucrose, and this was effective for at least a year (Powis 1986). This result was superior to all other restorative materials tested, including composite resins placed with the aid of enamel etching.

1.6.8 Early Studies on Clinical Applications

The expected clinical applications of glass-ionomer cements were first explored in a series of papers published in 1977 (McLean and Wilson 1977a, b, c), though there had been one early paper on this topic in 1974 (McLean and Wilson 1974). It was obvious at this time that these materials had a future as restorations with preventive properties, based on their features of adhesion and fluoride release. They were also seen to have scope for being used successfully as liners and bases (McLean and Wilson 1977a) and also for luting (McLean and Wilson 1974).

Glass-ionomer cements were considered well suited for use in gingival Class V lesions (McLean and Wilson 1977b). The property of adhesion was key to this, as it allowed minimal cavity preparation and the aesthetics of the cement when set made it acceptable for use in such locations. The earliest clinical results published were of a 3-year study in Class V restorations, where a failure rate of only 9 % was reported (McLean and Wilson 1977a). Other early studies generally confirmed these good results (Mount and Makinson 1982; Charbeneau and Bozell 1979; Lawrence 1979), though there was one that found a 43 % failure rate (Smales 1981). These poor results were from a study involving a variety of operators working in a dental hospital and were attributed to lack of experience with these materials (Smales 1981). It was the first indication that they were sensitive to handling in the clinical situation.

Other early clinical applications included Class III interproximal lesions (McLean and Wilson 1977a). A detailed study involving 332 restorations gave extremely promising results (Knibbs et al. 1986), with only a 5 % loss in 3 years, mainly due to abrasion. Only three specimens failed due to poor adhesion, which was a remarkable finding, and it was also observed that there was no recurrent caries observed with any of the restorations (Knibbs et al. 1986).

Fissure sealing was also suggested as an application for glass-ionomers quite early on in their development (McLean and Wilson 1974, 1977a), with the expectation that the good adhesion would provide an excellent seal and that the fluoride release would confer caries resistance. Later studies seem to have confirmed these ideas, though retention has been problematic, despite the generally good adhesion.

Early studies suggested that glass-ionomers were particularly suitable for restoring deciduous teeth (McLean and Wilson 1977a), and soon after, clinical reports appeared confirming this view (Saito 1978; Plant et al. 1977; Vliestra et al. 1978). Luting grade glass-ionomers were also shown to be effective in clinical studies from this time (Reisbick 1981; McComb 1982). In a variety of applications, glass-ionomers were shown to provide protection against secondary caries (Kidd 1978; Hicks et al. 1986), so that there was early evidence that they were able to protect from caries at the interface of the restoration with the tooth. They were also shown to reduce the occurrence of lesions in the adjacent enamel (Kidd 1978). This is an aspect of glass-ionomers in which there has been significant progress in the intervening years, with improved materials and innovative techniques playing their part. These more recent developments lie outside the scope of the present chapter, but it was apparent from the beginning that glass-ionomers were materials with potential for development and for deployment in novel ways. The earliest clinical studies demonstrated this versatility, and this has been confirmed by the numerous studies in subsequent years.

Biological testing showed that early glass-ionomers were acceptable for use in close proximity to the pulp, since the set cement exhibited no adverse effects in cell cultures (Dahl and Tronstad 1976; Meryon et al. 1983; Kawahara et al. 1979). Incompletely set cements were found to be more biologically active, with some possible indication of cytotoxicity (Dahl and Tronstad 1976; Meryon et al. 1983). However, later studies suggest that such effects are minimal in clinical situations (Oliva 1998).

Conclusion

The invention of glass-ionomer dental cements followed on from important and pioneering studies on the setting and structure of dental silicates. Armed with the knowledge won from these studies, Wilson and his team were able to make the key inventive steps and develop glass-ionomer cements as workable materials. Fundamental studies of these materials followed rapidly, and soon the essential features of their setting and maturation were established. Clinical applications were also developed early on. Later work has refined much of the details of our understanding of these materials, but the broad picture has changed very little. This is a tribute to the wisdom and insight of the early pioneers, especially their inventors Alan Wilson and Brian Kent, but also to those clinicians who identified the necessary techniques to make them successful and promoted them to the profession, most notably John McLean and Graham Mount. The place of glass-ionomers among current restorative dental materials owes much to them all.

References

Aboush YEY, Jenkins CBG. An evaluation of the bonding of glass-ionomer restoratives to dentine and enamel. Br Dent J. 1986;161:179–84.

Akitt JW. Multinuclear studies of aluminium compounds. Prog Nucl Magnet Spectr. 1989;21:1–149.

Asmussen E. Opacity of glass-ionomer cements. Acta Odont Scand. 1983;41:155–7.

Barry TI, Clinton DJ, Wilson AD. The structure of a glass ionomer cement and its relationship to the setting process. J Dent Res. 1979;58:1072–9.

Beagrie GS, Main JHP, Smith DC. Inflammatory reaction evoked by zinc polyacrylate and zinc eugenolate cements: a comparison. Br Dent J. 1972;132:351–7.

Beech DR. Improvement in the adhesion of polyacrylate cements to human dentine. Br Dent J. 1973;135:442–5.

Bertenshaw BW, Combe EC. Studies on polycarboxylates and related cements. I. Analysis of cement liquids. J Dent. 1972;1:13–6.

Bertenshaw BW, Combe EC. Studies on polycarboxylates and related cements. III. Molecular weight determination. J Dent. 1976;4:87–90.

Brannstrom M. Pretreatment before the placement of restorations. In: Dentine and pulp in restorative dentistry. Nacka: Dental Therapeutics; 1981. p. 93.

Brune D, Smith D. Microstructure and strength properties of silicate and glass ionomer cements. Acta Odontol Scand. 1982;40:389–96.

Causton BE. The physico-mechanical consequences of exposing glass ionomer cements to water during setting. Biomaterials. 1981;2:112–5.

Charbeneau GT, Bozell RR. Clinical valuation of a glass ionomer cement for restoring of cervical erosion. J Dent Res. 1979;98:936–9.

Connick RE, Poulsen RE. Nuclear magnetic resonance studies of aluminium fluoride complexes. J Am Chem Soc. 1957;79:5152–7.

Crisp S, Wilson AD. Reactions in glass ionomer cements. I. Decomposition of the powder. J Dent Res. 1974a;53:1408–13.

Crisp S, Wilson AD. Reactions in glass ionomer cements. III. The precipitation reaction. J Dent Res. 1974b;53:1420–4.

Crisp S, Wilson AD. Reactions in glass ionomer cements. V. Effect of incorporating tartaric acid in the cement liquid. J Dent Res. 1976;55:1023–31.

Crisp S, Pringuer MA, Wardleworth D, Wilson AD. Reactions in glass ionomer cements. II. An infrared spectroscopic study. J Dent Res. 1974;53:1414–9.

Crisp S, Ferner AJ, Lewis BG, Wilson AD. Properties of improved glass ionomer cement formulations. J Dent. 1975;3:125–30.

Crisp S, Lewis BG, Wilson AD. Characterization of glass-ionomer cements. 1. Long-term hardness and compressive strength. J Dent. 1976a;4:162–6.

Crisp S, Lewis BG, Wilson AD. Glass ionomer cements: chemistry of erosion. J Dent Res. 1976b;55:1032–41.

Crisp S, Lewis BG, Wilson AD. Characterization of glass-ionomer cements. 3. Effect of polyacid concentration on the physical properties. J Dent. 1977;5:51–6.

Crisp S, Abel G, Wilson AD. The quantitative measurement of the opacity of aesthetic dental filling materials. J Dent Res. 1979;58:1585–96.

Crisp S, Kent BE, Lewis BG, Ferner AJ, Wilson AD. Glass ionomer cement formulations. II. The synthesis of novel polycarboxylic acids. J Dent Res. 1980a;59:1055–63.

Crisp S, Lewis BG, Wilson AD. Characterization of glass-ionomer cements. 6. A study of erosion and water absorption in both neutral and acidic media. J Dent. 1980b;8:68–74.

Dahl BL, Tronstad L. Biological tests of an experimental glass ionomer (silicopolyacrylate) cement. J Oral Rehabil. 1976;55:1032–41.

De Witte AM, De Maeyer EA, Verbeeck RMH, Martens LC. Fluoride release profiles of mature restorative glass ionomer cements after fluoride application. Biomaterials. 2000;21:475–82.

Dollimore D, Spooner P. Sintering studies on zinc oxide. Trans Faraday Soc. 1971;67:2750–9.

Earl MSA, Ibbetson RJ. The clinical disintegration of a glass-ionomer cement. Br Dent J. 1986;161:287–91.

Earl MSA, Hume WR, Mount GJ. Effect of varnishes and other surface treatments on water movement across the glass-ionomer cement surface. Aust Dent J. 1985;30:298–301.

Elliot J, Holliday L, Hornsby PR. Physical and mechanical properties of glass-ionomer cements. Br Polym J. 1975;7:297–306.

Enderby JE, Nielson GW. The coordination of metal ions. In: Sykes AG, editor. Advances in inorganic chemistry, vol. 34. San Diego: Academic Press; 1989. p. 195–218.

Fleck H. The chemistry of oxyphosphate. Dent Items Interest. 1902:906–935, cited in Wilson [1].

Forsten L. Fluoride release from a glass ionomer cement. Scand J Dent Res. 1977;85:503–4.

Forsten L. Short- and long-term fluoride release from glass ionomers. Scand J Dent Res. 1991;99:241–5.

Foster JF, Dovey EH. Surgical cements of improved compressive strength containing stannous fluoride and polyacrylic acid. US Patent 3,856,737. 1974, cited in Wilson and Nicholson [14].

Guggenberger R, May R, Stephan KP. New trends in glass ionomer chemistry. Biomaterials. 1998;19:479–83.

Guida A, Towler MR, Wall JG, Hill RG, Eramo S. Preliminary work on the antibacterial effect of strontium in glass ionomer cements. J Mater Sci Lett. 2003;22:1401–3.

Hammond PW, Egan H. Weighed in the balance – a history of the laboratory of the government chemist. London: HMSO; 1992.

Hara M, editor. Polyelectrolytes. New York: Marcel Dekker; 1993.

Hembree JH, Andrews JT. Microleakage of several class V anterior restorative materials. J Am Dent Assoc. 1978;97:179–83.

Hicks MJ, Flaitz CM, Silverstone LM. Secondary caries formation *in vitro* around glass ionomer restorations. Quintessence Int. 1986;17:527–32.

Hien-Chi N, Mount G, McIntyre J, Tuisuva J, Von Doussa RJ. Chemical exchange between glass-ionomer restorations and residual carious dentine in permanent molars: an in vivo study. J Dent. 2006;34:608–13.

Hill EE, Lott J. A clinically focused discussion of luting materials. Aust Dent J. 2011;56 Suppl 1:67–76.

Hill RG, Wilson AD. Some structural aspects of glasses used in ionomer cements. Glass Technol. 1988;29:150–88.

Hornsby PR. Dimensional stability of glass-ionomer cements. J Chem Tech Biotechnol. 1980;30:595–601.

Hotz P, McLean JW, Sced I, Wilson AD. The bonding of glass ionomer cements to metal and tooth substrates. Br Dent J. 1977;142:41–7.

Iler RK. The polymerization of silica, chapters 3 and 6. In: The chemistry of silica. New York: Wiley-Interscience; 1979.

International Organization for Standardization (ISO). International standard for glass polyalkenoate cements. 1986. ISO7486.

Jorgensen KD. On the solubility of dental silicate cements. Acta Odont Scand. 1963;21:141–58.

Kakaboura A, Vougiouklakis G. Cements in orthodontics, Ch 11. In: Brantley W, Eliades G, editors. Orthodontic materials – scientific and clinical aspects. Stuttgart: Thieme; 2001.

Kawahara H, Imanashi Y, Oshima H. Biological evaluation of glass-ionomer cements. J Dent Res. 1979;58:1080–6.

Kent BE, Wilson AD. Dental silicate cements VIII. Acid–base aspect. J Dent Res. 1969;48:412–8.

Kent BE, Fletcher KE, Wilson AD. Dental silicate cements, XI. Electron probe studies. J Dent Res. 1970;49:86–92.

Kent BE, Lewis BG, Wilson AD. The properties of a glass-ionomer cement. Br Dent J. 1973;135:322–6.

Kent BE, Lewis BG, Wilson AD. Glass ionomer formulations. I. The preparation of novel fluoroaluminosilicate glasses high in fluorine. J Dent Res. 1979;58:1607–19.

Kidd EAM. Cavity sealing ability of composite resin and glass ionomer restorations: an assessment in vitro. Br Dent J. 1978;144:139–42.

Knibbs PJ, Plant CG, Pearson GJ. The use of a glass ionomer to restore Class III cavities. Rest Dent. 1986;2:42–8.

Kovarick RE. Restoration of posterior teeth in clinical practice: evidence base for choosing amalgam versus composite. Dent Clin North Am. 2009;53:71–6.

Kuhn AT, Setchell DJ, Teo CK. An assessment of the jet method for solubility measurements of dental cements. Biomaterials. 1984;5:161–8.

Lawrence LG. Cervical glass ionomer restorations: a clinical study. J Can Dent Assoc. 1979;45:58, 59, 62.

Levine RS, Beech DR, Garton B. Improving bond strength of polyacrylate cements to dentine. Br Dent J. 1977;143:275–7.

Long TE, Duke ES, Norling BK. Polyacrylic acid cleaning of dentin and glass ionomer bond strengths. J Dent Res. 1986;65(Special issue):345, Abstract 1583.

Lowenstein W. The distribution of aluminium in the tetrahedral of silicates and aluminates. Am Mineralog. 1954;39:92–6.

Lundall GEF, Hoffman JI. Outlines of methods of chemical analysis, Ch XIIC. New York: Wiley; 1938.

Maldonado A, Swartz ML, Phillips RW. An in vitro study of certain properties of a glass-ionomer cement. J Am Dent Assoc. 1978;96:785–91.

McComb D. retention of castings with glass ionomer cements. J Prosthet Dent. 1982;48:285–8.

McLean JW, Wilson AD. Fissure sealing and filling with an adhesive glass-ionomer cement. Br Dent J. 1974;136:269–76.

McLean JW, Wilson AD. The clinical development of the glass-ionomer cement. II. Some clinical applications. Aust Dent J. 1977a;22:120–7.

McLean JW, Wilson AD. The clinical development of the glass-ionomer cement. III. The erosion lesion. Aust Dent J. 1977b;22:190–5.

McLean JW, Wilson AD. The clinical development of the glass-ionomer cement. I. Formulations and properties. Aust Dent J. 1977c;22:31–6.

Meryon SD, Stephens PG, Browne RM. A comparison of the *in vitro* cytotoxicity of two glass ionomer cements. J Dent Res. 1983;62:769–73.

Mizrahi E, Smith DC. Direct cementation of orthodontic brackets to dental enamel. An investigation using zinc polycarboxylate cement. Br Dent J. 1969;127:371–410.

Mount GJ, Hume WR. Preservation and restoration of tooth structure. 2nd ed. Sandgate: Knowledge Books and Software; 2005.

Mount GJ, Makinson OF. Glass-ionomer restorative cements: clinical implications of the setting reaction. Oper Dent. 1982;7:134–41.

Ngo HG, Mount GJ, Peters MCRB. A study of glass-ionomer cement and its interface with enamel and dentin using a low-temperature, high-resolution scanning electron microscopic technique. Quintessence Int. 1997;28:63–9.

Nicholson JW. An infrared spectroscopic study of the interaction of metal salts with an acrylic acid/maleic acid copolymer. J Appl Polym Sci. 2000;78:1680–4.

Nicholson JW, Brookman PJ, Lacy OM, Wilson AD. Fourier transform infrared spectroscopic study of the role of tartaric acid in glass-ionomer cement. J Dent Res. 1988;76:1451–4.

Norman RD, Swartz MP, Phillips RW. Studies on the solubility of certain dental materials. J Dent Res. 1957;36:977–85.

Norman RD, Swartz MP, Phillips RW. Additional studies on the solubility of certain dental materials. J Dent Res. 1959;38:1025–37.

O'Reilly DE. NMR chemical shifts of aluminium: experimental data and variational calculations. J Chem Phys. 1960;32:1007–12.

Oliva A. Biocompatibility studies on glass ionomer cements by primary cultures of human osteoblasts. Biomaterials. 1998;17:1351–6.

Osborne JW, Swartz ML, Goodacre CJ, Pillips RW, Gale EM. A method for assessing the clinical solubility and disintegration of luting cements. J Prosthet Dent. 1978;40:413–7.

Paddon JM, Wilson AD. Stress relaxation studies on dental materials. I. Dental cements. J Dent. 1976;4:183–9.

Paffenbarger GC, Sweeney SJ, Isaacs A. A preliminary report on zinc phosphate cements. J Am Dent Assoc. 1933;20:1960–82.

Paffenbarger GC, Schoonover IC, Souder W. Dental silicate cements: physical and chemical properties and a specification. J Am Dent Assoc. 1938;25:32–87.

Phillips S, Bishop BM. An in vitro study of the effect of moisture on glass ionomer cement. Quintessence Int. 1985;16:175–7.

Pierce CN. Filling materials of oxide of zinc and glacial phosphoric acid. Dent Cosmos. 1879;21:696, cited in Wilson [1].

Plant CG. The effect of polycarboxylate containing stannous fluoride on the pulp. Br Dent J. 1970;135:317–21.

Plant CG, Shovelton DS, Vliestra JR, Wartnaby JM. The use of a glass ionomer cement in deciduous teeth. Br Dent J. 1977;143:271–4.

Powis DR. Unpublished report. 1986, cited in Wilson and McLean [68].

Powis DR, Folleras T, Merson SA, Wilson AD. Improved adhesion of a glass ionomer cement to dentin and enamel. J Dent Res. 1982;61:1416–22.

Prodger TE, Symonds M. ASPA adhesion study. Br Dent J. 1977;143:266–70.

Prosser HJ, Richards CP, Wilson AD. NMR spectroscopy of dental materials. II. The role of tartaric acid in glass-ionomer cements. J Biomed Mater Res. 1982;16:431–43.

Prosser HJ, Powis DR, Brant PJ, Wilson AD. Characterisation of glass-ionomer cements. 7. The physical properties of current materials. J Dent. 1984;12:231–40.

Prosser HJ, Powis DR, Wilson AD. Glass-ionomer cements of improved flexural strength. J Dent Res. 1986;65:146–8.

Ray KW. The behaviour of siliceous cements. J Am Dent Assoc. 1934;21:237–51.

Reisbick MH. Working qualities of glass ionomer cements. J Prosthet Dent. 1981;46:525–30.

Robinson AD. The life of a filling. Br Dent J. 1971;130:206–8.

Saito S. Characteristics of glass ionomer and its clinical application. 1. Relations between hardening reactions and water. Int J Dent Mater. 1978;8:1–16.

Schmidt W, Purrman R, Jochum P, Gasser O. Mixing compounds for glass-ionomer cements and use of a copolymer for preparing mixing components. Eur Pat App 24, 056. 1981, cited in Wilson and McLean [68].

Schoenbeck F. Process for the production of tooth material. US Patent N 897 160. 1980, cited in Wilson [1].

Skinner EW, Phillips RW. The science of dental materials. 5th ed. Philadelphia/London: W. B. Saunders; 1960.

Smales RJ. Clinical using of ASPA glass-ionomer cement. Br Dent J. 1981;151:58–60.

Smith DC. A new dental cement. Br Dent J. 1968;125:381–4.

Smith DC. A review of the zinc polycarboxylate cements. J Can Dent Assoc. 1971;37:22–9.

Smith DC. Composition and characteristics of dental cements, Ch 8. In: Smith DC, Williams DF, editors. Biocompatibility of dental materials, Biocompatibility of preventive dental materials and bonding agents, vol. II. Boca Raton: CRC Press; 1982.

Sorel S. Procedure for the formation of a very solid cement by the action of chloride on the oxide of zinc. C R Hebd Seances Acad Sci. 1855;41:784–5, cited in Wilson [1].

Steenbock P. Improvements in and relating to the manufacture of a material designed for the production of cement. Br Patent 174,558. 1904, cited in Wilson [1].

Stralfors A, Eriksson SE. The rate of dissolution of dental silicate cement. Odont Tidskrift. 1969;77:185–210.

Tarutani T. Polymerization of silicic acid: a review. Anal Sci. 1989;5:245–52.

Tay WM, Braden M. Fluoride ion diffusion from polyalkenoate (glass-ionomer) cements. Biomaterials. 1988;9:454–9.

Tay WM, Morrant GA, Borlace HR, Bultitude FW. An assessment of anterior restorations in vivo using the scanning electron microscope. Results after one year. Br Dent J. 1974;137:463–71.

Tay WM, Cooper IR, Morrant GA, Borlace HR, Bultitude FW. An assessment of anterior restorations in vivo using the scanning electron microscope. Results after three years. Br Dent J. 1979;146:71–6.

ten Cate JM, Buijs MJ, Miller CC, Exterkate RA. Elevated fluoride products enhance mineralisation of advanced enamel lesions. J Dent Res. 2008;87:943–7.

Turner D, Czarnecka B, Nicholson JW. The interaction of stannous fluoride with synthetic hydroxyapatite: modelling the anticaries effect. Ceram Silik. 2013;57:1–6.

Vliestra JR, Plant CG, Sovelton DS, Bradnock G. The use of glass ionomer cement in deciduous teeth. Br Dent J. 1978;145:164–6.

Voelker CC. Dental silicate cements in theory and practice. Dent Cosmos. 1916;36:1098–111, cited in Wilson [1].

Wasson EA, Nicholson JW. Studies on the setting of glass ionomer cements. Clin Mater. 1991;7:289–93.

Watts DC, Combe EC, Greener EH. Effect of storage conditions on the mechanical properties of polyelectrolyte cements. J Dent Res. 1979;58(Special issue C), Abstract No 18.

Wilson AD. Dental silicate cements VIII. Alternative liquid cement formers. J Dent Res. 1968;47:1133–6.

Wilson AD. Alumino-silicate polyacrylic acid cement. Br Polym J. 1974;6:165–79.

Wilson AD. The chemistry of dental cements. Chem Soc Rev. 1978;7:265–96.

Wilson AD. A hard decade's work: steps in the invention of the glass-ionomer cement. J Dent Res. 1996a;75: 1723–7.

Wilson AD. Acidobasicity of oxide glasses used in glass ionomer cements. Dent Mater. 1996b;12:25–9.

Wilson AD. A survey of dental practice in the use of silicate cements. Ministry of Technology Report. Br Dent J. 1969;127:7 (abstract).

Wilson AD, Batchelor RF. Dental silicate cements I. The chemistry of erosion. J Dent Res. 1967a;46:1075–85.

Wilson AD, Batchelor RF. Dental silicate cements, II. Preparation and durability. J Dent Res. 1967b;46:1425–32.

Wilson AD, Batchelor RF. Dental silicate cements III. Environment and durability. J Dent Res. 1968;47:115–20.

Wilson AD, Crisp S. Ionomer cements. Br Polym J. 1975;7:279–96.

Wilson AD, Kent BE. Dental silicate cements, V. Electrical conductivity. J Dent Res. 1968;47:463–70.

Wilson AD, Kent BE. The glass-ionomer cement, a new translucent cement for dentistry. J Appl Chem Biotechnol. 1971;21:313.

Wilson AD, Lewis BG. The flow properties of dental cements. J Biomed Mater Res. 1980;14:383–91.

Wilson AD, McLean JW. Glass-ionomer cement. Chicago: Quintessence Publishing; 1988.

Wilson AD, Mesley RF. Dental silicate cements VI. Infrared studies. J Dent Res. 1968;47:644–52.

Wilson AD, Nicholson JW. Acid base cements. Cambridge: The University Press; 1993.

Wilson AS, Kent KE, Batchelor RF. Dental silicate cements, IV. Phosphoric acid modifiers. J Dent Res. 1968;47:233–43.

Wilson AD, Kent BE, Batchelor RF, Scott BG, Lewis BG. Dental silicate cements XII. The role of water. J Dent Res. 1970a;49:307–14.

Wilson AD, Kent BE, Mesley RF, Miller RP, Clinton D, Fletcher KE. Formation of dental silicate cement. Nature. 1970b;225:272–3.

Wilson AD, Kent BE, Clinton D, Miller RP. The formation and microstructure of the dental silicate cement. J Mater Sci. 1972;7:220–38.

Wilson AD, Crisp S, Ferner AJ. Reaction in glass ionomer cements. IV. Effect of chelating co-monomers. J Dent Res. 1976;55:489–95.

Wilson AD, Crisp S, Abel G. Characterization of glass-ionomer cements. 4. Effect of molecular weight on physical properties. J Dent. 1977a;5:117–20.

Wilson AD, Crisp S, Lewis BG, McLean JW. Experimental luting cements based on the glass ionomer cements. Br Dent J. 1977b;142:117–22.

Wilson AD, Paddon JM, Crisp S. The hydration of dental cements. J Dent Res. 1979;58:1065–71.

Wilson AD, Crisp S, Prosser HJ, Lewis BG, Merson SA. Aluminosilicate glasses for polyelectrolyte cements. Ind Eng Chem Prod Res Dev. 1980;19:263–70.

Wilson AD, Crisp S, Paddon JM. The hydration of a glass-ionomer (ASPA) cement. Br Polym J. 1981; 13:66–70.

Wilson AD, Groffman DM, Kuhn AT. The release of fluoride and other chemical species from a glass-ionomer cement. Biomaterials. 1985;6:431–3.

Worner HK, Docking AR. Dental materials in the tropics. Aust Dent J. 1958;3:215–29.

Zachariasen WH. The atomic arrangement in glass. J Am Chem Soc. 1932;54:3841–51.

Physicochemical Nature of Glass-Ionomer-Based Materials and Their Clinical Performance

2

Michael F. Burrow

Abstract

This chapter outlines the physical and chemical properties of glass-ionomer (GIC) and resin-modified glass-ionomer cements. The latter part proceeds to summarise various aspects of their clinical performance.

It is noted that these materials are brittle in nature when fully matured or set. Glass-ionomer cements, due to the process of the setting reaction, reach their full strength about 24 h after the initial mixing. The resin-modified materials have an additional hydrophilic resin included that improves early strength and aesthetics but importantly reduces the initial sensitivity to water, allowing early finishing shortly after placement.

Application of a resin coating on the surface of GICs has shown some improvement in the fracture strength, but seems to be material dependent based on current evidence. The improvement in strength is thought to be due to the resin-filling surface defects and cracks where fracture may be initiated. Not all materials or studies have shown consistent outcomes for this coating method. There is limited evidence to suggest that the wear resistance may also be enhanced with the resin coating.

Ion release is also described in this chapter. This part shows that the initial release of ions, in particular fluoride, is high but tapers off to steady low-level release. The clinical benefits are still not well understood.

The latter part of the chapter summarises various aspects of the clinical performance of GICs. Studies of retention in non-carious cervical lesions are described, as well as recent work using the atraumatic restorative treatment (ART) technique. The last part outlines results from fissure sealant studies that tend to show poor retention of GIC sealants. However, even though retention may be limited, it appears that GICs can afford some long-lasting anticariogenic effects to the fissure system.

M.F. Burrow, BDS, MDS, PhD, DDSc, MEd
Restorative Dentistry, Melbourne Dental School,
The University of Melbourne, Carlton, VIC, Australia
e-mail: mfburrow@unimelb.edu.au

S.K. Sidhu (ed.), *Glass-Ionomers in Dentistry*, DOI 10.1007/978-3-319-22626-2_2

2.1 Introduction

As we move away from the age of silver amalgam restorations, the need for durable and biologically compatible long-lasting materials is becoming necessary. Never before has the situation been more important to have a dental material that can bond reliably to tooth structure, can potentially reduce biofilm formation and can also inhibit dental diseases as well as protect the tooth. The broad group of glass polyalkenoate (ionomer) cements is showing signs of being able to fulfil many of these qualities. In view of their properties and ease of use, they can be developed even further to become an increasingly useful group of materials to assist with overcoming the problems of dental disease management in such groups as paediatric, special-needs and elderly patients as well as routine caries management.

2.2 Composition and Classification

Glass-ionomer cements (GICs) are termed polyelectrolyte cements. The concept was first introduced in 1962 with the development of the zinc polycarboxylate cements made from a mixture of zinc oxide and polyacrylic acid. Polyacrylic acid was chosen as it was known to complex with calcium and potentially form hydrogen bonds with collagen (Smith 1998).

Glass-ionomer cement can be regarded as a composite material. Essentially, GICs are made up of a cross-linked polyacid matrix in which the fillers are the glass particles in the cement. In the resin-modified version of GIC (RM-GIC), the matrix also contains a polymer network of resinous materials throughout the set cement. The detailed differences will be described later in this chapter. The major categories in GICs are essentially the 'conventional' and 'resin-modified' GICs; the only difference is that the latter contains a polymerisable resin. It is generally accepted that RM-GICs have a higher toughness and better aesthetics than conventional materials (Xu and Burgess 2003). In addition, it appears that the greater resin content gives rise to a higher Weibull modulus compared with conventional GICs with regard to strength (McCabe 1998). Traditionally, GICs have been classified based on the publication of Wilson and McLean (1988). A modified version of the classification is outlined below, demonstrating the diversity of the GICs; hence, nowadays they can be better regarded as a 'group' of materials. In broad terms, the original classification is centred on the viscosity of the material and therefore its clinical uses. In 2009, Mount et al. proposed a revised classification of direct tooth-coloured restorative materials. This revision was brought about by the changes occurring in tooth-coloured filling materials where manufacturers blurred the boundaries between RM-GICs and resin composites due to further modifications of the materials. This revision was centred more towards how the setting cements reacted with tooth tissues. An emphasis was placed on the fact that glass-ionomer-based materials should have a distinct acid–base setting reaction that also incorporates an ion-exchange reaction with the underlying tooth structure. If this was not evident, then such materials should, ideally, not be called glass-ionomer cements even though the glass fillers may be almost identical to those found in glass-ionomer cements (Mount et al. 2009).

The generally accepted classification for GICs is outlined below, and it still relates closely to the viscosity of the unset cement.

2.2.1 Type 1: Luting and Bonding (RM-GIC Adhesive) Materials

These materials are used for the cementation of indirect restorations including crowns, bridges and orthodontic brackets. They are delivered as either conventional or resin-modified materials. The resin-modified materials can set with or without light polymerisation. These materials are either delivered as separate powder and liquid systems, encapsulated materials or nowadays even a paste/paste system (only the resin-modified materials). The luting cements are able to achieve a good thin film thickness in the order of 20 μm. The powder/liquid ratio can be in the order of 1.7:1 or increased to as much as 3.8:1 when the acid has been dehydrated to a powder form.

The other material in this group can be termed a RM-GIC adhesive. This material has only been available since the mid-1990s and has shown to be a useful alternative for bonding resin composite to tooth structure instead of with resin-based adhesives (Burrow and Tyas 1998). Only a couple of these adhesives are commercially available (Fuji Bond LC, GC Corporation, Japan; Riva Bond LC, SDI Ltd, Australia). Delivery can now be in the form of a hand-mixed powder and liquid or encapsulated. The mixed material is applied to the tooth as a thin layer using a micro-brush, similar to a resin-based adhesive.

2.2.2 Type 2: Restorative Materials

This group was originally classified into 'aesthetic' and 'nonaesthetic' materials and either conventional or resin-modified. More recently, many of these materials could be classified as being only Type 2, with the exception of the so-called reinforced materials that contain silver and are not tooth-coloured. The aesthetic and nonaesthetic subgroups are now almost eliminated,

The powder/liquid (P:L) ratio varies slightly amongst the currently available materials ranging from about 3.1:1 up to 3.6:1. The capsulated materials tend to have a higher powder/liquid ratio. The P:L ratio shows little variation whether the GIC is a conventional or resin-modified material.

The older classification included a second subgroup of a higher P:L ratio. These cements were stronger, set faster and could be trimmed and polished immediately after setting. It could be argued that some of the current GICs should still be placed in this subgroup. However, there are now other materials that set quickly and can be finished early and have good aesthetics but also a higher viscosity. Hence, the divisions of this classification have become less well defined. The lower P:L ratio conventional GICs have all but been replaced by the high-viscosity materials or by RM-GICs which provide the best aesthetics and acceptable strength. All of the restorative cements are radiopaque.

2.2.3 Type 3: Lining or Base Cements

These are either conventional or resin-modified and are either auto- or light-cured. More recent materials are presented in a paste/paste form for easier dispensing and application. These paste/paste materials are usually light-cured and resin-modified.

The original powder/liquid materials still exist and are widely available. These lining/base cements are most often used as a thin layer beneath restorations and serve as a thermal insulator or dentine replacement. However, the recent trend for dentine replacement is to use a restorative material (Type 2) in larger cavities due to their greater strength in association with the fast set allowing the restoration to be completed quickly.

Exceptions to the above materials now exist. Fissure sealant cements are usually low-viscosity, fast-setting and are typically conventional autocure materials. One manufacturer produces a high fluoride-releasing conventional GIC (Fuji VII, GC Corp, Japan) recommended for what has been termed as 'fissure protection' and has been reported in several research papers (Ganesh and Tandon 2006; Chen and Liu 2013). It has a powder/liquid ratio of 2:1. This GIC has also been recommended for use as a base due to its low viscosity and relatively high strength. Its initial introduction was aimed at stabilising caries lesions in patients with high risk of caries, i.e. as a 'temporary' cement.

A number of the newer materials that are claimed to be RM-GICs tend to have a very high resin content. Hence, the debate continues on what constitutes a true GIC, which led to the Mount et al. (2009) paper. The general consensus is that the mixed cement must be able to set in a dark environment to demonstrate the existence of an acid–base reaction which forms the matrix of the set cement. Those that do not meet this criterion are more like a resin composite with GIC glass particles and probably a little different for a polyacid-modified resin composite (PAMRC/ Compomer).

Another variation of RM-GICs has been the modification and incorporation of different filler particles. This came about after the successful application of using very small nanofillers in resin composite materials. In the case of resin composite materials, the use of nanotechnology was able to improve aesthetic outcomes without affecting the physical properties. This same concept was applied to an RM-GIC produced by 3M-ESPE, St Paul, MN, USA. It has been marketed as Ketac Nano or Ketac N-100 (Falsafi et al. 2014). This material has also been referred to as a 'nano-ionomer'. It still contains the fluoroaluminosilicate glass found in all GICs, with the addition of nanofillers which are not associated with the GIC setting reaction, but which have been coated and bond to the resin component of the cement. Debate continues whether this material is a 'true GIC' since it would seem that there is no typical acid–base reaction occurring. This material is delivered as a paste/paste system and relies on light polymerisation for setting to occur. However, it is claimed that there is also polycarboxylic acid copolymer present to contribute to the acid–base reaction with the fine aluminosilicate glass particles (Falsafi et al. 2014).

Another classification of GICs has also been used. This simplifies the materials into either conventional GICs or RM-GICs – the latter containing resin.

Within the conventional GICs, there are subgroups of the older materials that contain less reactive and larger glass particles and the newer more viscous and quicker setting cements that have more highly reactive and smaller glass particles. This latter group can be used as base or restorative materials and has a shorter setting time and increased strength. Some are now even being promoted for load-bearing restorations; however, the evidence still remains limited for other than small restorations.

Within the conventional GIC grouping are those materials that have been modified by the addition of a metal, typically silver. These materials can also be called admix GICs. Possibly, the most widely known material in this group is Ketac Silver (3M-ESPE, USA). This material is a 'cermet' where the silver and glass have been sintered together during the manufacturing process and then incorporated into the GIC powder. Other materials tend to have the silver separate from the fluoroaluminosilicate glass. They are not aesthetic materials, but have the advantage of increased wear resistance, but all other properties are a little different from other older conventional GICs. Typically, these GICs were used for posterior teeth or cores beneath crowns where there was sufficient tooth structure to support the GIC. With the advent of the high powder/liquid ratio viscous GICs that have improved strength and wear, the metal-modified materials are slowly being relegated to becoming a historical material.

The RM-GICs have tended not to vary greatly and have typically been the material of choice where aesthetics is important. Recently there has been the introduction of a more viscous, higher powder/liquid ratio RM-GIC, Fuji VIII (GC Corp, Tokyo, Japan), which chemically cures without the need of photoactivation. This latter material is regarded as an alternative to the high-viscosity conventional GICs where a slightly less soluble material is useful, e.g. in deep proximal box restorations.

2.3 Method of Delivery

The original GICs were delivered or dispensed as a separate powder and liquid. A scoop of specific volume and a bottle with a tip designed to dispense the correct drop size of liquid are still available in many parts of the world for both conventional GICs and RM-GICs (Fig. 2.1). The major disadvantages of this method is the potential variation that can occur if the powder is either packed too firmly into the scoop or if it too much air is incorporated due to shaking the bottle prior to dispensing. This will then give a powder/liquid ratio that is not ideal, thus leading to less than ideal handling and physical properties.

Due to the inconsistency of mix caused by dispensing the powder and liquid separately, the

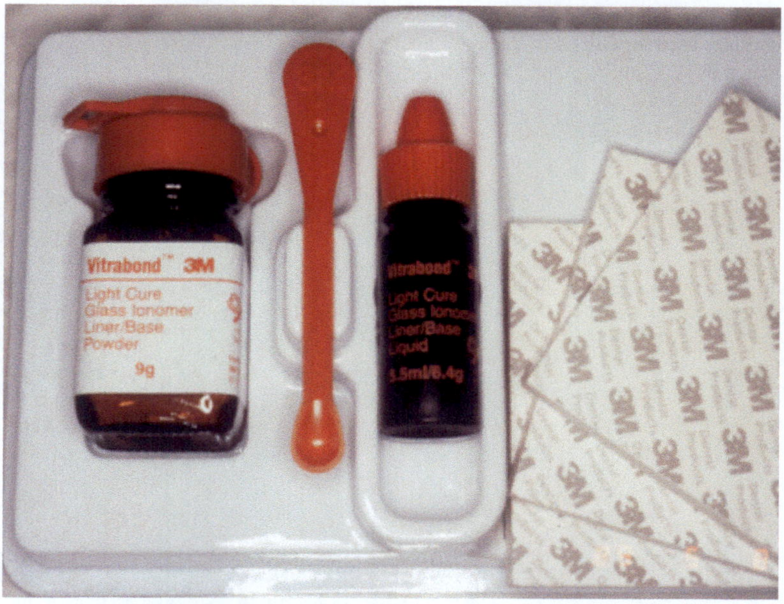

Fig. 2.1 A powder/liquid RM-GIC lining material. The scoop and bottle tip have been specifically designed for providing the correct powder/liquid ratio, but it is also important to ensure the powder has been 'fluffed up' in the bottle prior to filling the scoop

effect of varying mixing time and environmental influences such as ambient temperature and relative humidity, manufacturers developed capsulated GICs for both conventional and resin-modified materials. This provided practitioners with a high level of consistency of mix, the ideal viscosity for insertion into cavities and best physical and aesthetic properties and reduced the effects of temperature and humidity. Typically, each manufacturer has developed its own capsule design (Figs. 2.2 and 2.3), but essentially the method of use is very similar, i.e. activation of the capsule followed by mechanical mixing. The one great advantage of capsule use is the ease of inserting the viscous cement into cavity preparations in almost any part of the oral cavity.

More recently, there has been a further development by manufacturers to develop paste/paste systems. This is especially useful for those materials that are used as a thin lining over a cavity surface. The GIC is usually a RM-GIC but can be light-cured or chemically (self-)cured. By having a paste/paste system, again the best physical properties can be attained as well as being able to be dispensed in small quantities. Each manufacturer has developed its own system with some of those materials that were originally dispensed as a powder and liquid being modified to a paste/paste system, making it simpler to mix and use (Figs. 2.4 and 2.5).

2.3.1 Setting Reaction

The setting of GICs is via the attack of the glass filler particles by the acid liquid. Surface dissolution of glass particles releases metal ions such as calcium, strontium and aluminium into the newly created matrix which is formed by cross-linking with the polyacid (Cook 1983). This setting reaction is dependent on the component parts of the powder and liquid.

The filler portion is made up of a fluoroaluminosilicate glass which can range from 40 to 75 % by weight in the cement mix. The proportion of filler relates to the qualities required for the cement, for example, low-viscosity luting cements or fissure protection materials have less powder compared with high-strength and high-viscosity cements used as restorative materials that are likely to bear occlusal loading (Frankenberger et al. 1997). The set cement becomes a composite comprising unreacted glass fillers which are surrounded by a siliceous gel which is embedded in a matrix made up of the polyacid salt that is responsible for holding the

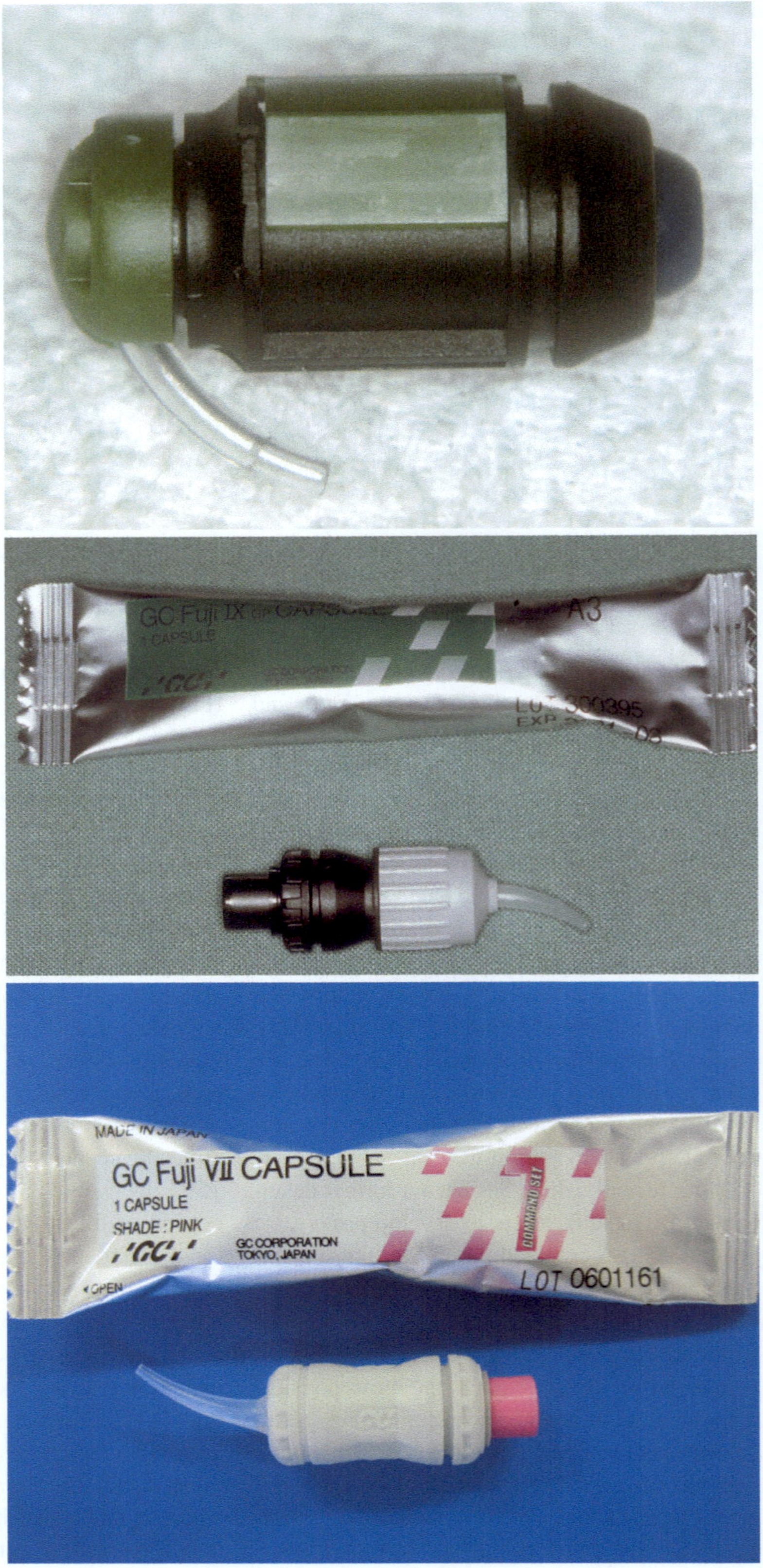

Fig. 2.2 Various types of capsules used for GIC materials

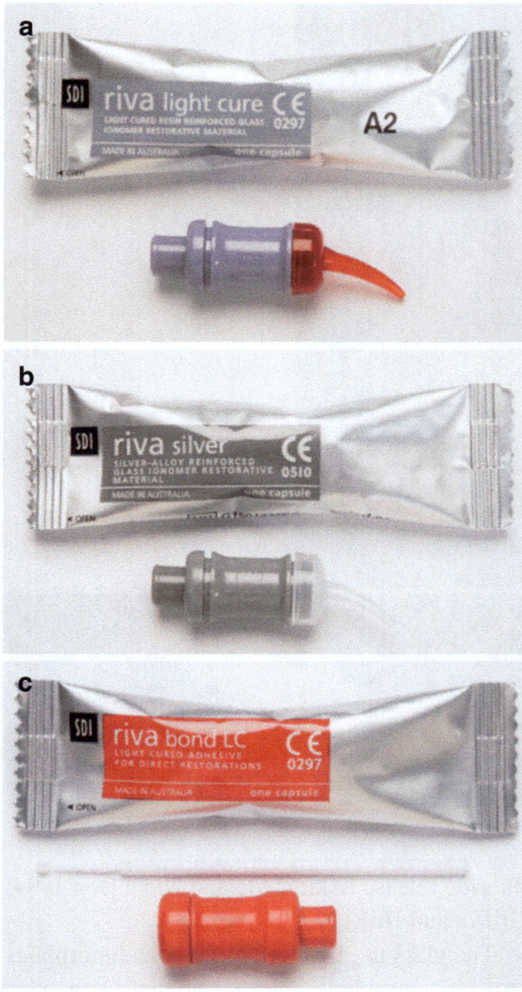

Fig. 2.3 Three different types of GICs delivered in capsule form: (**a**) a resin-modified GIC, (**b**) a silver-reinforced GIC and (**c**) a resin-modified GIC adhesive. Note that the last material is much more fluid and is applied to the tooth surface as a thin film to bond resin composite to the tooth surface. The material is mixed in an amalgamator which ensures a good consistency due to the manufacturer-controlled powder/liquid ratio

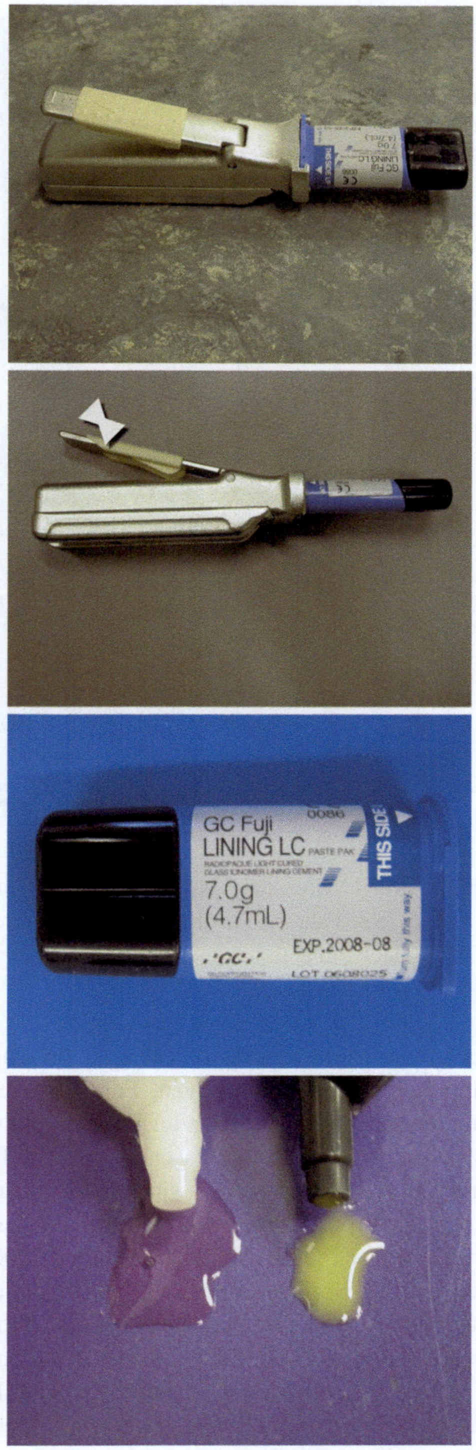

Fig. 2.4 Paste/paste dispenser for an RM-GIC lining material. Small equal amounts can be easily dispensed and mixed for placement in a small cavity. The quantity of material is varied by sliding the cream-coloured sleeve up and down the handle

set cement together (Watson et al. 2014). The component parts of the cement are described in more detail below.

2.3.1.1 Glass

The glass particles in GICs are more reactive than those found in resin composite materials. This has been achieved by incorporating fluorine into the glass. The original glass was based on the composition of $SiO_2–AlO_3–AlPO_4–NaAlF_6$

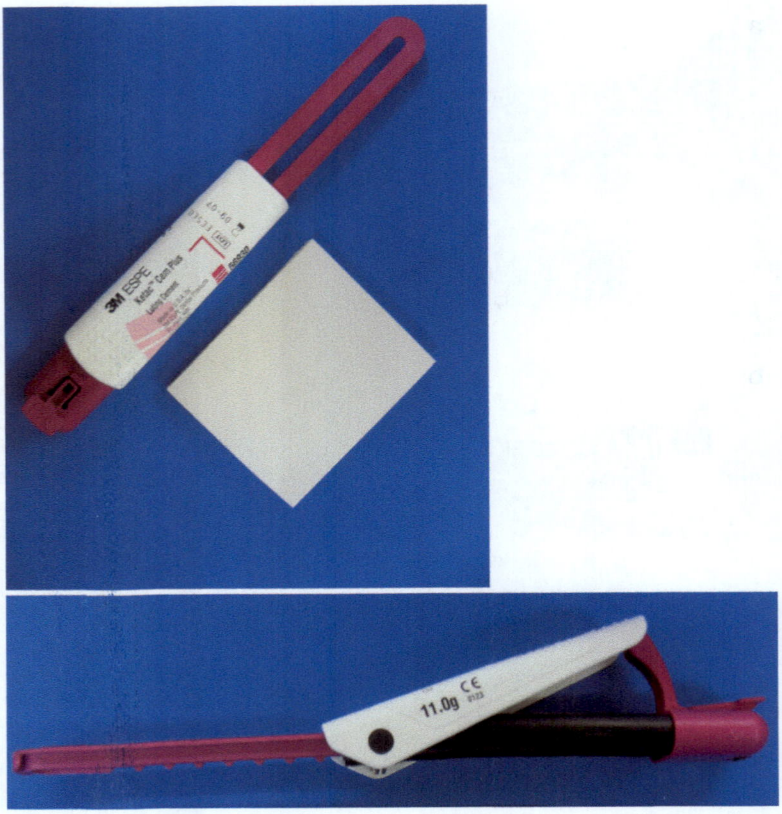

Fig. 2.5 Another type of RM-GIC paste/paste dispensing system. A 'clicker' system is used to dispense equal amounts of the paste from each half of the tubes

(Smith 1998). The early work by Wilson and McLean (1988) showed a ratio of 1:2 (or more) of Al_2O_3/SiO_2, and fluoride of up to 23 % was required for a viable GIC.

The original work when developing GICs was to use a glass made of calcium, fluorine, aluminium, silicon and oxygen. Further developments substituted the calcium with strontium and more recently zinc. Essentially, all GIC glasses have been based on a similar formula of calcium or strontium fluoroaluminosilicate glass (Shin-ichi et al. 2000; Zimehl and Hannig 2000; Nicholson 1998). The cements also contain other ions such as sodium, phosphorus, lanthanum, barium, boron and zinc. Strontium has been used to replace calcium and lanthanum to partially replace the aluminium, which gives the cement greater radiopacity. The composition of glasses has been extensively investigated but is beyond the scope of this book (De Barra and Hill 1998, 2000; Griffin and Hill 1999, 2000a, b). It would seem, however, that the Al:Si ratio is important to the glass composition, and this may influence the fluoride release (Akinmade and Nicholson 1994; Griffin and Hill 1999).

The glass in glass-ionomer has an amorphous structure in which microcrystalline structures seem to be present. The work by Schwieger et al. (2000)) using a model of the GIC setting reaction showed that the CaF_2 phase seemed to be preferentially leached to establish a silicon-rich surface on the glass which was greater than the size of the glass particles.

The inclusion of fluorine in GICs was not originally to impart an anticariogenic effect, but to aid the setting reaction of the GIC. It acts as a network disrupter allowing ion release necessary for the setting reaction. The final cement is formed by the cross-linking of the polyalkenoate matrix with strontium, calcium, aluminium and lanthanum ions. Silicon tends to remain nonreactive in the GIC reaction; it gives strength and stability to the set cement.

A recent paper showed that when the particle size of the glass is reduced, the reactivity of the particles is greatly increased with the same glass composition (De Caluwé et al. 2014). This also tends to decrease the setting time when 'nano-granular' particles replace the 'macrogranular particles'. Additional fluoride in the glass tends to decrease the setting time (De Caluwé et al 2014). The compressive strength increases as more nanogranular particles containing more fluoride are used.

2.3.1.2 Liquid

The other important component of the GIC is the liquid. The liquid is a polymeric acid having a carboxylate group(s), but it must be a lower molecular weight to prevent gelation. There are a broad range of acids that can be used, and each will provide some (Smith 1998) variation in the potential application of the set GIC (Mount 1990). The liquid can also contain water or tartaric acid. In addition, by increasing the number of carboxyl groups into the polymer chains, it also helps prevent gelation during setting, which imparts greater reactivity due to a greater number of carboxyl groups. This may also lead to increased cross-linking, thus enhancing the properties of the cement such as strength (Smith 1998). It appeared that larger-molecular-weight acids seemed to improve the overall physical strength of the cement (compressive strength, fracture toughness, etc.) (Fennel and Hill 2001a, b, c). In general, however, to achieve the ideal properties of the cement, some compromise must be made to the concentration of the liquid, which is usually limited to 50 % w/w.

The role of tartaric acid was investigated as the GICs were just starting to emerge as a clinically useful material (Wilson et al. 1976; Crisp and Wilson 1976). The inclusion of tartaric acid was shown to initially reduce the viscosity of the cement then rapidly increase it, almost leading to a 'snap' set (Prosser et al. 1982a, b). It seems that this action is due to the chelation of ions from the glass powder over the short term, which delays the formation of the gel stage of the cement. This leads to faster cross-linking of the polyacrylic acid component (Nicholson et al. 1988); hence, most GICs contain tartaric acid to improve the working time but reduce the setting time (Young et al. 2000).

It has also been shown that water is an important component in the setting reaction of GICs. It seems that the primary role of the water is to influence the acid–base reaction. The carboxylate groups dissociate allowing them to become active for ion transfer, and the water provides the medium for ion movement to the glass powder surface (Prentice 2005).

During the setting of the GIC, the amount of bound water in the matrix also increases. The matrix contains a degree of unbound water, hence the necessity for avoiding dehydration or desiccation (Small et al. 1998). This water transfer affords GICs the advantage of movement of ions (such as fluoride ions) that may reduce the damage caused in early caries attack. There is also some evidence indicating that ion uptake may occur from saliva leading to a surface hardening of the set cement surface (Okada et al. 2001).

2.3.2 Strength

Set glass-ionomer cements tend to be brittle materials. The final strength can be affected by a number of variables. The inclusion of resin into the cement seems to show improved strength but also tends to make the cement slightly less brittle in nature. This brittleness is one of the major reasons for GICs not being well suited for larger posterior load-bearing restorations.

During setting, GICs are sensitive to both moisture loss and uptake. Loss of water leads to dehydration of the cement that causes subsequent surface crazing and increased opacity. The consequences can thus be a weaker cement, a decrease in wear resistance and a loss of aesthetics. Recently, the high powder/liquid (P:L) ratio cements have shown some improvement in water sensitivity. These cements need to be protected during the 2 to 7 min of the initial set, depending on the product and whether it has been classified as a 'fast' or 'normal' set material. After this initial set, the high P:L ratio materials (e.g. Fuji IX GP, Fuji IX GP Fast, Ketac Molar, Ketac Molar Quick, Riva Self Cure Regular/Fast) can be trimmed under water spray without loss of strength or aesthetics. For the original conventional GICs, it was necessary to coat the cement with a waterproof material to prevent water uptake and weakening of the setting cement

Table 2.1 Examples of flexural and compressive strengths of glass-ionomer materials

Material	Type of GIC	Flexural strength (MPa)	Compressive strength (MPa)
Miracle Mix	Metal-reinforced	45	117 (21d)
Ketac Silver	Metal-reinforced	22.9 (7d)	211 (7d), 127 (21d)
Ketac Molar	Conventional high P:L ratio	44.1, 34.5 (24 h), 21.2 (7d)	86.2 (1 h), 177 (24 h), 232 (24 h), 301 (7d), 184 (21d)
Fuji IX/ Fuji IX Extra	Conventional high P:L ratio	33.3, (24 h), 20.2 (24 h)	99.5 (1 h), 83.3 (1 h), 166.7 (24 h), 201 (24 h), 168 (21d)
Riva	Conventional	23.9 (24 h)	126.5 (24 h), 200 (24 h)
Photac-Fil	Resin-modified	74.4 (7d)	243.5 (7d), 150 (21d)
Fuji II LC	Resin-modified	42.1, 49.6 (24 h), 71.1 (7d)	306 (7d), 166 (21d)

Based on data from McCabe (1998), Xie et al. (2000), Bapna et al. (2002), Xu and Burgess (2003), Kleverlaan et al. (2004), Bresciani et al. (2004), Bonifácio et al. (2009), Bonifácio et al. (2012) and Shiozawa et al. (2014)

for 24 h. It would seem that over time, the physical properties of conventional GICs tend to improve. The recent work by Shiozawa et al (2014) showed that five different GICs all tended to show an initial increase in compressive strength and surface hardness over the first 1–3 months of storage in deionised water. They then remained reasonably constant although slight decreases were observed (Table 2.1); this was product dependent. They showed that the surface quantities of Si, Sr, Na and F decreased over the period of 1 year. This demonstrated that there was some decrease in the surface integrity and hardness of the cements due to storage in the water. The decrease in surface hardness is contrary to that found by Okada et al (2001), who stored their samples in saliva and distilled water and used a time period limited to 40 days. This is equivalent to the early times noted for the increase in strength and hardness in Shiozawa et al.'s (2014) study. It can be useful to further assess the phenomenon of hardness or microhardness as it may have clinical implications for restorations subjected to occlusal loading. It can give some indication of the overall strength of the cement as well as surface changes when exposed to the various fluids GICs come in contact with during function.

Interestingly, one study examined Knoop hardness of a high-viscosity GIC that had been harvested from 10-year-old restorations (Zanata et al. 2011). The hardness was compared with the same material stored in water for up to 720 days. The outcomes for this study showed a similar increase in hardness which was no different from the laboratory-stored samples. The 10-year-old samples were similar in hardness to the water-stored specimens after 180 days. Energy dispersive X-ray diffraction (EDX) analysis showed that Ca was present in the cement which seemed to indicate that Ca from the oral cavity was able to diffuse into the cement.

The introduction of RM-GICs helped to overcome some of the initial dehydration problems of the conventional GICs. However, once set, the RM-GICs also show moisture sensitivity. If allowed to dehydrate, the surface crazes and becomes opaque. Hence, it is critical to maintain the water balance within the matrix of all GICs to ensure that the maximum strength possible is ensured as well as the best aesthetics.

One of the commonly mistaken concepts is that GICs do not shrink (Kim and Hirano 1999; Bryant and Mahler 2007). Both conventional GIC and RM-GIC shrink during setting. The shrinkage from the acid–base reaction portion of the set is slower, but not necessarily less than the shrinkage of the resin portion. In RM-GICs, shrinkage occurs more rapidly during the light-curing phase (Cheetham et al. 2014). In this case, the shrinkage from the acid–base component is minimal.

When it comes to the stress of the bond to the tooth, it is likely that GICs can resist some of these forces better when a resin composite restoration is placed. The cement goes through a rubbery gel stage during its set. This may assist with countering some of the stresses occurring from a light-polymerising resin composite which can be rapid and high depending on the type of composite used.

2.3.3 Fracture Toughness

As GICs are regarded as brittle and failure is related to material fracture, some researchers have focused on the fracture toughness of these and other tooth-coloured filling materials. This approach helps to characterise fracture resistance and provides some indication as to how much energy of loading is required to cause a material to fail. Several other studies have looked at this characteristic. In an approach to improve fracture toughness of GICs, resin coatings have been applied to the surface of GICs. Both conventional and resin-modified materials have been tested. It was previously shown that the application of a resin coating on the resin-modified materials generally showed an increase in toughness (Mitchell et al. 1999; Mitsuhashi et al. 2003; Ilie et al. 2012). In comparison with resin composite materials, several studies have shown that the conventional materials have the lowest fracture toughness, whereas the RM-GICs have 'comparable toughness' to the microfilled, flowable and nano-hybrid resin composites (Ilie et al. 2012) (Table 2.2).

Mitsuhashi et al. (2003) showed that there was a high correlation between the P:L ratio of conventional GICs and fracture toughness, whereas this pattern was not observed for RM-GICs. It seems that the resin component is able to increase toughness and perhaps fill in spaces where a crack may propagate more easily. One of the problems for fracture toughness measurement and comparison amongst research groups, however, is the test methodology used. The test method can lead to different outcomes as seen in Table 2.2.

Table 2.2 Fracture toughness of various GICs

Material	Type of GIC	Fracture toughness (K_{IC}, MPa $m^{1/2}$)
ChemFil Rock	Zinc-reinforced	0.99
Fuji IX GP Extra/ Fuji IX	Packable	0.8/0.53
Ketac Molar Quick Aplicap/Ketac Molar	Packable	0.85/0.48
EQUIA Fil	Resin-coated	1.21
Ketac Silver	Silver-reinforced (Cermet)	0.44
Ketac Fil	GIC	0.39
Fuji II LC	RM-GIC	1.16
Photac-Fil	RM-GIC	1.32

Based on data from Mitsuhashi et al. (2003) and Ilie et al. (2012)

2.3.4 Shear Punch Strength

Shear punch strength is another test method that has been used for comparison of materials and evaluation of coatings of GICs. This method is quite simple and gives some indication of how a cement behaves when it is loaded during function (Nomoto et al. 2001). Although not widely used, it has shown some interesting outcomes. The first shear punch strength evaluation was published in 1996 (Mount et al. 1996). This comprehensive study included conventional GIC and RM-GIC as well as a number of resin composite materials. The study was interesting in that it investigated 2-h strengths compared with 5-day strengths. They showed that for the conventional GICs, the strength showed a significant increase from the 2-h test to that of 5 days. In the case of the RM-GICs, which could be either light- or auto-cured, again it was noted that the strength increased significantly over the 5 days. If allowed to only auto-cure (i.e. no light exposure), the strength tended to be less at 5 days; hence, it would seem the light-curing aspect to curing is an essential step to achieve maximum strength. In fact, the Photac-Fil material (3M-ESPE, St Paul, MN, USA) tested at 5 days showed a lower strength than the 2-h light-cured strength. For the resin composite materials, the strength tended to increase by about 5–10 %, depending on the material, over the 5 days (Mount et al. 1996). This study was conducted prior to the introduction of the high-viscosity/high P:L ratio cements. Two later studies compared the strengths of GICs with and without resin coating (Bonifácio et al.

2012; Bagheri et al. 2013). These studies showed that in some cases, the coating was beneficial, whereas for other materials, there was little change. The interesting outcome from the study by Bagheri et al. (2013), where strengths were tested at 24 h, 4 and 8 weeks, was that irrespective of resin coating, the shear punch strengths were all observed to steadily increase over the 8 weeks of the study. In most materials, the shear punch strengths almost doubled. The effect of the coating seemed to be greater at the longer time periods after the cement had matured.

The influence of food-simulating solutions on the shear punch strength has also been evaluated (Bagheri et al. 2007; Kaur and Nandlal 2013). The solutions used were lactic acid, NaOH and coffee in one study (Bagheri et al. 2007) and citric acid, ethanol and heptane in another (Kaur and Nandlal 2013). In the first study, a RM-GIC was compared with other resin-based restorative materials, whilst in the latter study, a high-viscosity conventional GIC was assessed. The RM-GIC was shown to be strongly affected by the food-simulating solutions compared with the other resin-based materials. The same effect was also noted for the conventional GIC. It would therefore seem that GICs are more susceptible to the influence of various dietary solutions of varying pH, and this may result in some surface deterioration and weakening during clinical service.

Due to the brittle nature of GICs and their early sensitivity to water, an additional step is needed to protect the materials from water exposure in order to achieve their 'highest' strength. It was noted that the original cements had a soft 'opaque' surface layer if exposed to water too early; this was easily abraded and was quite unaesthetic (Norman et al. 1969). Other reports suggest that the newer high-strength conventional GICs may benefit from early water exposure (Leirskar et al. 2003; Wang et al. 2006).

2.3.5 Erosion

One of the important properties any restorative material must have is the ability to resist degradation from exposure to various fluids that will contact the set material in the oral cavity. The oral environment is very harsh, with restorative materials being exposed to a wide variation of temperatures and changes in acidity and alkalinity. In recent years, the loss of tooth structure due to erosive or acidic materials has become a significant issue (Kitasako et al. 2015). The matrix of the GIC is the most susceptible part of the set cement when exposed to acids. Acids such as acetic, citric and lactic have all been used to evaluate erosion (Crisp et al. 1980; Matsuya et al. 1984; Fukuzawa et al. 1987). One of the important aspects for preventing the effects of erosion is when laminate or sandwich restorations, which fill the gingival portion of deep posterior approximal restorations, are placed (van Dijken et al. 1999). The study by Scholtanus and Huysmans (2007) showed the erosive degradation of approximal lesions restored with a GIC.

As noted above, the conventional GICs are sensitive to water exposure shortly after placement. The water will damage and erode the surface of the GIC if it is left unprotected on insertion (Oilo 1984; Gemalmaz et al. 1998).

In the case of sandwich/laminate restorations, if a patient's oral hygiene is not adequate, then the biofilm may produce acid which can damage the surface of the set cement. This problem is exacerbated when the quantity of saliva is compromised and does not wash the acids away or have adequate buffering capacity. It has been shown (Nicholson et al 2000), however, that when GICs are exposed to lactic acid, the surrounding pH decreases initially, but as the GIC dissolves, the pH increases. Hence, GICs seem to exhibit a 'side effect' of being able to reduce the effects of acid attack by their own dissolution (Nicholson et al 2000). The Scholtanus and Huysmans (2007) study showed that this dissolution of conventional GIC has the beneficial effect of preventing caries initiation on susceptible adjacent tooth surfaces. It is most likely due to the constant exposure of a 'fresh' GIC surface that is able to release 'maximum' levels of fluoride ions into the surrounding environment and tooth structure. When erosion does occur, it is the matrix of the set cement that is most susceptible to damage (De Moor and Verveeck 1998; Patel et al. 2000).

RM-GICs are also susceptible to erosion. Water has been demonstrated to have an erosive effect on the surface of RM-GICs (Cattani-Lorente et al. 1999; Fano et al. 2004). It would appear that the amount of light irradiation, i.e. the duration of light curing, may have an influence on the degree of erosion of RM-GICs (Fano et al. 2004). They showed that an exposure time of less than 15 s resulted in cracking of the cement and a greater degree of erosion. The same study showed that the pH of the immersion solution also influenced the degree of erosion, which was also noted in the study by Czarnecka and Nicholson (2006). However, like the conventional GICs, when the degree of erosion does increase, the release of fluoride also increases (Carey et al. 2003), thus affording some benefit to assist with controlling demineralisation around cavity margins and adjacent teeth.

A recent study using pH cycling over a 35-day period using a cola drink and artificial saliva showed that both the conventional GIC and RM-GIC displayed greater amounts of erosion compared with amalgam and resin composite (Honório et al. 2008).

A study investigated the effects of erosion of a resin composite, conventional GIC and RM-GIC placed into root dentine cavities (Soares et al. 2012). It was observed that the acid erosion severely degraded the GIC surfaces but afforded the dentine at the cavity margins some protection against the erosive solution due to the ions released from the degrading GIC (Soares et al. 2012). Ion release has also been demonstrated in the study by Zalizniak et al. (2013) where GICs were exposed to various acid solutions. It was observed that ion release, particularly phosphate ions, seemed to be dependent on the type of acid the GICs were exposed to. The mechanism is still not well understood and needs further investigation.

Erosion also affects surface roughness. A study comparing resin composite and conventional GIC and RM-GIC showed large differences in surface roughness. Hence, it would seem that the addition of resin into RM-GICs may not provide a long-term benefit from the aspect of surface finish when exposed to an acidic solution (Hussein et al. 2014).

One of the areas which has so far not been investigated to any great extent is the influence of the new coating agents that are now used on GICs. These coating materials are resin-based and have been shown to increase the fracture toughness of the materials (Bagheri et al. 2010). However, little research has been conducted to determine whether these resin coatings or even the placement of a coat in the form of a resin-based adhesive or bonding resin will reduce the erosion. Unfortunately, this may also cause some reduction in the release of fluoride ions that may make the GICs less effective in reducing the caries experience or recurrence around margins or on adjacent teeth (Mazzaoui et al. 2000).

2.3.6 Abrasion

Often in association with erosion is abrasion of the softened GIC surface. Compared with resin composite materials, it has been reported that GICs have a much lower abrasion resistance. It is also known that due to the maturation of GICs during the setting process, their abrasion resistance is poor compared to the fully matured cement (Mount and Hume 2005). Although not aesthetic, it has been shown that the metal-reinforced GICs have a better abrasion resistance (Forss et al. 1991). With the introduction of the high powder/liquid ratio and small particle materials such as Fuji IX (GC Corp, Tokyo, Japan) or Ketac Molar (3M-ESPE, St Paul, MN, USA), it has been demonstrated that the wear (abrasion) can be reduced significantly (Kunzelmann et al. 2003).

Another means to increase abrasion resistance is also the concept of coating the GIC. To date, the research remains limited, similar to that for erosion resistance. One study using the resin glazing agent Bellfeel Brightener (Kanebo Ltd, Tokyo, Japan) when applied to a GIC surface showed a significant increase in surface hardness and thus more resistance to abrasion (Hotta and Hirukawa 1994). More recently, the use of proprietary resin coating agents, e.g. G-Coat Plus (GC Corp, Japan) in combination with the high-viscosity GIC, Fuji IX, has been marketed as EQUIA (GC Corp, Japan) or more recently as

EQUIA Forte Fil (GC Corp). The application of the coating as described previously has been shown to increase the strength of the GIC and increase its abrasion resistance. It is believed the resin is able to infiltrate the GIC surface, thus filling cracks and porosities (Lohbauer et al. 2011).

For the RM-GICs, the incorporation of the resin was not shown to improve the abrasion resistance. In fact, a number of studies have reported that the abrasion resistance is decreased and that the RM-GIC materials will abrade more rapidly than conventional GICs (Pelka et al. 1996; Momoi et al. 1997; Peutzfeldt et al. 1997; Xie et al. 2000; Sunnegårdh-Grönberg et al. 2002). The reason for this reduction in abrasion resistance is thought to be due to the glass particles being bonded loosely to the matrix in association with a nonuniform distribution of the glass particles throughout the set cement (Xie et al. 2000). When a polyacid-modified resin composite (PAMRC) was compared with an RM-GIC clinically, it was also noted that the abrasion resistance was lower for the RM-GIC (Chinelatti et al. 2004).

2.3.7 Adhesion

One of the great advantages of GICs is that they have become known for their ability to adhere to the moist cut tooth surface. This group of materials is able to bond to all parts of the tooth and carious tooth structure with a high degree of reliability and low technique sensitivity. Interestingly, however, there has not been as wide an evaluation of adhesive tests compared with resin-based adhesives. The original glass-ionomer cements were applied to smear layer-covered dentine. In the mid-1980s, workers started to consider how the adhesion of GICs might be improved (Lacefield et al. 1985). It was known from the work with phosphoric acid on enamel that adhesion for resin-based materials could be greatly enhanced. Various treatments such as polyacrylic acid, H_2O_2, citric acid or surface cleaning alone were tested. It was reported that the polyacrylic acid showed improved adhesion (Hinoura et al. 1986). Around 1990, manufacturers introduced conditioners such as Ketac Conditioner (3M-ESPE, St Paul, MN, USA) and GC Conditioner (GC Corp, Tokyo, Japan) for conditioning the dentine and enamel. It was shown that the use of these polyacrylic acid-based materials greatly enhanced the adhesion (Joynt et al. 1990; Tanumiharja et al. 2001). After such work, it became a routine practice to condition the dentine prior to GIC placement. These studies showed that the conditioning removed the smear layer but did not remove the smear plugs which 'protected' the dentine from becoming very wet. The tooth surface is not etched in the same way as acids such as phosphoric acid. This was the commencement of routine conditioning of tooth surfaces prior to placement of a GIC lining or restoration as opposed to etching for enamel and dentine with resin-based adhesives. Later work showed that removal of the smear layer could lead to better adaptation and bonding of the cement to the tooth surface. Another early study showed that this improved adhesion could be achieved with the use of maleic acid conditioning of dentine prior to the placement of Vitrebond (3M-ESPE, St Paul, MN, USA), which was one of the first resin-modified GICs to become available commercially (Watson 1990). Later Tyas showed that the use of polyacrylic acid conditioning clinically seemed to have little effect on restoration survival (Tyas 1993). This same outcome was shown in another study comparing 10 % polyacrylic acid conditioned and nonconditioned non-carious cervical lesions over a 4-year period. However, a slightly better retention rate was observed for the conditioned group, 15.6 % loss compared with 21.9 % loss in the nonconditioned group (van Dijken 1996a). Slightly later, a further study investigated the adhesion of a 'viscous' conventional GIC, Chem-Flex (Dentsply DeTrey GmbH, Konstanz, Germany), to dentine using different conditioning agents. These included 10 % polyacrylic acid (PAA) without rinsing, 10 % PAA with water rinsing, 25 % PAA with rinsing and 32 % phosphoric acid and a control of smear layer-covered dentine (Tay et al. 2001). Further to the bond study, this group also investigated the interface using transmission electron microscopy (TEM). It was shown that bond strengths after conditioning were much higher compared to the control. The TEM observations showed that the acidity of the GIC during setting was not able to alter the smear layer-covered control surface. However, when 10 % PAA was used as the conditioning agent, it was observed that the smear layer was removed and also partial demineralisation occurred up to 0.8 μm deep. An 'interphase' was noted between the tooth surface and cement (Tay et al. 2001). With the stronger acids or longer conditioning times, the depth of demineralisation increased. This interphase layer was also reported in the study by Tanumiharja et al. (2001), who investigated the interface using field emission scanning electron microscopy. They observed that this layer was resistant to attack by acidic and basic solutions and could range between 2.8 and 3.4 μm thick. A very similar phenomenon was noted when an RM-GIC was bonded to conditioned dentine. This study showed that using a conditioner provided a significant improvement in bond strengths. The interface of the RM-GIC and dentine also showed the acid–base resistant layer described by Tanumiharja et al. (2001). Subsequently, others observed that a hybrid-like layer similar to that formed by resin-based adhesives also formed (Cardoso et al. 2010).

With respect to RM-GICs, Coutinho et al. (2007) investigated several RM-GIC materials including an RM-GIC adhesive (Fuji Bond LC, GC Corp, Tokyo, Japan) as well as direct restorative materials (Photac-Fil and Vitrebond, 3M-ESPE, St Paul, MN, USA). They characterised the interfaces using transmission, scanning and field emission electron microscopy and atomic force microscopy. The tooth surfaces were either not conditioned or conditioned and treated with either a 20 % acrylic–maleic acid copolymer or 25 % polyacrylic acid. For the Fuji Bond LC conditioned samples, a very thin gel phase layer (0.5–1.0 μm thick) was observed above a sub-micrometre hybrid layer (Coutinho et al. 2007). This was also noted for the Photac-Fil but not the case for Vitrebond.

When conditioning did not take place, the gel phase was not observed, but partial demineralisation still occurred as in the conditioned groups. It would seem that when RM-GICs adhere to the tooth surface, it is a dual-type adhesive process. A thin hybrid layer is formed onto a partially demineralised surface with hydroxyapatite still remaining present in the collagen fibre matrix. Above this hybrid layer is a thin gel phase layer which has been identified previously as an 'absorption layer' (Sidhu and Watson 1998). Coutinho et al. (2007) showed that in the case of Vitrebond, it did not react in the same manner as the other RM-GICs tested. There was no sign of a hybrid layer or gel phase formation, but it did not seem to affect the bond. The other part of the bond seemed to be due to the reaction of polycarboxylic acid copolymers interacting with hydroxyapatite to form a chemical bond (Yoshida et al. 2000). This 'dual' adhesion process provides an answer as to why many clinical studies show such a high success of RM-GIC restorations.

With respect to surface treatments, recently some have advocated that a short etch with phosphoric acid on dentine and enamel will enhance the bond to tooth structure when an RM-GIC is used. Whilst there may be some logic to this concept, it should be remembered that even a short etch with phosphoric acid has the potential to remove all of the hydroxyapatite from the tooth surface. Based on the work of Coutinho et al. (2007), it would appear that this would then prevent the polycarboxylate groups from interacting chemically with calcium and thus potentially remove one of the modes of adhesion of the RM-GICs, namely, the chemical portion. This may also have long-term implications on adhesion since the bond would tend to be essentially micromechanical and be subject to degradation of the collagen similar to resin-based adhesives. Recently, Hamama et al. (2014) investigated the effect of a 5-s etch with phosphoric acid compared to conditioning with polyacrylic acid-based conditioners. They showed that in the short term (24 h), the bond strengths were little different, but later unpublished work by this group showed that the bonding outcomes for the etched group tended to decrease over time or became more variable (Hamama et al., unpublished). This may be an indication that the bond using a polyacrylic acid-based conditioner can lead to a more stable bond over the long term.

2.3.7.1 Adhesion to Composite and Repair

With the advent of the sandwich or laminate technique to restore deep approximal cavities, many have questioned the ability of GICs to bond to resin composite. There is little or no problem of bonding to composite with the RM-GICs since the HEMA in the cement, being a methacrylate, can easily adhere to resin-based adhesives or resin composite, which are also methacrylate-based materials. However, concern has been expressed with respect to the ability of the resin portion of the RM-GIC to adequately polymerise in deep cavities. Although the depth of cure has been poorly studied, the few studies available seem to consistently demonstrate that depth of cure is indeed an issue that must be carefully considered. The first paper by Mount et al. (2002) concluded that 'cavities more than 3 mm deep' should be filled incrementally. The shade of the material was also an influencing factor for the depth of cure. A later study also made the same recommendation (Roberts et al. 2009). It would therefore seem that for cavities extending onto the root face, a conventional high powder/liquid ratio GIC is possibly the most reliable material to use. However, the issue remains of being able to achieve adhesion to the overlying resin composite.

The first study to investigate long-term adhesion of conventional GICs with recent etch-and-rinse and self-etch adhesives was that of Zhang et al. (2011). They showed that effective bonding could be achieved with any of the adhesives tested which included etch-and-rinse, self-etch and all-in-one systems. One potential issue was the effect of the phosphoric acid on the GIC surface causing microcracks that seemed to influence the long-term adhesion. The self-etch materials, however, showed quite stable adhesion over the 6 months of the test. Another study that included a conventional GIC was that of Navimipour et al. (2012). They investigated the adhesion of a conventional GIC and RM-GIC to resin composite using either phosphoric acid or Er,CR:YSGG laser for etching the GICs for 15 s. Both treatments showed improvements of bond strengths with the RM-GIC showing higher bond strengths compared with the conventional material. A further study compared RM-GIC and conventional GIC with an etch-and-rinse adhesive and acidic all-in-one adhesive (Pamir et al. 2012). This group concluded that both GICs bonded well to either adhesive, but an etch time of 30 s was recommended. The study by Zhang et al. (2011) contradicts this, as the impression was that stronger and longer etching can possibly damage the matrix of the underlying cement and weaken its cohesive strength. Generally, it was considered that the self-etch materials may provide a more reliable bond and reduce the possibility of damaging the underlying GIC. Recent studies on bonding an RM-GIC to resin composite with a variety of adhesives showed successful bonding (Kasraie et al. 2013; Boruziniat and Gharaei 2014). However, caution must still be exercised with respect to the depth of cure.

The other aspect in this section is the repair of GIC restorations. Very little work has been undertaken to determine if previously placed GIC restorations can be successfully repaired by the addition of new GIC. Only one study seems to have been published investigating the bonding of RM-GIC or resin composite to 4-day-old RM-GIC (Maneenut et al. 2010). The surfaces were treated with or without acid etch. The bond of the new RM-GIC was lower and slightly more variable in comparison with that of the resin composite. This study recommended that when addition to existing RM-GIC is warranted, the addition of resin composite is preferable (Maneenut et al. 2010). A very recent study (Welch et al. 2015) has investigated almost the same scenario as Maneenut et al. This latter study used roughening, roughening and etching or roughening, etching and the addition of a resin-based adhesive. It was concluded that the addition of the resin-based adhesive to a roughened and etched surface produced the best outcomes (Welch et al 2015). The conclusions concurred with the former study of preferably bonding resin composite to the RM-GIC when a repair is needed.

2.3.8 Ion Release

One of the major points all practitioners will mention about their reason for selection of a GIC material is the release of ions, particularly fluoride. Certainly this is a great advantage of GICs since it affords them the ability to alter the environment round the material. This allows potentially healing and/or preventing early caries attack, as well as aiding the healing of deep caries lesions in prepared cavities which have not had all the carious tissue excavated. Research is moving towards developing GICs to be able to release or supply other ions or compounds, and this is discussed elsewhere in this book. The first cements to show the effect of fluoride release and thus prevent re-initiation of caries were the silicate cements. The source of the fluoride from GICs is the glass particles. Unfortunately, it is still unclear how much fluoride is actually needed to prevent the initiation of caries. The paper by Randall and Wilson (1999) indicated that the clinical evidence was unclear with respect to the prevention of caries in teeth restored with GIC.

Some of the original work conducted on fluoride release from GICs was done by Forsten (1990, 1995). His work of 1990 was based on some of the original conventional GICs where fluoride release was evaluated from 24 h up to 8 weeks. This was the pioneering work on this important topic. It was shown that the release of fluoride was highest in the first 24 h whilst the cement was still maturing, with a large reduction in the first week, followed by a more steady decline over the 8 weeks of the study. Fluoride was still detectable at 8 weeks but at very low levels. When analysed from the aspect of cumulative release, it was noted that the amounts of fluoride detected was very much material dependent. Interestingly, Forsten also investigated the fluoride release after exposing the cements to running water for up to 22 months. Again even at 22 months, fluoride ions were still being released from the cements which were detected at about 1 part per million. The only material that did not show release of the fluoride ion was the cermet material, Ketac Silver (3 M-ESPE, USA). When exposed to an acidic solution, a greater level of fluoride was identified (Forsten 1990). Forsten followed this work up to 5 years later with an evaluation of RM-GIC fluoride release as well as uptake. This study initially observed fluoride release for up to 1 month. Again it was shown there was a high initial burst of fluoride at 24 h with a greatly reduced release by 1 month (Forsten 1995). Another aspect of the research was to determine whether 9-month-old RM-GIC specimens, which had been in running water, could take up fluoride if stored in a 50 ppm fluoride-containing solution for 1 week. He showed that even after 9 months, fluoride could still be detected, but specimens stored in the fluoride-containing solution showed a much greater release for the following week. This was probably the first paper to indicate that GICs could be 'recharged' with fluoride. Furthermore, it was also shown that in an acidic environment, the level of fluoride release increased (Forsten 1995). This fluoride release occurred due to erosion of the GIC, as discussed in the previous sections, where 'fresh' GIC that has F ions in abundance would be continually exposed. In a later review paper, Forsten noted that the fluoride release was a little different between the conventional GIC and RM-GIC. Forsten's work also noted that the other fluoride-releasing materials such as PAMRC did not respond in the same way to the recharging process (Forsten 1998).

A more recent paper investigated the fluoride release from RM-GICs (Vitremer, 3M-ESPE; Fuji II LC, GC Corp), including an RM-GIC containing nanofillers (Ketac Nano, 3M-ESPE) and a flowable PAMRC (Dyract Flow, Dentsply), when exposed to solutions of different pHs (4, 5.5 and 7) (Moreau and Xu 2010). Fluoride release was measured up to 84 days post-setting. This study showed an initial high release of fluoride which was again material dependent. It was noted that the PAMRC and nanofilled RM-GIC released significantly less fluoride than the other two RM-GICs tested. During the first 2–3 weeks, the lower pH solutions led to greater release of fluoride, but by days 70–84, the rate of release was no different amongst the 3 different pH solutions. Figure 2.6 illustrates the typical pattern of cumulative fluoride ion release, whilst Fig. 2.7 shows the typical rate of fluoride release for these types of material.

A previous study investigated the recharge and release of fluoride in a number of GICs at varying pH (Markovic et al. 2008). In this study, NaF solution was used for recharge, but there was no mention of surface deterioration as a

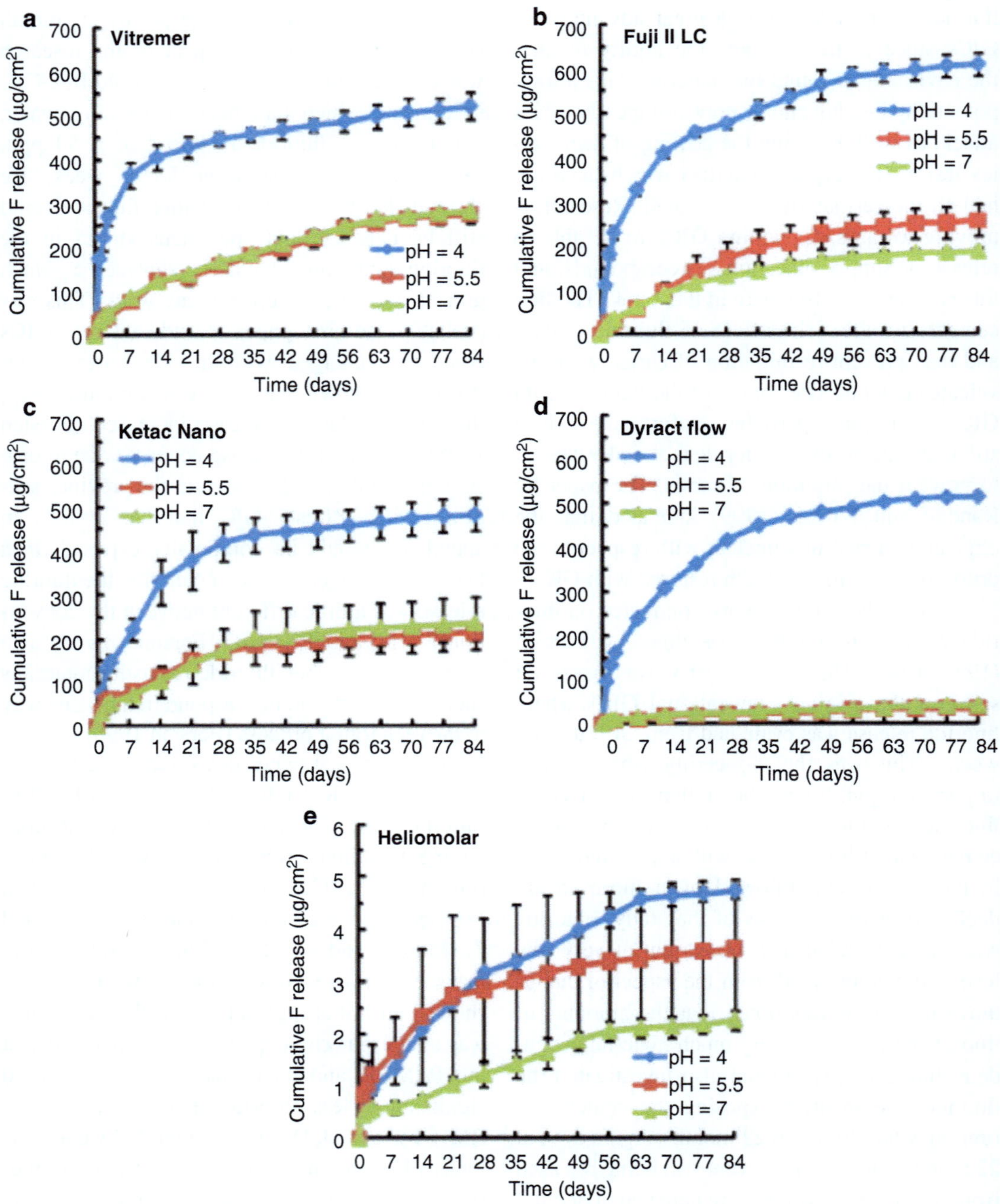

Fig. 2.6 This figure provides an illustration of the typical pattern shown for cumulative fluoride ion (F) release per specimen area (μg/cm²) from various tooth-coloured restorative materials: (**a**) Vitremer, (**b**) Fuji II LC, (**c**) Ketac Nano, (**d**) Dyract Flow and (**e**) Heliomolar. Each value is mean ± sd. The F release was higher in pH 4 solution than in pH 5.5 or pH 7 (Reprinted from Moreau and Xu (2010). With permission from Elsevier)

function of the NaF exposure, but rather attributed recharging to the effects of the acidic environment. A very low pH of 2.5 was used as one of the test solutions. When specimens were placed in the NaF solution, it was noted that the surface fluoride content increased. They also concluded that fluoride release was related to the degradation of the cement, and the concentration of the

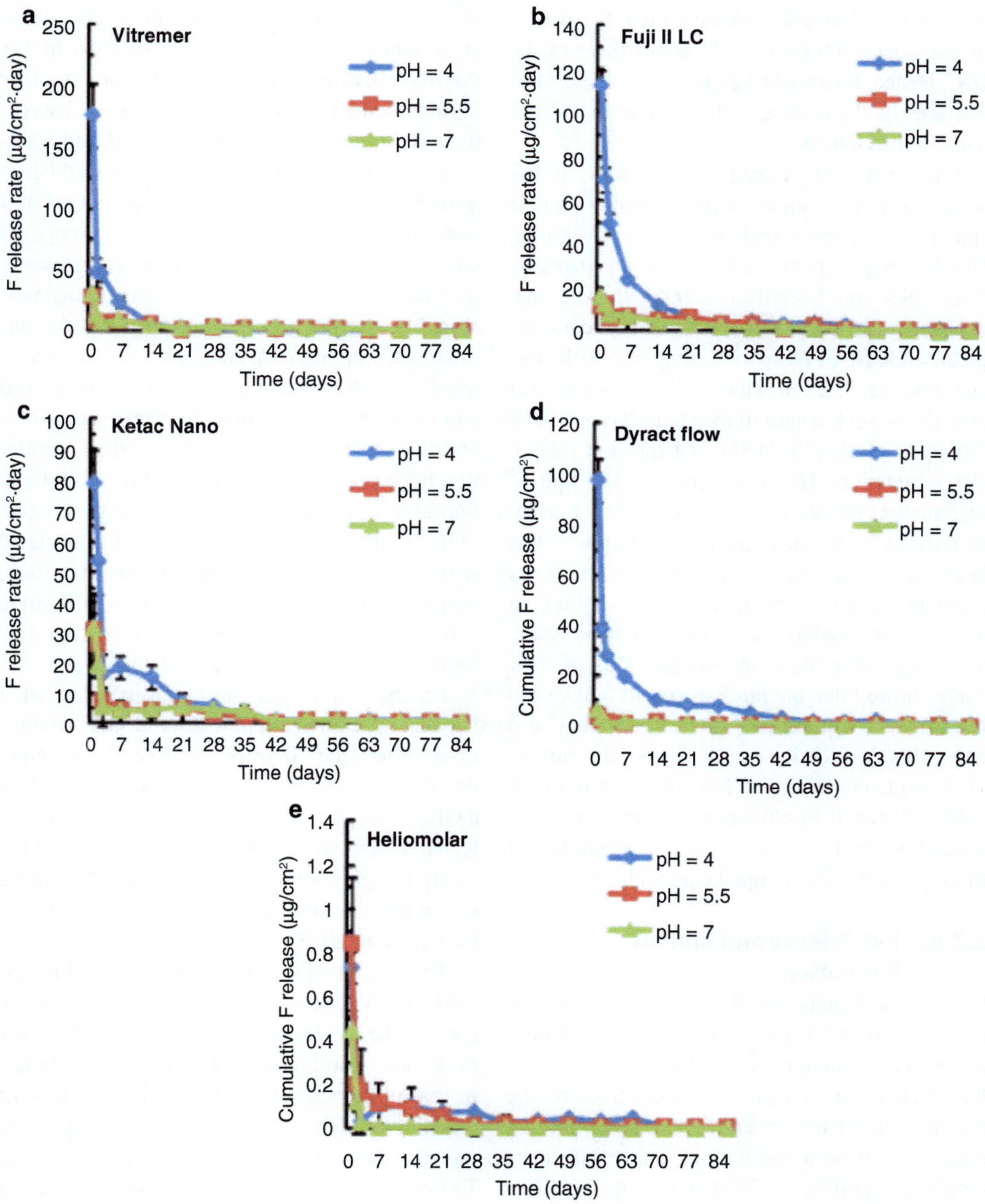

Fig. 2.7 This figure illustrates the typical pattern of release of F ions over time: an initial high burst of ions with a rapid drop within the first week and then a steady low level thereafter. F release rate, which is the F release per specimen surface area per day, is shown for (**a**) Vitremer, (**b**) Fuji II LC, (**c**) Ketac Nano, (**d**) Dyract Flow and (**e**) Heliomolar. Each value is mean ± sd (Reprinted from Moreau and Xu (2010). With permission from Elsevier)

fluoride at the surface was related to the surface media and pH. It seems that all the GICs tested could be recharged, and this was influenced by the pH, with better recharge occurring at a lower pH (Markovic et al. 2008). It would appear that the recharge process is a surface interaction as shown by Hadley et al. (2001) who investigated ion distribution in two GICs. They noted that when exposed to a KF solution, the GICs have a higher concentration of F on the surface of the GIC. Hence, it cannot be expected for these fluoride ions on the surface to diffuse into the deeper parts of the cement.

GICs not only release fluoride ions. It has been shown in a number of papers that other ions can also be released such as calcium, strontium, aluminium, phosphorus and silicon. The paper by Czarnecka and Nicholson (2006) showed that exposure of two RM-GICs to lactic acid caused a greater release of these ions compared with storage in water. The ion release did vary somewhat over the 6-week length of the study. The work by Zalizniak et al. (2013) showed that ion release also seemed to be dependent on the type of organic acid that the GIC was exposed to. Further work needs to be undertaken to explain why this is so, but it may relate to the valency of the acids used: lactic, citric and hydrochloric. Billington et al. (2006) undertook a comprehensive study analysing ion release and uptake. Part of their study showed that the mechanisms of uptake and release were still not well understood. They also noted that fluoride ions could disrupt the surface of fluoride-containing GICs (Billington et al. 2006). Hence, it would seem that further study is needed to better understand the dynamics of these processes of ion uptake and release.

2.3.8.1 Ion Release and Biofilm Formation

One of the benefits of the fluoride ion release is to assist with preventing demineralisation around cavity margins and adjacent teeth. Work has been done to determine the effect of the fluoride release and its effect on the biofilm that may develop on a restoration or at cavity margins (Al-Naimi et al. 2008; Chau et al. 2015). The study by Al-Naimi et al. (2008) compared a number of GICs, a PAMRC, a fluoride-releasing composite (Giomer, Shofu Dental Corp, Kyoto, Japan) and a resin composite. They measured fluoride release and showed that the GICs released more fluoride than the other materials. Biofilm was grown on the material surfaces at pH 3.8 or 7.1 in saliva. It was demonstrated that the biofilm growth was greatest in neutral conditions with much less growth in acidic conditions (Al-Naimi et al. 2008). This study showed that the higher fluoride-releasing GICs did not seem to alter biofilm growth. However, the confocal observations did not state if they used a live/dead staining technique, which would have provided better information as to whether the biofilm on the GICs was any different in characteristics compared with the other materials. The more recent study by Chau et al. (2015) shows different outcomes. Five different GICs, both conventional and resin-modified, were used together with a hydroxyapatite disc as the control material. This study used a mono-culture of *S mutans* to investigate a 94-h biofilm. Their results showed a negative correlation between acid production by the biofilm and fluoride release. It was also shown that the volume of the 94-h old biofilms was negatively correlated with the mean rate of fluoride release. Therefore, it appears from this work that if enough fluoride is released, it may 'decrease the virulence of cariogenic biofilms' (Chau et al. 2015).

Another interesting study investigated what happens to cavity margins around GIC restorations after the fluoride release is severely depleted. Several restorative materials, including a GIC, were placed in cavities and then were subjected to acid attack. The results showed that the cavity margins were indeed protected by uptake of the fluoride into the surrounding tooth tissue (Shiiya et al. 2012).

This uptake of fluoride in the surrounding tissues and the changes in biofilm growth indicate one of the potential advantages of GICs over most other tooth-coloured restorative materials in that placement of GICs may be one way of reducing initiation of breakdown of cavity-restoration margins through carious demineralisation. The review by Wiegand et al. (2007) describes the release and uptake of fluoride and its influence on caries and antibacterial activity. It was concluded that clinically, there remains a paucity of data from prospective clinical trials to provide a definitive answer to this issue. Hence, more clinical evaluation data are needed to better understand this point. This conclusion is similar to the findings 8 years previously of Randall and Wilson (1999).

2.4 Clinical Performance

The most important aspect of any material is how it performs clinically. More data have been published in recent years, but it still remains limited and not well standardised. There is now a lot of information from ART-based studies, but large prospective studies are scarce. The ART-based trials will be dealt with separately from those where GICs are used in a more 'conventional' manner.

The two reviews comparing the long-term survival of cervical restorations against resin-based adhesives and glass-ionomer cements both concluded that the GICs still achieve the highest survival rates (Peumans et al. 2005, 2014). Sidhu (2010) has also published a review of the clinical performance of RM-GICs. The paper by Hickel and Manhart (2001) investigated the longevity of materials in posterior teeth. They included GICs in this review although the authors stated that GICs are not considered for load-bearing restorations. They reported failure rates of between 1.4 and 14.4 % for GICs. The major reason for failure was noted to be due to caries and bulk failure. The studies reported in the Hickel and Manhart (2001) review are no longer contemporary and do not reflect current outcomes or materials.

2.4.1 Clinical Evaluation of GICs Placed in Non-carious Cervical Lesions

When testing the adhesive ability and longevity of GICs from the standpoint of clinical evaluations, it is the restoration of non-carious cervical lesions (NCCL) that has been the most common. The shape of NCCL is typically non-retentive, the lesions are quite prevalent and they occur in non-load-bearing regions. Hence, they are ideal for evaluating the adhesive qualities of a material. Table 2.3 summarises several studies over time with respect to retention of GICs and RM-GICs in NCCLs. Most studies investigated RM-GICs in this cavity configuration because of the improved aesthetics compared with many conventional GIC materials, particularly the earlier ones. The length of studies is quite variable with short studies of 12 months' duration up to a few more comprehensive studies of 10 or more years in length. Many studies include a GIC, or more commonly an RM-GIC, for comparison or as a control material when evaluating new resin-based adhesives. This is due to the fact that restorations of NCCLs with a GIC or RM-GIC are often associated with good outcomes from the aspect of restoration retention. The figures in Table 2.3 show that the failure rates of these restorations remain quite low even for the longer-term studies. The studies of 10 and 13 years in length showed a failure of 76 % or annual failure rate of 2.7 %. This attests to the very good retention of GICs and RM-GICs when placed in NCCLs. The quality of the dentine of these lesions usually tends to be hypermineralised and sclerosed. This type of dentine is ideal for bonding of a GIC-based material as the mineral content is high, ensuring good chemical adhesion to the tooth surface.

Retention of a restoration is possibly the most important criterion. However, other factors such as marginal breakdown and surface characteristics of the material must also be evaluated as these will have a significant impact on the aesthetic quality of a restoration which, from a patient's perspective, is the most important. The short study by Maneenut and Tyas (1995) showed marginal staining was beginning quite early in about five restorations of the 20 for each material they evaluated. They also noted darkening of the restorations. The 10-year study by Matis et al. (1996) indicated that about 87 % of the GIC restorations were rated alpha with no or minimal staining, whilst the resin-based material, Cervident (SS White Corp, Boston, USA), showed no discolouration. Interestingly though, when the parameter of marginal adaptation was examined, the GICs performed slightly better with an 81–87 % alpha rating compared with only 75 % for the resin-based material. These older GICs all showed surface roughness developing, with only 53–67 % of restorations showing an alpha rating after 10 years, compared with the resin-based material having a 100 % alpha rating. These changes did not appear to be tooth

Table 2.3 Retention rates of GICs in various clinical evaluations in non-carious cervical lesions

Authors	No. of restorations (patients)	Type of GIC	Alternative material	Retention rate	Study duration
Maneenut and Tyas (1995)	60 (13 patients)	RM-GIC (3 materials, 20 restorations each)	Nil	RM-GICs: 100 %	1 yr
Matis et al. (1996)	120 at baseline; 36 at 10 yrs (30 patients at baseline; 18 patients at 10 yrs)	GIC (2 materials, but 1 GIC had 2 subgroups: finished immediately or delayed)	1 Resin composite (RC)	GICs: 76 % (67–83 %) RC: 17 %	10 yrs
Brackett et al. (1999)	68 at baseline, 58 at 2 yrs (29 patients at baseline)	GIC and RM-GIC (34 restorations each)	Nil	GIC: 93 % RM-GIC: 93 %	2 yrs
Ermis (2002)	100 (30 patients at baseline)	RM-GIC (1 material, 20 restorations)	PAMRCs (4 materials, 20 restorations each)	RM-GIC: 95 % PAMRCs: 84–90 %	2 yrs
Özgünaltay and Önen (2002)	98 (24 patients)	RM-GIC (1 material, 50 restorations)	RC (1 material, 48 restorations)	RM-GIC: 98 % RC: 95 %	3 yrs
Loguercio et al. (2003)	32 (12 patients)	RM-GIC (1 material, 16 restorations)	PAMRC (1 material, 16 restorations)	RM-GIC: 93 % PAMRC: 79 %	5 yrs
Franco et al. (2006)	70 (30 patients)	RM-GIC (1 material, 35 restorations)	RC (1 material, 35 restorations)	RM-GIC: 96 % RC: 52 %	5 yrs
Burrow and Tyas (2007)	92 (20 patients)	RM-GIC (1 material, 31 restorations)	RC (2 materials, 61 restorations)	RM-GIC: 97 % RC: 83.5 % (77–90 %)	3 yrs
Van Dijken and Pallesen (2008)	270 at baseline; 215 at 13 yrs (88 patients at baseline; 68 patients at 13 yrs)	RM-GIC (1 material, 49 restorations)	RC (1 material, 5 adhesives, 221 restorations)	Annual loss rate – RM-GIC: 2.7 % RCs: 2.8–13 %	13 yrs
Santiago et al. (2010)	70 (30 patients)	RM-GIC (1 material, 35 restorations)	RC (1 material, 35 restorations)	RM-GIC: 100 % RC: 79 %	2 yrs
Jyothi et al. (2011)	80 (32 patients)	RM-GIC (1 material, 40 restorations)	Giomer (1 material, 40 restorations)	RM-GIC: 87.5 % RC: 87.5 %	1 yr
Perdigão et al (2012)	92 (33 patients)	RM-GIC (1 conventional, 1 nanofilled, 31 restorations each)	RC (1 material, 31 restorations)	RM-GICs: 100 % RC: 93 %	1 yr
Namgung et al. (2013) (retrospective)	479 (131 patients; initially evaluated from 564 restorations, only 479 included in study)	GIC (74 restorations), RM-GIC (23 restorations)	RC (377 restorations)	Survival of GICs: 11.5 yrs RC: 10.4 yrs	–
Folwaczny et al. (2000) (including carious lesions)	197 (37 patients)	RM-GIC (2 materials, 51 and 31 restorations = 82 altogether)	RC (1 material, 36 restorations) PAMRC (1 material, 79 restorations)	RM-GIC: 92 % RC: 100 % PAMRC: 91 %	2 yrs

or arch position related. A slightly later study evaluated an RM-GIC and resin composite over 3 years (Özgünaltay and Önen 2002). At 3 years, only 59 % of the RM-GIC (Vitremer, 3M-ESPE) restorations had an alpha rating for marginal discolouration, whilst the resin composite, Z100 (3M-ESPE), had a 93 % alpha rating. Regarding marginal adaptation, it was almost the same for

Vitremer at 95 % and the composite at 93 %. This study shows that resin composite seems to exhibit better long-term outcomes based on these two parameters. Another study of 5 years' duration compared Vitremer with a resin composite (Franco et al. 2006). Interestingly, this study showed a combined 100 % alpha and bravo rating for marginal discolouration for both material types. However, marginal integrity was 76 % alpha and bravo rating for the resin composite compared with 85 % for the RM-GIC. The 3-year study by Burrow and Tyas (2007) compared two resin composites with an RM-GIC. This study showed minimal marginal staining amongst all of the materials tested. Although colour and shape of the restorations remained good, it was noted that the RM-GIC did show some loss of surface texture, but it was not enough to elicit concerns from patients. However, the RM-GIC had the greatest retention at 97 %. The most recent retrospective study (Namgung et al. 2013) indicated that the resin composite performed better than the GIC from the aspects of marginal discolouration and adaptation. Care is needed when interpreting these outcomes, as the number of resin composite restorations was much higher than the GIC restorations. It seemed, however, in this case, that the resin composites were performing better overall. The 2-year study evaluating restoration of carious lesions showed some slightly different outcomes to the non-carious cervical lesions (Folwaczny et al. 2000). This study compared a resin composite, PAMRC and two RM-GICs. They examined marginal integrity on both the enamel and cementum sides of the restoration. The resin composite showed alpha ratings of 88 % for enamel and 100 % for cementum, 73 and 85 %, respectively, for the PAMRC. As for the RM-GICs, the ratings were 70.6 and 58.8 for Fuji IILC (GC Corp) compared with 62.5 and 33.3 % for Photac-Fil (3M-ESPE). This study showed quite large variations, for example, marginal discolouration showed large variations between the two GICs. The GICs also did not perform particularly well with regard to surface integrity of the restorative material. Only 10 % of Photac-Fil and 23.5 % of Fuji II LC were given an alpha rating compared with 100 % for the resin composite and 95 % for the PAMRC (Folwaczny et al. 2000). These outcomes differ from the non-carious study outcomes and may reflect the different oral conditions of this group of patients. Little evidence exists relating to restoration survival and the oral environment, and it would seem important to know how a patient's oral environment may influence the longevity and marginal quality of restorations.

2.4.2 Other Clinical Studies

The section above relates to a specific type of restoration, namely, NCCLs; however, GICs are not exclusively used for restoration of cervical lesions. They have also been recommended for the restoration of small approximal lesions in anterior teeth. The development of high powder/liquid ratio materials, also referred to as high-viscosity GICs, in association with the ART method for treatment of caries lesions has led to the use of GICs being extended to treatment of occlusal caries, as well as small posterior approximal load-bearing restorations. This section will summarise some of the work published in this area.

The original clinical work published on GIC use and survival was that of Mount (1997) where he outlined successful use of GICs by himself and others over 20 years since their inception.

One early retrospective study examined 42 restorations, half treated with resin composite and the other half with conventional GIC (de Araujo et al. 1998). This study examined restorations that had been placed for 24 months. Criteria such as aesthetics, anatomic form, staining and marginal leakage were classified into three groups. Most of the restorations were rated as either satisfactory or acceptable for all the criteria for both materials. By 24 months, the aesthetics remained acceptable for all the resin composite restorations, but in the case of the GIC, there was a steady decrease in acceptable restorations (equivalent to a beta rating), although it was only 23 % of the total. The outcome for staining was similar, but from the aspect of marginal leakage, both materials performed well (de Araujo et al.

1998). Another study comparing a total of 152 restorations of either resin composite, PAMRC or RM-GIC in anterior approximal restorations over 3 years reported that the resin composite and PAMRC 'performed significantly better' than the RM-GIC. The RM-GIC was observed to have changed colour slightly, but the quality of the surface of the RM-GIC decreased significantly (van Dijken 1996b).

A more recent practice-based study examined the performance of a 'reinforced' GIC (Fuji IX, GC Corp) in occlusal and 2-surface posterior approximal cavities (Burke et al. 2007). This study provides some insight into the clinical success centred in 'real-world' practices. Altogether, 67 occlusal and 102 posterior approximal restorations were evaluated over a mean restoration age of 25 months (range 5–56 months). Of all the restorations examined, 98 % were observed to be present and intact. No further caries was observed, and three had fractured and were replaced with another GIC restoration. The only factor amongst marginal adaptation, marginal discolouration and surface roughness that most notably changed with time was the surface roughness. It was concluded that over the 2 years of this study, the reinforced GIC restorations were 'performing satisfactorily' (Burke et al. 2007).

The coating of GICs for protection and increased fracture resistance has not been clinically evaluated widely. This method is now promoted as a technique to restore occlusal caries lesions. Recently a 3-year clinical trial reported the longevity of a high-viscosity GIC (Fuji IX, GC Corp) with and without the nanofilled resin coating G-Coat Plus (GC Corp) in comparison with a hybrid resin composite (Diem et al. 2014). Just over 80 restorations were initially placed for each method; however, at the end of the 3 years, only 69 GIC restorations, 65 coated-GIC and 64 resin composite restorations were evaluated. The results reported 'moderate wear' on 7 % of restorations with little difference between each method. Surface chipping and cracking was noted on 3 % of the coated-GIC and 2 % of resin composite restorations. With respect to wear, the GIC showed consistent wear more than the adjacent enamel over the 3 years. The coated-GIC showed slightly less wear but more than the resin composite which showed the least wear. In conclusion, the authors believed the coated-GIC was showing a trend of less wear than the uncoated-GIC. Their guarded conclusion was that the 'G-Coat Plus gave some protection against wear' (Diem et al. 2014). It is clear that more evidence is needed to determine whether this coating in association with the high powder/liquid GIC can be used in other than small occlusal restorations. If this is the case, careful monitoring for wear should be undertaken.

2.4.3 ART Restorations and Their Performance

As the ART method has developed and been studied, there are now an increasing number of studies evaluating the success of this commonly used public health method. Initially developed for caries management in countries where dental facilities may be limited, the technique is now seeing greater usage in many different clinical settings (Frencken 2010). One of the earlier studies over 12 months compared the ART method with conventional caries removal as well as amalgam restorations (Yip et al. 2002). This study evaluated 149 restorations in total, i.e. 60 restorations were placed for each of the GIC groups using either ART or conventional methods, and a further 29 restorations for dental amalgam. The GIC was also extended into any pits and fissures (as a sealant) not included in the small cavity preparations. This short study showed no failures in either the amalgam or GIC; the only issue noted was when GIC was extended into fissures, it was rapidly lost. They also noted some wear of the GIC with an increase in marginal discrepancies being noted in comparison with the amalgam. It was concluded that the high-viscosity GIC may be suitable for clinical use in small occlusal restorations (Yip et al. 2002).

Another recent study compared conventional rotary caries removal methods and restoration with resin composite to ART preparation using GIC. This study was also of 12 months' duration, but the treatment was provided to patients with disabilities (Molina et al. 2014). A total of 298 carious lesions were restored in primary and permanent teeth, of which 182 used ART and the remaining 116 were conventional cavity preparations. The survival rates of the ART restorations in primary and permanent teeth were both 98 %. Interestingly, the ART restorations showed a better survival rate at 12 months compared with the conventional method using resin composite. The authors noted that longer-term data are now needed to further support the evidence base for the use of ART and GICs in the treatment of special-needs patients (Molina et al. 2014). This does, however, demonstrate where this technique has now extended beyond its original intention and seems to be proving a successful technique and philosophy.

Other studies have evaluated the success of using ART for restoration of not only occlusal but also posterior approximal restorations. A small study of only 6 months' duration placed 60 ART restorations in children (Cefaly et al. 2005). There were 36 occlusal and 24 posterior approximal restorations. Over this short period of time, all occlusal restorations survived; however, the posterior approximal restorations showed a 100 % success rate for the RM-GIC, Fuji VIII (GC Corp), but only 92 % for the highly viscous GIC, Ketac Molar (3M-ESPE) (combined 96 %). This study was of a very short duration, but it does point to the potential problem and weakness of these GICs that when subjected to loading in a larger restoration not wholly supported by tooth structure, it does seem to lead to a higher failure rate. Hence, case selection is an important aspect to ensure restoration survival. Following on from this, a much larger and longer trial has reported the 3- and 6-year survival of ART restorations in small and large 1- and 2-surface restorations, although most restorations were placed in occlusal cavities (Holmgren et al. 2000; Lo et al. 2007). The study, as with most clinical evaluations, was not able to review all the restorations placed. At 3 years, 92 % of the small occlusal, 76 % of the large occlusal and 57 % of the approximal restorations were deemed satisfactory (Holmgren et al. 2000). By the end of 6 years, the survival outcomes were 76 % for the small occlusal and 59 % for the large restorations (Lo et al. 2007). This shows that the ART method for small restorations can provide a good outcome. However, when the restoration becomes larger, the evidence for GIC would seem to indicate that it is still not suitable for larger load-bearing situations (Lo et al. 2007).

Another study evaluated anterior approximal restorations using ART over 4 years with an RM-GIC in 117 restorations placed in 67 patients (Jordan et al. 2011). By the end of the study, only 76 of the original 117 restorations could be evaluated. At the 4-year recall, 13 restorations were lost with 10 restorations in 5 patients exhibiting secondary caries. In percentage terms, 28 % of the reviewed restorations did not need any intervention, 17 % needed minor intervention such as repair and 20 % were in need of replacement, with 35 % lost to follow-up (Jordan et al. 2011). The annual failure rate was determined at 4.9 %. For all the evaluation criteria of the restorations such as surface quality, marginal integrity and discolouration, all restorations showed deterioration over the life of the study.

A number of studies have been centred on using ART for paediatric patients and the treatment of primary teeth. The study by Hilgert et al. (2014) compared ART using a high-viscosity GIC with conventional treatment using dental amalgam. This study was quite large in that the initial numbers of restorations were 386 ART restorations (116 single surface, 270 multiple surface) compared with 364 amalgam (conventional) restorations (105 single surface, 259 multiple surface). The results showed that there was no significant difference between the ART or conventional methods of restoration. The 3-year survival rates were, however, better for the multiple surface amalgam (64.7 %) compared with the ART restorations (56.4 %). Furthermore, 20 % of the ART failures were due to marginal defects. From the aspect of overall cumulative survival, there was no significant difference between the two methods. However, the single-surface restorations lasted longer than the multiple surface restorations (Hilgert et al. 2014).

A further recent study on primary molars compared two techniques for approximal ART restorations over 18 months (Bonifácio et al. 2013). The methods here were the use of a single layer of the recommended P:L ratio compared with a 2-layer method which involved placing a

1:2 P:L ratio 'flowable' layer directly on the tooth surface which was then overlaid with the recommended P:L ratio material. Altogether, 208 cavities were restored. The cumulative survival of all restorations was calculated to be 68 % at 18 months (Bonifácio et al. 2013). There was no difference between the two groups. The authors concluded that the modification of the technique did not improve survival and further work was needed to enhance the long-term outcomes using ART for restoring primary teeth.

With the introduction of the nanofilled RM-GIC, two studies have reported the use of this material. The first used the ART method and compared the nanofilled material with a conventional high-viscosity GIC in primary molars (Konde et al. 2012). One hundred restorations in 50 patients were inserted and evaluated over 12 months. At 6 months, three patients were excluded due to secondary caries detected around the restorations. It was noted that slightly more patients had secondary caries in the conventional GIC group, but the numbers were quite small so these results should be viewed with some caution. It did show, however, that the new nanofilled material was performing as well as, if not slightly better than, the conventional GIC. Another study comparing the nanofilled material used conventional methods for cavity preparation and restoration. The nanofilled RM-GIC was compared with another RM-GIC for restoring single surfaces. Thirty restorations of each were placed and evaluated over 2 years (Abo-Hamar et al. 2015). In this study, the two materials performed in a similar manner. From the aspect of recurrent caries, the traditional RM-GIC performed marginally better at 2 years. Most other parameters showed little difference between the two materials. It was concluded that the nanofilled material was no better than the conventional RM-GIC (Abo-Hamar et al. 2015).

2.4.4 Sealants

The other clinical aspect of GIC use is as fissure sealants or fissure protection. More recently, GIC has been promoted as an excellent material for use as an 'ART sealant'. Frencken (2014) recently published a 'start-of-the-art' piece on ART sealants. He outlined that meta-analyses had shown that there was no clear evidence suggesting either glass-ionomer or resin-based sealants were better than the other. The potential advantage of the ART sealant is that no specialised dental facilities are needed and the rate of dentine carious lesion development using this technique was approximately 1 % in the first 3 years (Frencken 2014).

A 3-year clinical evaluation of 400 GIC sealants compared a conventional and resin-modified GIC placed in first permanent molars (Pereira et al. 2003). The retention rates of the sealants were low by the end of the 3 years, but the caries incidence was much lower than the control teeth. The RM-GIC seemed to perform slightly better than the conventional material in terms of retention.

A small study compared the retention of GIC and resin sealants in teeth with and without preparation over 24 months (Dhar and Chen 2012). Twenty-five teeth were sealed with each of the techniques, i.e. resin or GIC, with or without preparation. For the glass-ionomer, 100 % sealant loss occurred in the no-treatment group compared with 60 % in the prepared teeth. In the resin-sealed group, 80 % of sealants were lost by 24 months compared with 32 % for the prepared group. With respect to caries incidence, the GIC group showed 4 % (prepared) and 8 % (unprepared) caries occurrence compared with 16 % (prepared) and 12 % (unprepared) for the resin group (Dhar and Chen 2012). This outcome shows that even though the GIC may be lost completely, there seems to be remaining benefit with respect to the prevention of caries. This study also showed that tooth preparation was not a wise choice as it increased the caries susceptibility.

With respect to caries risk, a 2-year study investigated the effect of a high fluoride-releasing conventional GIC as a sealant, comparing it with a resin-based sealant. One hundred and fifty teeth were sealed in 57 children (Chen and Liu 2013). The retention rate of the GIC at 2 years was 31 % for the low caries-risk group and 44.5 % for the high-risk group, compared with the resin sealant which was 77 % for the low-risk group and 63 % for the high-risk group. With regard to caries rates, no difference was noted between the two risk groups for either material (Chen and Liu 2013). Even though no difference was noted, it is perhaps interesting to note that even though the failure rate of the GIC was higher, this did not lead to a greater caries experience. A larger and longer study may provide more robust evidence.

Another 2-year study comparing a high fluoride-releasing GIC with an ormocer composite sealant in 200 teeth has been reported (Guler and Yilmaz 2013). Again, the retention rates for the resin-based sealant were much higher than the GIC. However, the caries experience for the GIC (16 %) was half that of the resin-based material (32 %). The outcomes of this study are contradictory to the previous study. This study concluded that 'the GIC may be better for preventing occlusal caries' (Guler and Yilmaz 2013).

A recent paper investigated the effect of a fluoride-releasing resin sealant and ART GIC sealant over 2 years in 280 children (383 molars) (Liu et al 2014). The results showed that the proportion of molars with dentine caries was 7.3 % for the ART sealant and 3.9 % for the resin-based sealant. Life table survival analysis at 2 years showed that the retention of the resin sealant was statistically higher at 73 % compared with the ART sealant at 50 %. From the aspect of caries not developing, there was no difference between the materials at 93 % (ART) and 96 % (resin). Liu et al. (2014) concluded that the effectiveness of both materials was no different and hence the ART sealant was a 'good alternative' where dental facilities are not available or limited. Hence again, even though retention is poorer for the GIC, there seems to be a growing pool of evidence that teeth treated with GIC sealants seem to have some preventive effect occurring even though the fissure system is exposed to the oral cavity.

Conclusions

GICs have now become a routine part of clinical practice for restorations, luting cements and lining materials. The strength and wear resistance of the recent materials has markedly improved over the last 10 or so years. The first major improvement was the incorporation of resins into the GIC; however, these materials were still not strong enough to withstand occlusal loading. The recent innovation of coating materials with a resin-based agent seems to have provided a major advance for use of higher powder/liquid ratio materials in the restoration of small load-bearing restorations.

The methods of delivery have also undergone major changes. Capsule systems have much improved allowing reliable mixing and dispensing directly into cavities in almost any location in the oral cavity. These systems have also reduced the porosity of the set cement, which has often been a problem with the older GICs. We are likely to see further modifications in delivery systems as manufacturers make further advances in both conventional GIC and RM-GICs.

GICs, particularly the resin-modified version, have been shown to be an excellent long-lasting restorative material for restoration of cervical lesions. In addition, because GICs are moisture tolerant and bond well to tooth structure, they remain an excellent material for restoring deep cavities where the dentine may be moist or adjacent to gingival tissues where moisture control is more difficult to achieve. The recent developments in conventional GICs with the resin coating agents are beginning to show that the GICs may become a good alternative for small, conservative occlusal restorations. However, the strength of GICs still limits their use for load-bearing restorations. Hence, they are still not recommended for larger restorations that are exposed to direct loading during function.

The release of ions such as fluoride and also the ability to probably slow down biofilm formation make the GICs useful materials for a variety of patient groups such as high caries-risk and special-needs patients. Further advances will also most likely improve treatment outcomes for these groups in the future years.

It is likely that as GICs are further developed, the potential exists for them to become a truly universal, tooth-coloured restorative material able to control caries initiation, heal early lesions and perhaps repair already damaged tooth structure from caries.

References

Abo-Hamar SE, El-Desouky SS, Abu Hamila AA. Two-year clinical performance in primary teeth of nano-filled versus conventional resin-modified glass-ionomer restorations. Quintessence Int. 2015;46:381–8.

Akinmade AO, Nicholson JW. Development of glasses for novel polyphosphonate dental cements. Br Ceram T. 1994;93:85–90.

Al-Naimi OT, Itota T, Hobson RS, McCabe JF. Fluoride release for restorative materials and its effect on biofilm formation in natural saliva. J Mater Sci Mater Med. 2008;19:1243–8.

Bagheri R, Tyas MJ, Burrow MF. Comparison of the effect of storage media on hardness and shear punch strength of tooth-colored restorative materials. Am J Dent. 2007;20:329–34.

Bagheri R, Azar MR, Tyas MJ, Burrow MF. The effect of aging on the fracture toughness of esthetic restorative materials. Am J Dent. 2010;23:142–6.

Bagheri R, Taha NA, Azar MR, Burrow MF. Effect of G-coat plus on the mechanical properties of glass-ionomer cements. Aust Dent J. 2013;58:448–53.

Bapna MS, Gadia CM, Drummond JL. Effects of aging and cyclic loading on the mechanical properties of glass ionomer cements. Eur J Oral Sci. 2002;110: 330–4.

Billington RW, Williams JA, Pearson GJ. Ion processes in glass ionomer cements. J Dent. 2006;34:544–55.

Bonifácio CC, Kleverlaan CJ, Raggio DP, Werner A, de Carvalho RC, van Amerongen WE. Physical-mechanical properties of glass ionomer cements indicated for atraumatic restorative treatment. Aust Dent J. 2009;54:233–7.

Bonifácio CC, Werner A, Kleverlaan CJ. Coating glass-ionomer cements with a nanofilled resin. Acta Odont Scand. 2012;70:417–7.

Bonifácio CC, Hesse D, de Oliveira RR, Bönecker M, Raggio DP, van Amerongen WE. Survival rate of approximal-ART restorations using a two-layer technique for glass ionomer insertion. Clin Oral Investig. 2013;17:1745–50.

Boruziniat A, Gharaei S. Bond strength between composite resin and resin modified glass ionomer using different adhesive systems and curing techniques. J Conserv Dent. 2014;17:150–4.

Brackett WW, Gilpatrick RO, Browning WD, Gregory PN. Two-year clinical performance of a resin-modified glass-ionomer restorative material. Oper Dent. 1999;24:9–13.

Bresciani E, Barata Tde J, Fagundes TC, Adachi A, Terrin MM, Navarro MF. Compressive and diametral tensile strength of glass ionomer cements. J Appl Oral Sci. 2004;12:344–8.

Bryant RW, Mahler DB. Volumetric contraction in some tooth-coloured restorative materials. Aust Dent J. 2007;52:112–7.

Burke FJ, Siddons C, Cripps S, Bardha J, Crisp RJ, Dopheide B. Clinical performance of reinforced glass ionomer restorations placed in UK dental practices. Br Dent J. 2007;203, E2. discussion 40–1.

Burrow MF, Tyas MJ. Clinical evaluation of a resin-modified glass-ionomer adhesive system. Oper Dent. 1998;23:290–3.

Burrow MF, Tyas MJ. Clinical evaluation of three adhesive systems for the restoration of non-carious cervical lesions. Oper Dent. 2007;32:11–5.

Cardoso MV, Delme KIM, Mine A, Neves AA, Coutinho E, De Moor RJG, Van Meerbeek B. Towards a better understanding of the adhesion mechanism of resin-modified glass-ionomers by bonding to differently prepared dentin. J Dent. 2010;38:921–9.

Carey CM, Spencer M, Give RJ, Eichmiller EC. Fluoride release from a resin-modified glass-ionomer cement in a continuous flow system. Effect of pH. J Dent Res. 2003;82:829–32.

Cattani-Lorente MA, Dupuis V, Payan J, Moya F, Meyer JM. Effect of water on the physical properties of resin-modified glass ionomer cements. Dent Mater. 1999;15:132–7.

Cefaly DF, Barata TJ, Tapety CM, Bresciani E, Navarro MF. Clinical evaluation of multisurface ART restorations. J Appl Oral Sci. 2005;13:15–9.

Chau NP, Pandit S, Cai JN, Lee MH, Jeon JG. Relationship between fluoride release rate and anti-cariogenic biofilm activity of glass ionomer cements. Dent Mater. 2015;31:e100–8.

Cheetham JJ, Palamara JE, Tyas MJ, Burrow MF. A comparison of resin-modified glass-ionomer and resin composite polymerisation shrinkage stress in a wet environment. J Mech Behav Biomed Mater. 2014;29:33–41.

Chen XX, Liu XQ. Clinical comparison of Fuji VII and a resin sealant in children at high and low risk of caries. Dent Mater J. 2013;32:512–8.

Chinelatti MA, Ramos RP, Chimello DT, Palma-Dibb RG. Clinical performance of a resin-modified glass ionomer and two polyacid modified resin composites in cervical lesion restorations; 1-year follow-up. J Oral Rehabil. 2004;31:251–7.

Cook WD. Degradative analysis of glass ionomer polyelectrolyte cements. J Biomed Mater Res. 1983;17:1015–27.

Coutinho E, Yoshida Y, Inoue S, Fukuda R, Snauwaert J, Nakayama Y, De Munck J, Lambrechts P, Suzuki K, Van Meerbeek B. Gel phase formation at resin-modified glass ionomer/tooth interfaces. J Dent Res. 2007;86:656–61.

Crisp S, Wilson AD. Reactions in glass ionomer cements: V. Effect of incorporating tartaric acid in the cement liquid. J Dent Res. 1976;55:1023–31.

Crisp S, Lewis BG, Wilson AD. Characterization of glass ionomer cements. 6. A study of erosion and water absorption in both neutral and acidic media. J Dent. 1980;8:68–72.

Czarnecka B, Nicholson JW. Ion release by resin-modified glass ionomer cements into water and lactic acid solutions. J Dent. 2006;34:539–43.

de Araujo MA, Araujo RM, Marsilio AL. A retrospective look at esthetic resin composite and glass-ionomer Class III restorations: a 2-year clinical evaluation. Quintessence Int. 1998;29:87–93.

De Barra E, Hill RG. Influence of alkali metal ions on the fracture properties of glass polyalkenoate (ionomer) cements. Biomaterials. 1998;19:495–502.
De Barra E, Hill RG. Influence of glass composition on the properties of glass polyalkenoate cements. Part III: Influence of fluorite content. Biomaterials. 2000;21:563–9.
De Caluwé T, Vercruysse CW, Fraeyman S, Verbeeck RM. The influence of particle size and fluorine content on aluminosilicate glass on the glass ionomer cement properties. Dent Mater. 2014;30:1029–38.
De Moor RJ, Verveeck RM. Effect of acetic acid on the fluoride release profiles of restorative glass ionomer cements. Dent Mater. 1998;14:261–8.
Dhar V, Chen H. Evaluation of resin based and glass ionomer based sealants placed with or without preparation – a two year clinical trial. Pediatr Dent. 2012;34:46–50.
Diem VT, Tyas MJ, Ngo HC, Phuong LH, Khanh ND. The effect of a nano-filled resin coating on the 3-year clinical performance of a conventional high-viscosity glass-ionomer cement. Clin Oral Invest. 2014;18:753–9.
Ermis RB. Two-year clinical evaluation of four polyacid-modified resin composites and a resin-modified glass-ionomer cement in class V lesions. Quintessence Int. 2002;33:542–8.
Falsafi A, Mitra SB, Oxman JD, Ton TT, Bui HT. Mechanisms of setting reactions and interfacial behaviour of a nano-filled resin-modified glass ionomer. Dent Mater. 2014;30:632–43.
Fano L, Fano V, Ma W, Wang X, Zhu F. Hydrolytic degradation and cracks in resin-modified glass-ionomer cements. J Biomed Mater Res Part B Appl Biomater. 2004;69:87–93.
Fennel B, Hill RG. The influence of poly(acrylic) acid molar mass and concentration on the properties o polyalkenoate cements. Part I – compressive strength. J Mater Sci. 2001a;36:5193–202.
Fennel B, Hill RG. The influence of poly(acrylic) acid molar mass and concentration on the properties of polyalkenoate cements. Part II: young's modulus and flexural strength. J Mater Sci. 2001b;36:5177–83.
Fennel B, Hill RG. The influence of poly(acrylic) acid molar mass and concentration on the properties o polyalkenoate cements. Part III – fracture toughness and toughness. J Mater Sci. 2001c;36:5185–92.
Folwaczny M, Loher C, Mehl A, Kunzelmann KH, Hinkel R. Tooth-colored filling materials for the restoration of cervical lesions; a 24-month follow-up study. Oper Dent. 2000;25:251–8.
Forss H, Seppa I, Lappalainen WR. In vitro abrasion resistance and hardness of glass ionomer cements. Dent Mater. 1991;7:36–9.
Forsten L. Short- and long-term fluoride release from glass ionomers and other fluoride-containing filling materials in vitro. Scand J Dent Res. 1990;98:179–85.
Forsten L. Resin-modified glass ionomer cements: fluoride release and uptake. Acta Odont Scand. 1995;53:222–5.
Forsten L. Fluoride release and uptake by glass-ionomers and related materials and its clinical effects. Biomaterials. 1998;19:503–8.
Franco EB, Benetti AR, Ishikiriama SK, Santiago SL, Lauris JRP, Jorge MFF, Navarro MFL. 5-year clinical performance of resin composite versus resin modified glass ionomer restorative system in non-carious cervical lesions. Oper Dent. 2006;31:403–8.
Frankenberger R, Sindel J, Kramer N. Viscous glass-ionomer cements: a new alternative to amalgam in the primary dentition? Quintessence Int. 1997;28:667–76.
Frencken JE. The ART, approach using glass-ionomers in relation to global oral health care. Dent Mater. 2010;26:1–6.
Frencken JE. The state-of-the-art of ART sealants. Dent Update. 2014;41:119–20. 122–4.
Fukuzawa M, Matsuya S, Yamane M. Mechanism of erosion of glass-ionomer cements in acidic buffer solution. J Dent Res. 1987;66:1770–4.
Ganesh M, Tandon S. Clinical evaluation of FUJI VII sealant material. J Clin Pediatr Dent. 2006;31:52–7.
Gemalmaz D, Yoruc B, Ozcab M, Alkumru HN. Effect of early water contact on solubility of glass ionomer luting cements. J Prosthet Dent. 1998;80:474–8.
Griffin SG, Hill RG. Influence of glass composition on the properties of glass polyalkenoate cements. Part I: Influence of aluminium to silicon ratio. Biomaterials. 1999;20:1579–86.
Griffin SG, Hill RG. Influence of glass composition on the properties of glass polyalkenoate cements. Part II: influence of phosphate content. Biomaterials. 2000a;21:399–403.
Griffin SG, Hill RG. Influence of glass composition on the properties of glass polyalkenoate cements. Part IV: influence of fluorine content. Biomaterials. 2000b;21:693–8.
Guler C, Yilmaz Y. A two-year clinical evaluation of glass ionomer and ormocer based fissure sealants. J Clin Pediatr Dent. 2013;37:263–7.
Hadley PC, Milella E, Gerardi C, Hill RG, Billington RW. Distribution of fluoride in glass ionomer determined using SIMS. Biomaterials. 2001;22:1563–9.
Hamama HH, Burrow MF, Yiu C. Effect of dentine conditioning on adhesion of resin-modified glass ionomer adhesives. Aust Dent J. 2014;59:193–200.
Hickel R, Manhart J. Longevity of restorations in posterior teeth and reasons for failure. J Adhes Dent. 2001;3:45–64.
Hilgert LA, de Amorim ZRG, Leal SC, Mulder J, Creugers NHJ, Frencken JE. Is high-viscosity glass-ionomer-cement a successor to amalgam for treating primary molars? Dent Mater. 2014;30:1171–8.
Hinoura K, Moore BK, Phillips RW. Influence of dentin surface treatments on the bond strengths of dentin-lining cements. Oper Dent. 1986;11:147–54.
Holmgren CJ, Lo ECM, Hu D, Wan H. ART restorations and sealants placed in Chinese school children – results after three years. Community Dent Oral Epidemiol. 2000;28:314–20.
Honório HM, Rios D, Fransisconi LF, Magalhães AC, Machado MA, Buzalaf MA. Effect of prolonged

erosive pH cycling on different restorative materials. J Oral Rehabil. 2008;35:947–53.

Hotta M, Hirukawa H. Abrasion resistance of restorative glass-ionomer cements and a light-cured surface coating. Oper Dent. 1994;19:42–6.

Hussein TA, Bakar WZ, Ghani ZA, Mohamad D. The assessment of surface roughness and microleakage of eroded tooth-colored dental restorative materials. J Conserv Dent. 2014;17:531–5.

Ilie N, Hickel R, Valceanu AS, Huth KC. Fracture toughness of dental restorative materials. Clin Oral Invest. 2012;16:489–98.

Jordan RA, Hetzel P, Franke M, Markovic L, Gaengler P, Zimmer S. Class III atraumatic restorative treatment (ART) in adults living in West Africa – outcome after 48 months. Community Dent Oral Epidemiol. 2011;39:164–70.

Joynt RB, Davis EL, Wieczkowski G, Pierce L. Effect of dentinal pretreatment on bond strength between glass-ionomer and dentin. Oper Dent. 1990;15:173–7.

Jyothi NJ, Annapurna S, Kumar AS, Venugopal P, Jayashankara CM. Clinical evaluation of giomer and resin-modified glass ionomer cement in class V noncarious lesions: An in vivo study. J Conserv Dent. 2011;14:409–13.

Kasraie S, Shokripour M, Safari M. Evaluation of micro-shear bond strength of resin modified glass-ionomer to composite resins using various bonding systems. J Conserv Dent. 2013;16:550–4.

Kaur H, Nandlal B. Effect of dietary solvents on the strength of nanocomposite, compomer, glass ionomer cement: An in vitro study. J Conserv Dent. 2013;16:527–31.

Kim YG, Hirano S. Setting shrinkage and hygroscopic expansion of resin-modified glass ionomer in experimental cylindrical cavities. Dent Mater J. 1999;18:63–75.

Kitasako Y, Sasaki Y, Takagi T, Sadr A, Tagami J. Age-specific prevalence of erosive tooth wear by acidic diet and gastroesophageal reflux in Japan. J Dent. 2015;43:418–23.

Kleverlaan CJ, van Duinen RN, Felizer AJ. Mechanical properties of glass ionomer cements affected by curing methods. Dent Mater. 2004;20:45–50.

Konde S, Rais S, Jaiswal D. Clinical evaluation of a new art material: nanoparticulated resin-modified glass ionomer cement. J Int Prev Community Dent. 2012;2:42–7.

Kunzelmann KH, Burkle V, Bauer C. Two-body and three-body wear of glass ionomer cements. Int J Paediatr Dent. 2003;13:434–40.

Lacefield WR, Reindl MC, Retief DH. Tensile bond strength of glass-ionomer cement. J Prosthet Dent. 1985;53:194–8.

Leirskar J, Nordbø H, Mount GJ, Ngo H. The influence of resin coating on the shear punch strength of a high strength auto-cure glass ionomer. Dent Mater. 2003;19:87–91.

Liu BY, Xiao Y, Chu CH, Lo EC. Glass ionomer ART sealant and fluoride-releasing resin sealant in fissure caries prevention – results from a randomized clinical trial. BMC Oral Health. 2014;145:54.

Lo EC, Holmgren CJ, Hu D, van Palenstein HW. Six-year follow up of atraumatic restorative treatment restorations placed in Chinese school children. Community Dent Oral Epidemiol. 2007;35:387–92.

Loguercio AD, Reis A, Barbosa AN, Roulet JF. Five-year double-blind randomised clinical evaluation of a resin-modified glass ionomer and a polyacid-modified resin in noncarious cervical lesions. J Adhes Dent. 2003;5:323–32.

Lohbauer U, Krämer N, Siedschlag G, Schubert EW, Lauerer B, Müller FA, Petschelt A, Ebert J. Strength and wear resistance of a dental glass-ionomer cement with a novel nanofilled resin coating. Am J Dent. 2011;24:124–8.

Maneenut C, Tyas MJ. Clinical evaluation of resin-modified glass ionomer restorative cements in cervical 'abrasion' lesions: One –year results. Quintessence Int. 1995;26:739–43.

Maneenut C, Sakoolnamarka R, Tyas MJ. The repair of resin-modified glass-ionomer cements. Dent Mater. 2010;26:659–65.

Markovic DLJ, Petrovic BB, Peric TO. Fluoride content and recharge ability of five glass ionomer dental materials. BMC Oral Health. 2008;8–21.

Matis BA, Cochran M, Carlson T. Longevity of glass-ionomer restorative materials: results of a 10-year evaluation. Quintessence Int. 1996;27:373–82.

Matsuya S, Matsuya Y, Yamamoto Y, Yamane M. Erosion process of glass ionomer cement in organic acids. Dent Mater J. 1984;3:210–9.

Mazzaoui SA, Burrow MF, Tyas MJ. Fluoride release from glass ionomer cements and resin composites coated with a dentin adhesive. Dent Mater. 2000;16:166–71.

McCabe JF. Resin-modified glass-ionomers. Biomaterials. 1998;19:521–7.

Mitchell CA, Douglas WH, Cheng YS. Fracture toughness of conventional, resin-modified and composite luting cements. Dent Mater. 1999;15:7–13.

Mitsuhashi A, Hanaoka K, Teranaka T. Fracture toughness of resin-modified glass ionomer restorative materials: effect of powder/liquid ratio and powder particle size reduction on fracture toughness. Dent Mater. 2003;19:747–57.

Molina G, Faulks D, Mazzola I, Mulder J, Frencken JE. One year survival of ART and conventional restorations in patients with disability. BMC Oral Health. 2014;14:49.

Momoi Y, Hirosaki K, Kohno A, McCabe JF. In vitro toothbrush-dentifrice abrasion of resin-modified glass ionomers. Dent Mater. 1997;13:82–8.

Moreau JL, Xu HH. Fluoride releasing restorative materials: effects of pH on mechanical properties and ion release. Dent Mater. 2010;26:e227–35.

Mount GJ. Polyacrylic cements in dentistry. Am J Dent. 1990;3:79–84.

Mount GJ. Longevity in glass-ionomer restorations: review of a successful technique. Quintessence Int. 1997;28:643–50.

Mount GJ, Hume WR. Preservation and restoration of tooth structure. 2nd ed. Queensland: Knowledge Boos and Software; 2005.

Mount GJ, Makinson OF, Peters MC. The strength of auto-cured and light-cured materials. The shear punch test. Aust Dent J. 1996;41:118–23.

Mount GJ, Patel C, Makinson OF. Resin modified glass-ionomers: strength, cure depth and translucency. Aust Dent J. 2002;47:339–43.

Mount GJ, Tyas MJ, Ferracane JI, Nicholson JW, Berg JH, Simonsen RJ, Ngo HC. A revised classification for direct tooth-coloured restorative materials. Quintessence Int. 2009;40:691–7.

Namgung C, Rho YJ, Jin BH, Lim BS, Cho BH. A retrospective clinical study of cervical restorations: longevity and failure-prognostic variables. Oper Dent. 2013;38:376–856.

Navimipour EJ, Oskoee SS, Oskoee PA, Bahari M, Rikhtegaran S, Ghojazadeh M. Effect of acid and laser etching on shear bond strength of conventional and resin-modified glass-ionomer cements to composite resin. Lasers Med Sci. 2012;27:305–22.

Nicholson JW. Chemistry of glass-ionomer cements – a review. Biomaterials. 1998;19:485–94.

Nicholson JW, Brookman PJ, Lacy OM, Wilson AD. Fourier transform infrared spectroscopic study of the role of tartaric acid in glass ionomer cements. J Dent Res. 1988;67:1451–4.

Nicholson JW, Aggarwal A, Czarnecka B, Limanowska-Shaw H. The rate of change of pH of lactic acid exposed to glass-ionomer dental cements. Biomaterials. 2000;21:1989–93.

Nomoto R, Carrick TE, McCabe JF. Suitability of a shear punch for dental restorative materials. Dent Mater. 2001;17:415–21.

Norman RD, Swartz ML, Phillips RW, Virmani R. A comparison of the intraoral disintegration of three dental cements. J Am Dent Assoc. 1969;78:777–82.

Oilo G. Early erosion of dental cements Scan. J Dent Res. 1984;92:539–43.

Okada K, Tosaki S, Hirota K, Hume WR. Surface hardness change of restorative filling materials stored in saliva. Dent Mater. 2001;17:34–9.

Özgünaltay G, Önen A. Three-year clinical evaluation of a resin modified glass-ionomer cement and a composite resin in non-carious class V lesions. J Oral Rehabil. 2002;29:1037–41.

Pamir T, Sen BH, Evcin O. Effects of etching and adhesive applications on the bond strength between composite resin and glass-ionomer cements. J Appl Oral Sci. 2012;20:636–42.

Patel M, Tawfik H, Myint Y, Brocklehurst D, Nicholson JW. Factors affecting the ability of dental cements to alter pH of lactic acid solutions. J Oral Rehabil. 2000;27:1030–3.

Pelka M, Ebert J, Schneider H, Kramer N, Petschelt A. A comparison of two- and three-body wear of glass ionomers and composites. Eur J Oral Sci. 1996;104:132–7.

Perdigão J, Dutra-Corrêa M, Saraceni SHC, Ciaramicoli MT, Kiyan VH. Randomised clinical trial of two resin-modified glass ionomer materials: 1-year results. Oper Dent. 2012;37:591–601.

Pereira AC, Pardi V, Mialhe FL, Meneghim Mde C, Ambrosano GM. A 3-year clinical evaluation of glass-ionomer cements used as fissure sealants. Am J Dent. 2003;16:23–7.

Peumans M, Kanumulli P, De Munck J, Van Landuyt P, Van Meerbeek B. Clinical effectiveness of contemporary adhesives: a systematic review. Dent Mater. 2005;21:864–81.

Peumans M, De Munck J, Mine A, Van Meerbeek B. Clinical effectiveness of contemporary adhesives for the restoration of non-carious cervical lesions. A systematic review. Dent Mater. 2014;30:1089–103.

Peutzfeldt A, Garcia-Godoy F, Asmussen E. Surface hardness and wear of glass ionomers and compomers. Am J Dent. 1997;10:15–7.

Prentice LH. Investigations into the mechanical properties and curing characteristics of dental glass-ionomer cements. PhD thesis, University of Melbourne; 2005.

Prosser HJ, Jerome SM, Wilson AD. The effect of additive on the setting properties of a glass-ionomer cement. J Dent Res. 1982a;61:1195–8.

Prosser HJ, Richards CP, Wilson AD. NMR spectroscopy of dental materials. II. The role of tartaric acid in glass-ionomer cements. J Biomed Mater Res. 1982b;16:431–45.

Randall RC, Wilson NH. Glass-ionomer restoratives: a systematic review of secondary caries treatment effect. J Dent Res. 1999;78:628–37.

Roberts HW, Berzins DW, Charlton DG. Hardness of three resin-modified glass-ionomer restorative materials as a function of depth and time. J Esthet Restor Dent. 2009;21:262–72.

Santiago SL, Passos VF, Vieira AH, Navarro MF, Lauris JR, Franco EB. Two-year clinical evaluation of resinous restorative systems in non-carious cervical lesions. Braz Dent J. 2010;21:229–34.

Scholtanus JD, Huysmans MC. Clinical failure of class-II restorations of a highly viscous glass-ionomer material over a 6-year period: a retrospective study. J Dent. 2007;35:156–62.

Schwieger M, Groning P, Schlapbach L, Höland W, Rheinberger V. Thermal and chemical properties of a glass in the SiO2-CaOF system for dental applications. J Therm Anal Calorim. 2000;60:1009–18.

Shiiya T, Mukai Y, Ten Cate JM, Teranaka T. The caries-reducing benefit of fluoride-release from dental restorative materials after fluoride release has ended. Acta Odontol Scand. 2012;70:15–20.

Shin-ichi K, Atsuhiro T, Michiko H. GC Dental Ind Corp, assignee. Glass powder for dental glass ionomer cement. US Patent 6136737. 2000.

Shiozawa M, Takahashi H, Iwasaki N. Fluoride release and mechanical properties after 1-year storage of recent restorative glass ionomer cements. Clin Oral Investig. 2014;18:1053–60.

Sidhu SK. Clinical evaluations of resin-modified glass-ionomer restorations. Dent Mater. 2010;26:7–12.

Sidhu SK, Watson TF. Interfacial characteristics of resin-modified glass-ionomer materials: a study on fluid permeability using confocal fluorescence microscopy. J Dent Res. 1998;77:1749–59.

Small ICB, Watson TF, Chadwick AV, Sidhu SK. Water sorption in resin-modified glass-ionomer cements – an in vitro comparison with other materials. Biomaterials. 1998;19:545–50.

Smith DC. Development of glass- ionomer cement systems. Biomaterials. 1998;19:467–78.

Soares LE, Lima LR, Vieira LS, Do Espírito Santo AM, Martin AA. Erosion effects on chemical composition and morphology of dental materials and root dentin. Microsc Res Tech. 2012;75:703–10.

Sunnegårdh-Grönberg K, Peutzfeldt A, van Dijken JW. Hardness and in vitro wear of a novel ceramic restorative cement. Eur J Oral Sci. 2002;110:175–8.

Tanumiharja M, Burrow MF, Cimmino A, Tyas MJ. The evaluation of four conditioners for glass ionomer cements using field-emission scanning electron microscopy. J Dent. 2001;29:131–8.

Tay FR, Smales RJ, Ngo H, Wei SH, Pashley DH. Effect of different conditioning protocols on adhesion of a GIC to dentin. J Adhes Dent. 2001;3:153–67.

Tyas MJ. The effect of dentine conditioning with polyacrylic acid on the clinical performance of glass ionomer cement. Aust Dent J. 1993;38:46–8.

van Dijken JW. Four-year evaluation of the effect of 10% polyacrylic acid or water rinsing treatment on retention of glass polyalkenoate cement. Eur J Oral Sci. 1996a;104:64–6.

van Dijken JW. 3-year clinical evaluation of a compomer, a resin-modified glass ionomer and a resin composite in Class III restorations. Am J Dent. 1996b;9:195–8.

van Dijken JW, Pallesen U. Long-term retention of etch-and-rinse and self-etch adhesives and a resin-modified glass ionomer cement in non-carious cervical lesions. Dent Mater. 2008;24:915–22.

van Dijken JW, Kieri C, Carlén M. Longevity of extensive class II open-sandwich restorations with a resin-modified glass-ionomer cement. J Dent Res. 1999;78:1319–25.

Wang XY, Yap AU, Ngo HC. Effect of early water exposure on the strength of glass ionomer restoratives. Oper Dent. 2006;31:584–9.

Watson TF. A confocal microscope study of some factors affecting adaptation of a light-cured glass ionomer to tooth tissue. J Dent Res. 1990;69:1531–8.

Watson TF, Atmeh AR, Sajini S, Cook RJ, Festy F. Present and future of glass-ionomers and calcium-silicate cements as bioactive materials in dentistry; biophotonics-based interfacial analyses in health and disease. Dent Mater. 2014;30:50–61.

Welch D, Seesengood B, Hopp C. Surface treatments that demonstrate a significant positive effect on the shear bond strength of repaired resin-modified glass ionomer. Oper Dent. 2015;40:403–9.

Wiegand A, Buchalla W, Attin T. Review on fluoride-releasing restorative materials – fluoride release and uptake characteristics, antibacterial activity and influence on caries formation. Dent Mater. 2007;23: 343–62.

Wilson AD, McLean JW. Glass-ionomer cement. Chicago: Quintessence Publishing; 1988.

Wilson AD, Crisp S, Ferner AJ. Reactions in glass-ionomer cements: IV. Effect of chelating comonomers on setting behavior. J Dent Res. 1976;55:489–95.

Xie D, Brantley WA, Culbertson BM, Wang G. Mechanical properties and microstructures of glass ionomer cements. Dent Mater. 2000;16:129–38.

Xu X, Burgess JO. Compressive strength, fluoride release and recharge of fluoride releasing materials. Biomaterials. 2003;2451–61.

Yip KH, Smales RJ, Gaol W, Peng D. The effects of two cavity preparation methods on the longevity of glass ionomer restorations: an evaluation after 12 months. J Am Dent Assoc. 2002;133:744–51.

Yoshida Y, Van Meerbeek B, Nakayama Y, Snauwaert J, Hellemans L, Lambrechts P, Vanherle G, Wakasa K. Evidence of chemical bonding at biomaterial-hard tissue interfaces. J Dent Res. 2000;79:709–14.

Young AM, Sherpa A, Pearson G, Schottlander B, Waters DN. Use of Raman spectroscopy in the characterisation of the acid–base reaction in glass-ionomer cements. Biomaterials. 2000;21:1971–9.

Zalizniak I, Palamara JE, Wong RH, Cochrane NJ, Burrow MF, Reynolds EC. Ion release and physical properties of CPP-ACP modified GIC in acid solutions. J Dent. 2013;41:449–54.

Zanata RL, Magalhães AC, Lauris JR, Atta MT, Wang L, Navarro MF. Microhardness and chemical analysis of high-viscous glass-ionomer cement after 10 years of clinical service as ART restorations. J Dent. 2011;39:834–40.

Zhang Y, Burrow MF, Palamara JE, Thomas CDL. Bonding to glass ionomer cements using resin-based adhesives. Oper Dent. 2011;36:618–25.

Zimehl R, Hannig M. Non metallic restorative materials based on glass ionomer cements – recent trends and developments. Colloid Surf A. 2000;163:55–62.

The Benefits and Limitations of Glass-Ionomer Cements and Their Use in Contemporary Dentistry

3

Geoffrey M. Knight

Abstract

Since the advent of glass-ionomer cement as a dental restorative material, the number of clinical applications has steadily increased as both the efficiency and improved clinical outcomes for patients have been realized.

Glass-ionomer cements provide tooth-coloured restorations with a low technique sensitivity. They bond chemically to sound and caries-affected tooth structure and release levels of fluoride that protect cavosurface margins from recurrent caries attack. In a clinical environment, a more predictable bond is achieved by pretreating teeth with 37 % phosphoric acid than 20 % polyacrylic acid.

The ion exchange layer between glass-ionomer cement and dentine facilitates the remineralization of caries-affected dentine into fluorapatite that provides a caries-resistant base beneath a glass-ionomer cement restoration or lining.

Auto-cure glass-ionomer cements can be used to restore carious lesions in a tooth where the cusps are not undermined and the restoration does not involve a high-wear area such as a centric stop. Resin-modified glass-ionomer cements should be limited as restorative materials to sites that are not subject to occlusal forces, and photo-curing is able to penetrate to the base of the restoration to minimize any residual unpolymerized HEMA.

Photo-cured resin-modified glass-ionomer cements are well suited as lining materials, luting agents and dental adhesives. As dental adhesives, resin-modified glass-ionomer cements eliminate the effects of polymerization shrinkage stress of composite resins and provide a caries-resistant zone around the perimeter of the restoration.

When composite resins and auto-cure glass-ionomer cements are combined to form a “sandwich restoration”, the use of a resin-modified

G.M. Knight, BDSc, MSc, MBA, PhD
Private Practice, Brighton, VIC, Australia
e-mail: geoffbds@dentalk.com.au

S.K. Sidhu (ed.), *Glass-Ionomers in Dentistry*, DOI 10.1007/978-3-319-22626-2_3

glass-ionomer cement adhesive as a "co-cure" intermediary between the two materials provides a time-efficient technique that effectively triples the bond strength between glass-ionomer cement and composite resin.

Since the advent of glass-ionomers as a dental restorative material, the number of clinical applications has steadily increased as dentists have discovered both the efficiency and improved clinical outcomes for patients that can be achieved with this material.

3.1 Clinical Benefits

From a clinician's point of view, glass-ionomer cements have a low technique sensitivity and can be efficiently applied over a wide range of clinical situations. There is also a popular perception amongst dentists that glass-ionomer cements protect teeth from recurrent caries more than composite resins (Forsten et al. 1994). The caries protection ability of glass-ionomer cements is now well established in the dental literature (McComb et al. 2002; Hicks et al. 2003).

3.1.1 Adhesion

Glass-ionomer cements chemically bond to tooth structure by ionic bonding. Although relatively weak compared to the mechanical bond strengths of resin-based adhesives, glass-ionomer cements will bond to both sound and (slightly less strongly) to caries-affected tooth structure (Lenzi et al. 2013).

3.1.2 Ion Exchange Layer and Fluorapatite Formation

The ion exchange layer between glass-ionomer cement and dentine in fact extends further into both tooth structure and the glass-ionomer cement than first observed (Wilson and McLean 1988). Electron probe microanalysis (EPMA) studies have shown penetration of over 75 μm of calcium and phosphorous ions into glass-ionomer cements and fluoride, strontium and aluminium ions into dentine, after two weeks of placing an auto-cure glass-ionomer overlay (Knight et al. 2007a). It can be postulated that the depth and amount of ion exchange could be expected to increase further over time. The penetration of fluoride ions into the dentine facilitates the transformation of carbonated apatite to fluorapatite (Fig. 3.1).

3.1.3 Fluoride Release

EPMA studies have demonstrated in vitro that fluoride released from glass-ionomer cements into demineralized dentine penetrates deeply into the underlying dentine at concentrations of about 5000 ppm (Ngo et al. 2006). Aqueous fluoride concentrations as low as 600 ppm have been shown to inhibit fluoride-resistant *Streptococcus mutans* bacteria (Brown et al. 1980) (Fig. 3.2).

3.1.4 Remineralization

The penetration of strontium, calcium and fluoride from glass-ionomer cements into dentine (Knight et al. 2007a, b) indicates that these ions are available to assist with remineralization of any demineralized dentine remaining beyond the restorative interface.

The combination of dentinal tubular fluid and ion penetration from auto-cure glass-ionomer cements into demineralized dentine creates an environment that predisposes to fluorapatite formation and increase in hardness of the demineralized tooth structure (Fig. 3.3).

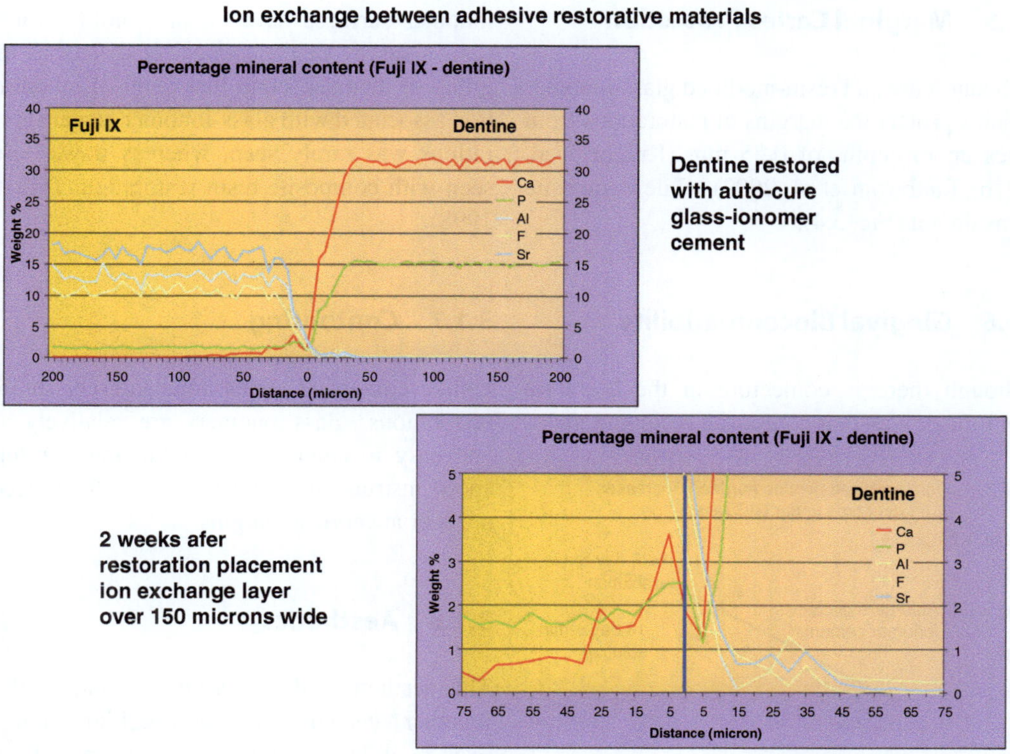

Fig. 3.1 Shows specific ion penetration between glass-ionomer cement and dentine after 2 weeks (Courtesy of Dr. Geoff Knight)

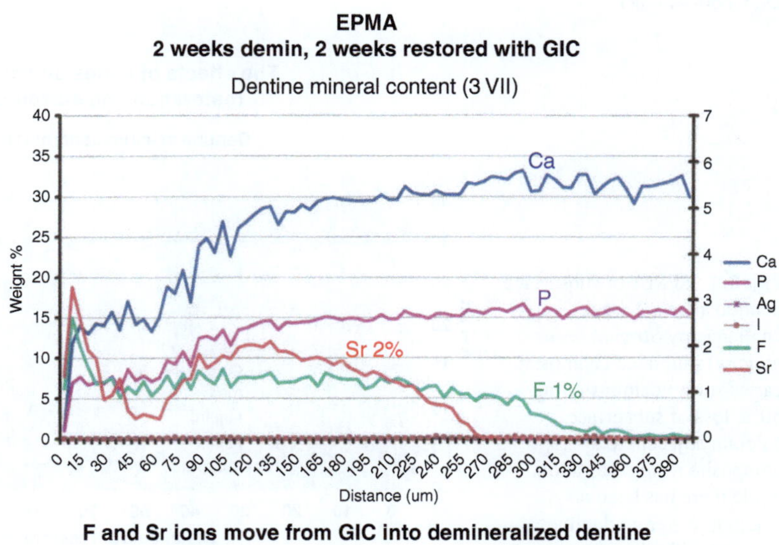

Fig. 3.2 This specimen was demineralized in an demineralizing solution (mimicking caries) onto which an auto-cure glass-ionomer cement restoration was placed. The specimen was examined 2 weeks after placement of the glass-ionomer. EPMA measurement of ion penetration from glass-ionomer cement into demineralized dentine. Note the concentration of fluoride ions at 1 % (about 5000 ppm) to the depth of demineralization, 300 µm into the dentine (Courtesy of Dr. Geoff Knight)

3.1.5 Marginal Caries Protection

Both auto-cure and resin-modified glass-ionomer cements protect the margins of restorations from caries up to depths of 0.25 mm (Knight et al. 2007b; Tantbirojn et al. 2009) while composite resins do not (Fig. 3.4).

3.1.6 Gingival Biocompatibility

Although there is conjecture in the literature about the effects that composite resin and glass-ionomer surfaces have on oral biofilm formation, a survey of the clinical observations of a group of dentists found that gingival inflammation associated with glass-ionomer cement restorations was rarely seen, whereas it was often seen with composite resin restorations (Forsten 1998).

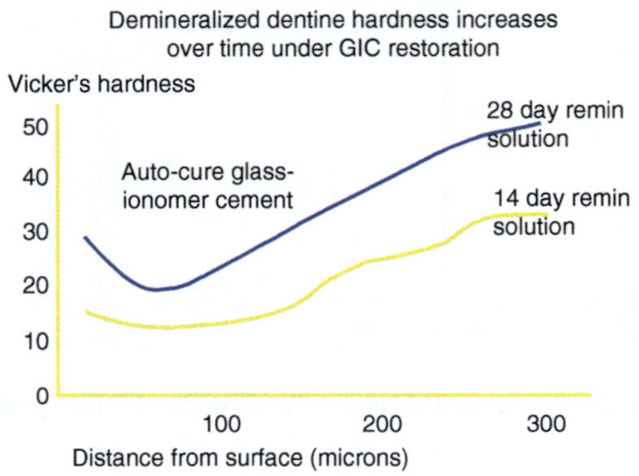

Fig. 3.3 Increase in Vickers hardness of demineralized dentine in a remineralizing solution of artificial saliva (to simulate the oral cavity) under a glass-ionomer cement restoration between 14 and 28 days (Courtesy of Dr. Geoff Knight)

3.1.7 Contouring

Unlike composite resins, amalgams or indirect restorations, glass-ionomers are relatively soft and easy to contour with either low- or high-speed instruments, especially in difficult access areas or at cervical margins.

3.1.8 Aesthetics

The aesthetics of the newer auto-cure glass-ionomer cements are approaching that of resin-modified glass-ionomer cements. In the aesthetic zone, requiring high aesthetics, composite resins are better suited. However, beyond this zone, most clinicians find that the aesthetics of glass-ionomer cements meet their patient's requirements.

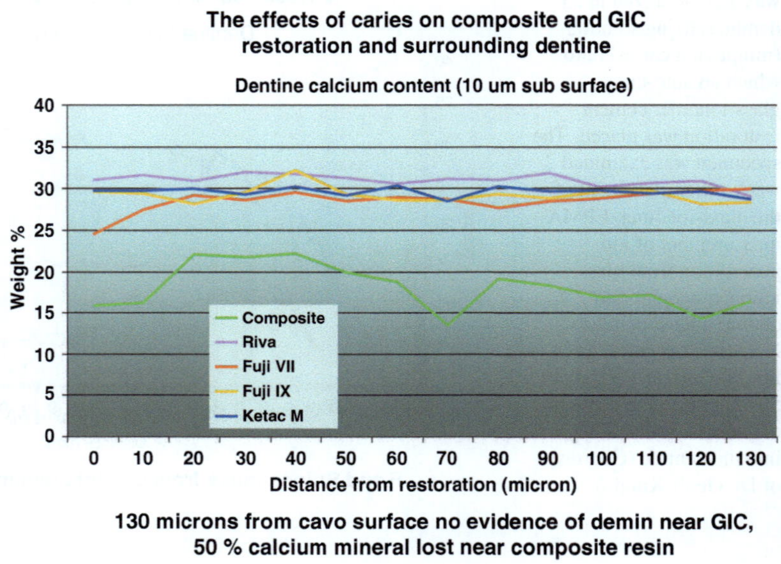

Fig. 3.4 EPMA of subsurface dentine after a 2-week challenge by *Streptococcus mutans* (simulated chemostat caries study) demonstrating 50 % loss of subsurface calcium adjacent to a composite resin restoration, while there has been no calcium loss from dentine restored with glass-ionomer cements (Courtesy of Dr. Geoff Knight)

3.2 Limitations of Glass-Ionomer Cements

3.2.1 Wear Resistance

The low wear resistance of glass-ionomer cements is often cited as a reason to exclude them as an occlusal restorative material. While the surface wear of resin-modified glass-ionomer cements clinically is significant, the restorative auto-cure glass-ionomer cements have an excellent record of low occlusal wear and marginal integrity, providing that they are not placed over occlusal surfaces that involve centric stops (Knight 1992; Lazaridou et al. 2015).

3.2.2 Buffering Oral Acids

Glass-ionomer cements act as buffers to changes in oral pH that will cause their slow degradation in areas where saliva is unable to wash oral acids away. This can result in the surfaces of the glass-ionomer cements being degraded and lost (Nicholson et al. 2000).

In such circumstances, when glass-ionomer cement and composite resin are placed to form an "open-sandwich" restoration, the glass-ionomer cement component of the restoration can be "washed out" to create the effect of proximal recurrent caries. This is possibly the reason why clinicians suggest that they observe proximal caries associated with these restorations (Tyas 2005). While caries may not be a problem, food packing certainly is, and the use of "open-sandwich" restorations should be discouraged as a clinical procedure and a "closed-sandwich" restoration should be placed instead (Figs. 3.5 and 3.6).

3.2.3 Residual HEMA (2-Hydroxyethylmethacrylate)

Resin-modified glass-ionomer (RMGIC) restorations have relatively good aesthetics. However, they should be limited to shallow restorations,

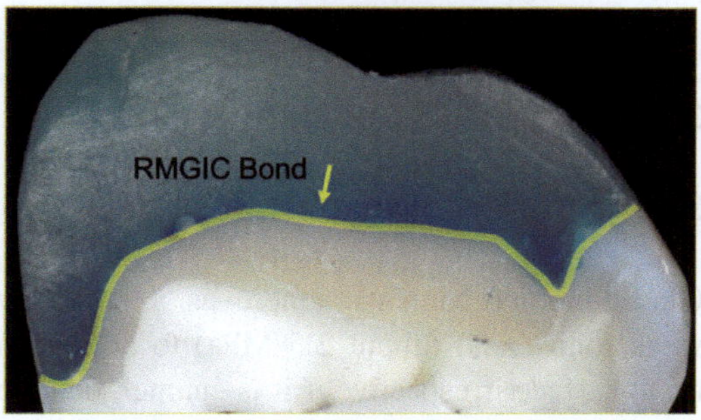

Fig. 3.6 Shows a "closed-sandwich" proximal restoration that prevents loss of proximal glass-ionomer cement (Courtesy of Dr. Geoff Knight)

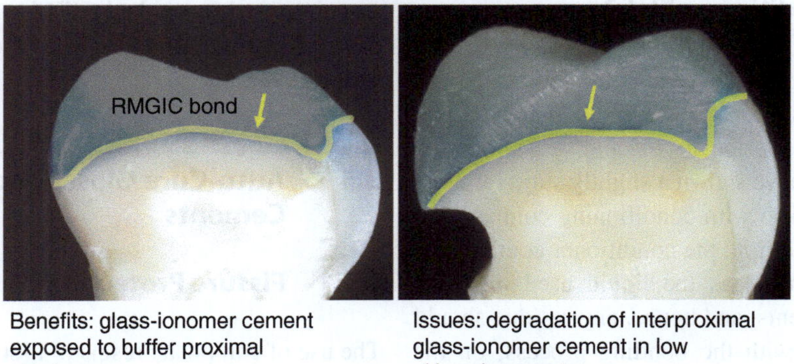

Fig. 3.5 Demonstrates the potential consequences of interproximal plaque acids on the glass-ionomer cement in an "open-sandwich" restoration (Courtesy of Dr. Geoff Knight)

away from occlusal loads as they have poor wear resistance, e.g. in cervical restorations.

Furthermore, these materials are quite opaque compared to composite resins, and there is limited penetration of light to the base of RMGIC restorations during photo-curing that can leave unpolymerized HEMA remaining at the restorative interface. This predisposes to water uptake from the tooth into the restoration and penetration of unpolymerized HEMA from the restoration into the dentinal tubules and eventually into the pulp (Watson 1997).

Light-cured resin-modified adhesives and luting agents, however, are applied as thin films over tooth surfaces that will result in much higher levels of polymerization of the HEMA upon photo-curing.

3.3 Clinical Applications

3.3.1 Surface Preparation

Glass-ionomer cements adhere as a relatively weak ionic bond (about 2.5 MPa) to any clean tooth surface irrespective if it is enamel, dentine or cementum and sound or carious (Lenzi et al. 2013). The bond strength may be enhanced by removing the surface bioload using either conditioning for 10 s with 20 % polyacrylic acid or etching for 5 s with 37 % phosphoric acid (Van Meerbeek et al. 2003).

3.3.2 Condition or Etch?

Traditionally, manufacturers have instructed clinicians to condition teeth with 20 % polyacrylic acid for 10 s prior to placing glass-ionomer cements and have shown a slightly superior bond achieved in vitro with conditioning compared to etching. In addition, the conditioner contains the same components as the liquid used in glass-ionomer cements, and hence, any residue should not interfere with the bonding process; on the other hand, it is said that etching removes mineral content from dentine that reduces the bond strength (McLean 1992).

Much of this published work has been carried out in vitro, and there are significant clinical differences when applied to the oral environment.

Firstly, most hand-pieces are oiled prior to autoclaving, resulting in a spray of oil over the tooth surface from the hand-piece during cavity preparation. The bond strength of dentine surfaces contaminated with oil and conditioned with polyacrylic acid is half that of a non-contaminated surface (Matos et al. 2008). However, etching removes the oil from the dentine surface; dentine with oil contamination that has been etched has the same bond strength as etched non-contaminated dentine (Matos et al. 2008).

Furthermore, a recent paper has shown that RMGIC bonding agents are equally effective, irrespective of whether they are etched or conditioned (Hamama et al. 2014).

Finally, as the fluoride ions from a glass-ionomer cement penetrate the etched dentine surface and combine with dentinal tubular fluid, the dentine will remineralize to form a caries-resistant layer of fluorapatite.

3.4 Auto-Cure or Resin-Modified Glass-Ionomer Cements?

Auto-cure glass-ionomer cements are better suited as restorative materials than resin-modified glass-ionomers as they have better occlusal wear and do not have the problems associated with residual HEMA found at the base of resin-modified glass-ionomer cement restorations.

3.5 Auto-Cure Glass-Ionomer Cements

3.5.1 Fissure Protection

The use of composite resins to fissure seal occlusal surfaces deemed to be at risk from caries has long been advocated by many in the dental profession.

As teeth form in a "biological soup", when they first erupt into the mouth, the hydroxyl apatite crystals are contaminated with carbonate groups that make them more prone to acid breakdown at a higher pH than teeth that have been erupted for some time. After eruption, the outer layers of apatite are subjected to a series of demineralization and remineralization cycles, which in the presence of fluoride, will form a layer of fluorapatite crystals that require a lower pH for demineralization and hence are more caries resistant than a newly erupted tooth (Chow and Vogel 2001).

Sealing a fissure with composite resin on a recently erupted tooth prevents the transformation from carbonated apatite to fluorapatite, leaving the tooth potentially more susceptible to caries if the seal was lost. A tooth that has been in the mouth and subjected to multiple demineralization and remineralization cycles will be far more resistant to microbial attack.

Protecting a fissure with auto-cure glass-ionomer cement has the benefit of, firstly, demineralizing the outer apatite crystals due to the low pH of the uncured glass-ionomer. Secondly, after curing when the pH returns to neutral and in the presence of a high concentration of fluoride ions, demineralized apatite crystals will remineralize as fluorapatite.

Eventually, when the glass-ionomer has worn from the surface, the remaining enamel will be able to resist caries attack as well, if not better, than a mature tooth that has been subjected to multiple remineralizing cycles in a high-fluoride environment.

3.5.1.1 Technique

- Etch the surface to be protected for 5 s with 37 % phosphoric acid, wash and dry thoroughly.
- Isolate the tooth with cotton rolls.
- Apply an auto-cure glass-ionomer over the surface and "puddle" into the fissures with a disposable mini-brush.
- Place a 3 x 2 cm film of a "freezer bag" over the surface and have the patient close in maximum intercuspation. This will force the glass-ionomer into the fissures and maximize the amount that can exist within the occlusion, substantially increasing the area to be protected and the time the glass-ionomer will remain upon the occlusal surface before being worn away (Fig. 3.7).

3.5.2 Management of Cervical Hypersensitivity

The low-viscosity auto-cure glass-ionomer cements are well suited for protection from cervical hypersensitivity by isolating the tooth sur-

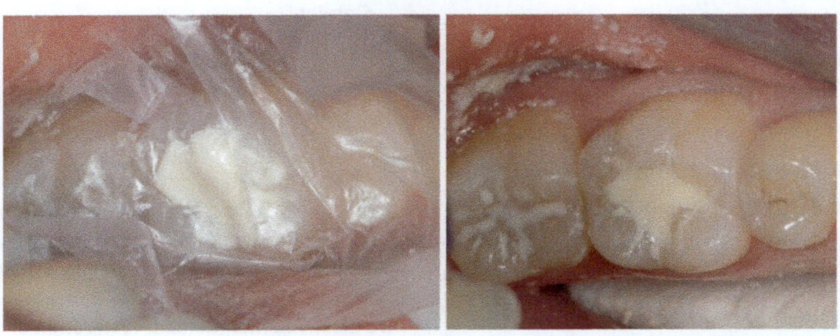

Fig. 3.7 Placement of a 3 × 2 cm piece of freezer bag over a glass-ionomer cement when fissure sealing will force the cement into the fissures and defines the occlusal envelope allowing the maximum amount of glass-ionomer cement coverage of the occlusal surface (Courtesy of Dr. Geoff Knight)

face from the oral environment and releasing fluoride that may well further help encourage desensitization.

3.5.2.1 Technique

- Clean the surface to be treated ideally with 37 % phosphoric acid for 5 s; depending upon the level of sensitivity, this may require prior administration of a local anaesthetic.
- Isolate the area with cotton rolls.
- Mix the low-viscosity auto-cure glass-ionomer and place the unset material on a mixing pad.
- Using a small disposable mini-brush, paint over the relevant areas identified with the hypersensitivity. Distribution of the glass-ionomer cement may be aided by blowing air gently into the interproximal spaces.
- Allow the glass-ionomer to cure.
- A second application of the glass-ionomer may occasionally be required.

3.5.3 Luting Cements

Both auto-cure and resin-modified glass-ionomer cements can be used as luting cements. They are radiopaque and have reasonable adhesion (about 10 MPa) and a relatively high-fluoride release that protects margins from recurrent caries (Tantbirojn et al. 2009).

Auto-cure luting cements have a film thickness of about 20 μm and resin-modified luting cements as low as 10 μm.

Auto-cure luting cements are suitable for metal-based restorations or posts. Resin-modified luting cements have similar properties and benefit from a controlled setting time.

Resin-modified luting cements will bond to both metallic and ceramic surfaces at bond strengths of about 7 MPa. Resin-modified luting cements are best applied to translucent restorations that will facilitate photo-cure polymerization of the HEMA within the cement.

3.6 Auto-Cure Glass-Ionomer Cement as a Restorative Material

The choice of the type of restoration technique depends upon the site of the lesion and the state of the tooth to which it is to be applied. If the lesion occurs in a region of a tooth where the surrounding cusps are well supported and not involving a centric stop, a wear-resistant glass-ionomer cement restoration may be used. When adjacent cusps are undermined and susceptible to occlusal loads, or if the centric stops occur on the occlusal surface, then a composite resin or combined composite resin/glass-ionomer cement restoration may be more appropriate (Figs. 3.8 and 3.9).

3.6.1 Occlusal Restorations with Supported Cusps: OI-Type Cavity

These are small cavities that do not involve centric stops and can be placed using auto-cure glass-ionomers.

Cavity classification

Site	Supported cusps I	Unsupported cusps II	Missing cusps III
Occlusal "O"			
Proximal "P"			
Cervical "C"			

Based upon the site and anatomical integrity of the surrounding tooth

Fig. 3.8 This table, developed by the author, shows a classification for restorations based upon the site of a lesion and the anatomical integrity of the surrounding tooth structure; i.e. if the surrounding cusps are supported and centric stops not involved, then a wear-resistant auto-cure glass-ionomer cement restoration is indicated: if surrounding cusps are not supported, then a composite resin or glass-ionomer composite "sandwich" restoration is required (Courtesy of Dr. Geoff Knight)

Occlusal cavity with supported cusps

Site	Supported cusps I	Unsupported cusps II	Missing cusps III
Occlusal "O"	●		
Proximal "P"			
Cervical "C"			

Type "OI" cavity restored with auto-cure glass-ionomer cement

Fig. 3.9 Traditional Class I cavity: this classification is for a small occlusal cavity with well-supported surrounding cusps suitable for placing a wear-resistant auto-cure glass-ionomer cement. OI-type cavity (Courtesy of Dr. Geoff Knight)

Caries removal for a small occlusal cavity restored with auto cure-glass-ionomer cement

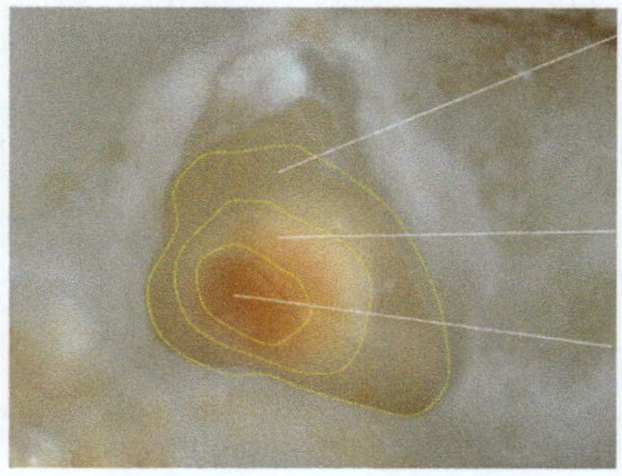

Fig. 3.10 Cavity preparation. Remove caries to just above the infected dentine layer as shown, leaving a 0.5 mm layer of carious dentine at the base of the preparation surrounded by affected (remineralizable) dentine. Prepare a moat around the periphery of the cavity into sound dentine using a no. 3 round bur (Courtesy of Dr. Geoff Knight)

3.6.1.1 Technique

- Caries removal: as glass-ionomer cements release bactericidal levels of fluoride, a conservative preparation to just above the affected dentine layer is recommended, leaving a 0.5 mm layer of carious dentine at the base of the preparation (Knight et al. 2007a; Ngo et al. 2006; Brown et al. 1980).
- Cavity preparation is completed by preparing a moat around the dentino-enamel junction using a size no. 3 round slow-speed bur to aid retention and assure a biological seal into sound dentine. This acts as a further preventive measure against recurrent caries.
- After cavity preparation, etch the preparation for 5 s with 37 % phosphoric acid (to remove hand-piece oil and other debris), wash and dry with oil-free air.
- Isolate with cotton rolls.
- Place the glass-ionomer cement into the cavity (preferably with a capsule) from the base of the cavity upwards to minimize air inclusions and to slightly overfill the cavity.
- Place a 3 x 2 cm piece of "freezer bag" over the restoration and ask the patient to close into maximum intercuspation until the glass-ionomer cement cures. This forces the glass-ionomer cement into the cavity and creates an occlusal matrix that minimizes contouring of the cured restoration.
- In small cavities, the only adjustment required can be done with a sharp excavator.
- In larger restorations that involve more of the occlusal surface, it may be necessary to contour the inclined planes of the restoration parallel to those of adjacent teeth to compensate for lateral and protrusive movements of the mandible during mastication
- Covering the restoration with an isolating varnish film is a matter of the clinician's choice (Fig. 3.10).

3.6.2 Occlusal Restorations with Unsupported Cusps: OII-Type Cavity

These cavities involve more of the occlusal surface such that cusps are either unsupported or involve centric stops. Glass-ionomer cement restorations do not have the shear strength to support these cusps and are subject to high levels of wear on surfaces involving centric stops. In such circumstances, the preferred restorative technique is a "sandwich" technique, described by John McLean, where glass-ionomer cement

Occlusal cavity with unsupported cusps

Site	Supported cusps I	Unsupported cusps II	Missing cusps III
Occlusal "O"		●	
Proximal "P"			
Cervical "C"			

Type "OII" cavity restored with auto-cure glass-ionomer cement with composite resin overlay

Fig. 3.11 Traditional Class I cavity: this classification is for a larger occlusal cavity when the surrounding cusps are unsupported or the restoration involves a centric stop indicating a composite resin or glass-ionomer composite "sandwich" restoration. OII-type cavity (Courtesy of Dr. Geoff Knight)

Occlusal cavities with unsupported cusps

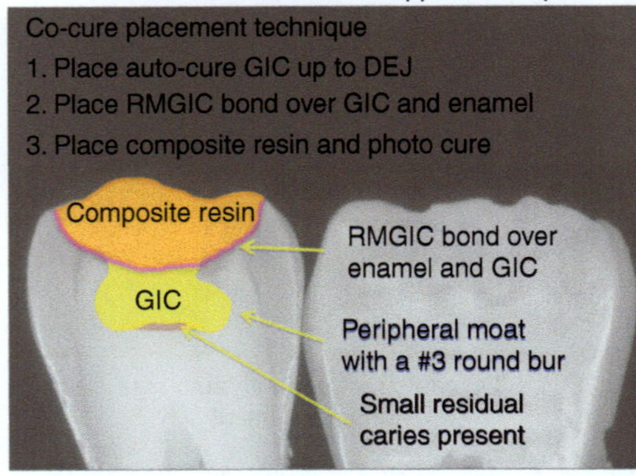

Fig. 3.12 During cavity preparation, the cusps are protected by forming a cusp overlay on the occlusal surface. The technique of bonding composite resin to auto-cure glass-ionomer cement with resin-modified glass-ionomer cement bonding adhesive is called "co-curing", enabling chemical adhesion of about 7 MPa between the two materials (Knight et al. 2006) (Courtesy of Dr. Geoff Knight)

replaces dentine and composite resin replaces enamel (McLean 1992) (Fig. 3.11).

3.6.2.1 Technique

- Caries removal is similar as for a small occlusal restoration: leave 0.5 mm layer of carious dentine and prepare a moat into sound dentine around the dentino-enamel junction using a no. 3 round bur.
- As the cusps are unsupported, it is advisable to protect them using an occlusal overlay preparation with a high-speed large round diamond bur.
- After cavity preparation, etch the preparation for 5 s with 37 % phosphoric acid (to remove hand-piece oil and other debris), wash and dry with oil-free air.
- Isolate with cotton rolls.
- Place the glass-ionomer cement into the cavity (preferably using a capsule), filling from the base of the cavity upwards to minimize air inclusions up to the dentino-enamel junction.
- Prepare a resin-modified glass-ionomer adhesive bond and either wait until the auto-cure glass-ionomer has set or place the bond directly over the uncured glass-ionomer and the exposed cavosurface margin walls (Knight et al. 2006). (This procedure is called "co-curing" and discussed later within this chapter.)
- Insert an increment of composite resin over the freshly set or unset glass-ionomer to slightly overfill the cavity.
- Burnish the margins with a ball burnisher.
- Place a 3 x 2 cm piece of "freezer bag" over the restoration and ask the patient to close into maximum intercuspation onto the uncured composite resin.
- While the patient remains in occlusion, photo-cure the restoration from the buccal aspect for 5 s.
- Ask the patient to open and photo-cure for a further 10 s.

If the composite resin has been placed onto the uncured glass-ionomer, the heat generated from the polymerization of the composite will initiate a cascade setting reaction within the glass-ionomer cement, causing a complete cure within 40 s (Knight et al. 2006) (Fig. 3.12).

- As these restorations involve most of the occlusal surface, it will be necessary to contour the inclined planes of the restoration parallel to those of adjacent teeth to compensate for lateral and protrusive movements of the mandible during mastication.
- After contouring, polish the composite resin to a high gloss to minimize patient discomfort and plaque accumulation (Fig. 3.13).

3.6.3 Proximal Restorations with Supported Cusps: PI-Type Cavity

These restorations are usually associated with unrestored proximal caries.

Breaking through the marginal ridge destroys the structural integrity of the tooth and weakens cusps that eventually lead to fracture.

A "tunnel" or slot restoration will maintain this structural integrity and is the most conservative and efficient way to manage such lesions (Knight 1992). If the lesion is visible on either the facial or lingual aspect of the tooth, slot (Morand and Jonas 1995) restorations are preferable; if the lesion is not visible, then a tunnel restoration is indicated (Knight 1984; Hunt 1984). As neither of these restorative techniques involve a centric stop, both are suitable for restoration by auto-cure glass-ionomer cements (Fig. 3.14).

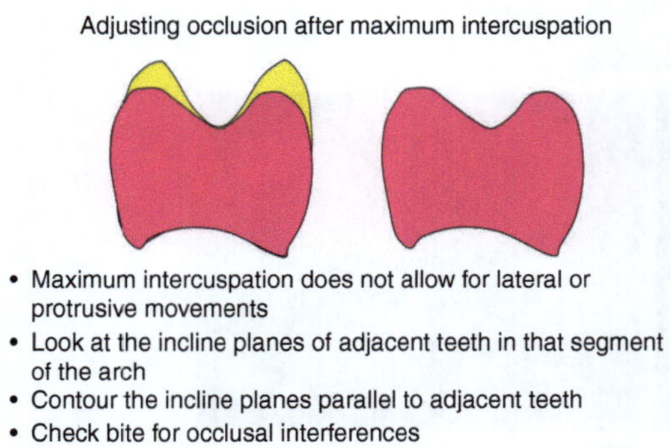

Fig. 3.13 Following photo-curing of the occlusal surface, the inclined planes of the restoration require to be contoured parallel to the inclined planes of adjacent teeth to facilitate lateral and protrusive movements within the dentition (Courtesy of Dr. Geoff Knight)

Proximal lesion with supported cusps

Site	Supported cusps I	Unsupported cusps II	Missing cusps III
Occlusal "O"			
Proximal "P"	●		
Cervical "C"			

Type "PI" cavity restored with auto-cure glass-ionomer cement

Fig. 3.14 Traditional Class II cavity: this classification is for initial proximal lesions (irrespective of size) where the marginal ridge remains intact and surrounding cusps are supported, indicating a wear-resistant auto-cure glass-ionomer cement restoration. PI-type cavity (Courtesy of Dr. Geoff Knight)

3.6.3.1 Technique

Slot Restorations

- Access the lesion where it is visible with a water-cooled high-speed bur.
- Use a slow-speed round bur (nos. 3 to 6 depending on the extent of caries) to conservatively remove the carious dentine, leaving the affected dentine if practicable.
- Prepare a moat around the dentino-enamel junction into sound dentine with a no. 3 round bur at the perimeter of the cavity to aid retention and ensure a biological seal into sound dentine to prevent recurrent caries.
- Etch the preparation for 5 s, wash and dry the preparation.
- Isolate with cotton rolls.
- Insert a sectional matrix or Mylar strip into the proximal area and wedge the matrix against the preparation with a suitably sized GP point.
- Mix a capsulated auto-cure glass-ionomer cement and insert to the depth of the preparation.
- Slowly extrude the glass-ionomer cement into the cavity, withdrawing the capsule to avoid air bubbles until the cavity is slightly overfilled.
- Fold the matrix band or Mylar strip over the exposed part of the preparation and hold in place until the glass-ionomer has cured.
- Remove the GP point and matrix or Mylar strip and remove any flash of glass-ionomer that may be present.
- Covering the restoration with an isolating varnish film is a matter of the clinician's choice (Figs. 3.15, 3.16 and 3.17).

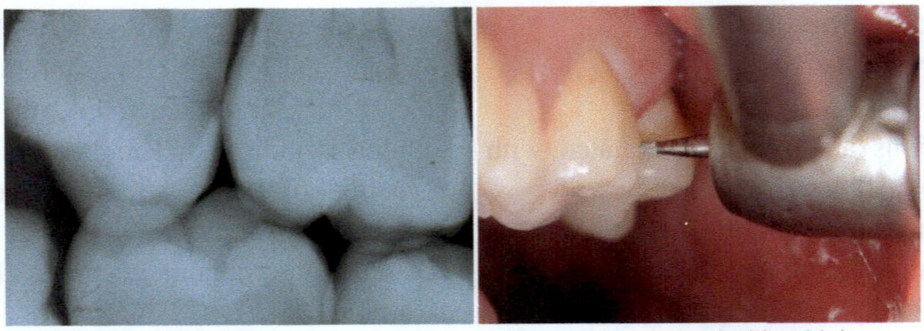

Fig. 3.15 Slot preparation when the lesion is visible from the buccal aspect using a high-speed bur, taking care to avoid the adjacent proximal tooth surface (Courtesy of Dr. Geoff Knight)

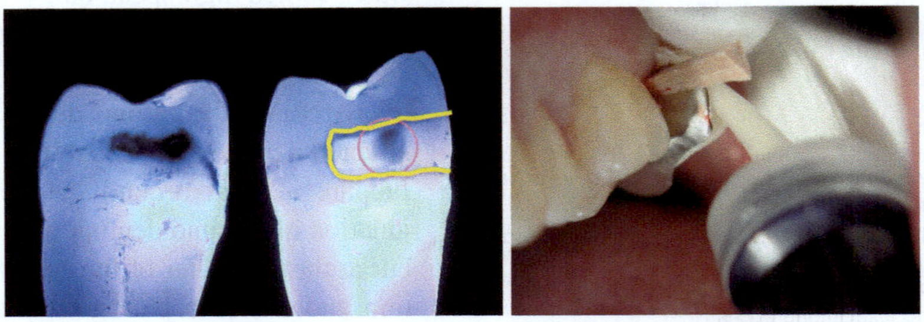

Fig. 3.16 After initial caries removal with a slow-speed round bur, a moat is prepared around the perimeter of the slot with a no. 3 round bur into sound dentine. The nozzle of the GIC capsule is inserted to the depth of the cavity and cement slowly extruded as the nozzle is withdrawn (Courtesy of Dr. Geoff Knight)

Fig. 3.17 The completed restoration maintaining the structural integrity of the tooth (Courtesy of Dr. Geoff Knight)

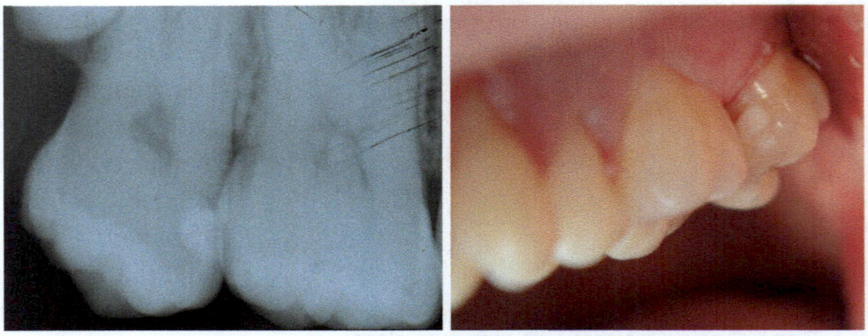

Tunnel Restorations

- Prepare a "T" cavity in the enamel above the lesion with a water-cooled high-speed bur 2 mm in from the marginal ridge, extending 2 mm facially, 2 mm lingually and 2 mm over the occlusal surface. This will conservatively maximize both mechanical and visual access to the preparation.

- Choose a slow-speed round bur depending on the size of the lesion and start removing dentine above the lesion by running the bur along the dentino-enamel margin until the lesion is reached.
- Once the caries has been accessed, gently loop the bur around the proximal lesion, staying at the dentino-enamel junction and limiting tooth removal to tactile detectable softened dentine.
- Run the bur around the enamel margins of the proximal cavitation to remove any unsupported enamel.
- With a no. 3 round bur, create a moat into sound dentine at the dentino-enamel junction, starting either facially or lingually and running the bur below the cavitated enamel and up the other side of the preparation to biologically seal the restoration, preventing recurrent caries.
- Etch with 37 % phosphoric acid for 5 s, wash and dry the preparation.
- Isolate with cotton rolls.
- Insert a Mylar strip into the interproximal space and withdraw it facially until there is about 0.5 cm extending beyond the lingual aspect of the tooth.
- With a pair of scissors, cut away the facial strip, leaving about 0.5 cm of it protruding.
- Firmly wedge the proximal matrix against the preparation with a suitably sized GP point.
- Mix a capsulated auto-cure glass-ionomer cement and insert to the depth of the preparation.
- Slowly extrude the glass-ionomer cement into the cavity, withdrawing the capsule to avoid air bubbles until the cavity is slightly overfilled.
- Ask the patient to commence closing slowly into maximum intercuspation and just prior to tooth contact; fold the matrix over the occlusal aspect of the cavity using a periodontal probe or a similar plastic instrument.
- The patient should remain closed in this position until the glass-ionomer cement has set.
- When the glass-ionomer cement has set, remove the GP point and the matrix band along with any flash visible on the proximal surfaces.
- Minimal contouring to remove occlusal interferences is usually required.
- Covering the restoration with an isolating varnish film is the clinician's choice (Figs. 3.18, 3.19, 3.20 and 3.21).

3.6.4 Proximal Restorations with Unsupported Cusps (Fig. 3.22)

Soon after auto-cure glass-ionomer cements first started to be used as a restorative material, McLean advocated the concept of a "sandwich"

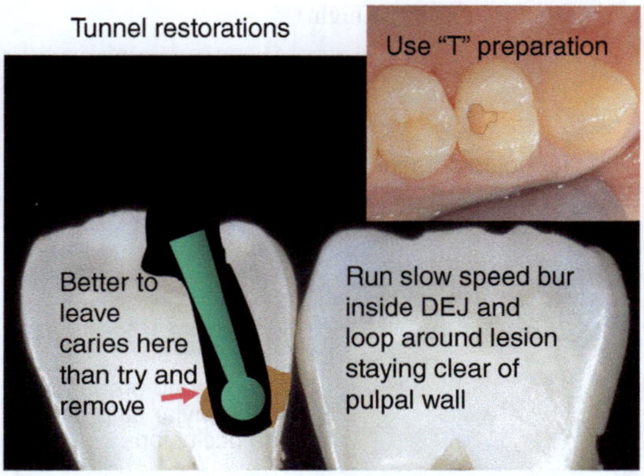

Fig. 3.18 Prepare a conservative "T" preparation in the enamel with a high-speed diamond bur. Following this, access the lesion with a slow-speed round bur running along the dentino-enamel junction until the caries is reached, looping the bur slightly below the point where the lesion has broken through the enamel (Courtesy of Dr. Geoff Knight)

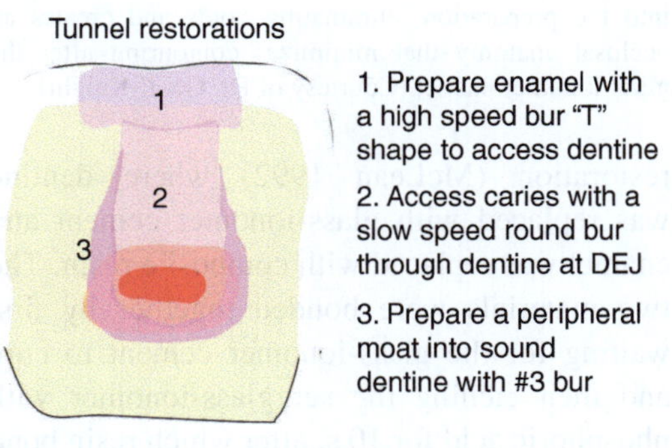

Fig. 3.19 After removing caries around the lesion along the dentino-enamel junction, take a no. 3 round slow-speed bur and prepare a moat into sound dentine at the perimeter of the preparation (Courtesy of Dr. Geoff Knight)

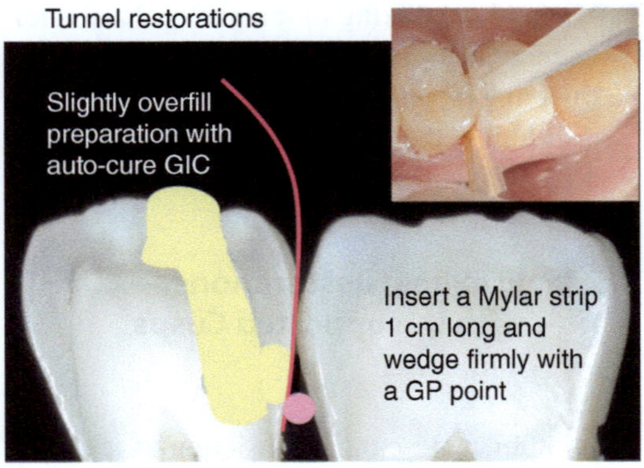

Fig. 3.20 Insert a 1-cm-long Mylar strip interproximally and wedge it firmly with a GP point followed by slightly overfilling the cavity with auto-cure glass-ionomer cement (Courtesy of Dr. Geoff Knight)

Proximal lesion with unsupported cusps

Site	Supported cusps I	Unsupported cusps II	Missing cusps III
Occlusal "O"			
Proximal "P"		●	
Cervical "C"			

Type "PII" cavity restored with auto-cure glass-ionomer cement and composite resin overaly

Fig. 3.22 Traditional Class II cavity: this classification is for proximal lesions where the marginal ridge is no longer present; cusps are unsupported, indicating a composite resin or glass-ionomer composite "sandwich" restoration. PII-type cavity (Courtesy of Dr. Geoff Knight)

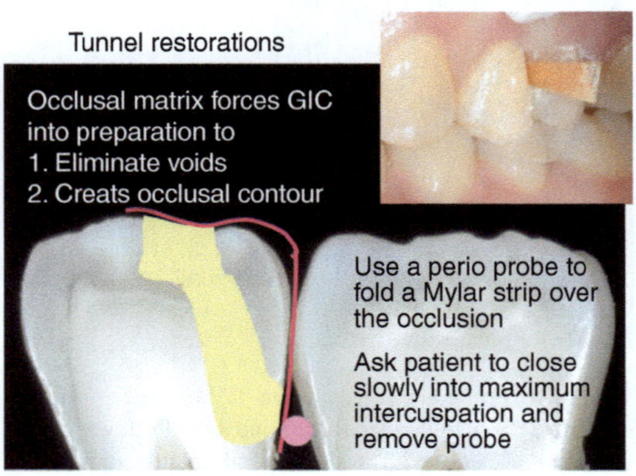

Fig. 3.21 Ask the patient to close slowly into maximum intercuspation and just prior to contact; fold the Mylar strip over the occlusal surface with a periodontal probe or similar instrument. This forces the glass-ionomer cement into the preparation, eliminating voids and creates an occlusal anatomy that minimizes contouring after the glass-ionomer has set (Courtesy of Dr. Geoff Knight)

restoration (McLean 1992) where dentine was replaced with glass-ionomer cement and enamel was replaced with composite resin. The two materials were bonded together by first waiting for the glass-ionomer cement to cure and then etching the set glass-ionomer with phosphoric acid for 10 s, after which resin bond was applied to the glass-ionomer surface followed by composite resin. The weak resulting bond was in the order of 2 MPa (Knight et al. 2006) and prone to debonding in areas where moderate tensile forces were applied to the restoration. A much higher bond can be achieved between auto-cure glass-ionomer cements by placing a layer of resin-modified glass-ionomer cement adhesive between the glass-ionomer and composite resin.

This resin-modified bonding system can be applied to the auto-cure glass-ionomer cement either before or soon after the glass-ionomer cement has cured to achieve a bond strength of about 7 MPa (Knight et al. 2006), which is the bond strength at cohesive failure of auto-cure glass-ionomer cement. In other words, the bond achieved in this manner is greater than the forced required for cohesive failure of the glass-ionomer cement.

When the composite resin is applied to the uncured glass-ionomer cement and subsequently photo-cured, the exothermic setting reaction of the composite resin heats up the surface of the auto-cure glass-ionomer and causes a cascade setting reaction within the glass-ionomer, significantly reducing the setting time and thus the clinical time required to place the restoration (Knight et al. 2006). This procedure is called "co-curing" and is discussed in depth later within this chapter.

"Open-sandwich" restorations may lead to food packing and are generally clinically unsatisfactory (Welbury and Murray 1990). A "closed-sandwich" technique is preferred where a layer of auto-cure glass-ionomer cement is laid down as a base but not extending onto the proximal surfaces. A thin layer of resin-modified cement bonding agent is present at the margins to afford some protection from recurrent caries, and the glass-ionomer cement remains available to help arrest proximal caries if they proceed past the layer of overlying composite resin.

With these factors in mind, the technique for placing a closed-sandwich restoration is described below.

3.6.4.1 Technique

- Access the lesion with a water-cooled high-speed bur.
- If caries are present, use a slow-speed round bur (nos. 3 to 6 depending on the extent of caries) to conservatively remove the carious dentine, leaving the affected dentine.
- Prepare a moat around the dentino-enamel junction into sound dentine with a no. 3 round bur to form a biological seal. This is particularly important on the floor of the proximal box where dentinal tubules run parallel to the cavity floor. Creation of a moat means that the ends of the dentinal tubules will be blocked with either auto-cure glass-ionomer or a resin-modified dentine bonding agent.
- If bleeding is present on the proximal gingivae, a small amount of a saturated solution of trichloroacetic acid (TCA) may be applied with a periodontal probe onto the tissues as a powerful haemostatic agent. When using this product, clinicians are advised to have an antidote of a saturated solution of sodium bicarbonate on hand in case any acid is inadvertently spilled onto the patient's skin, where it will cause an uncomfortable and long-lasting caustic burn.
- Etch the preparation with 37 % phosphoric acid for 5 s, wash and dry.
- Isolate with cotton rolls.
- Prior to applying a proximal matrix, place a layer of auto-cure glass-ionomer cement over the dentinal surfaces up to the dentino-enamel junction. If no enamel is present on the proximal floor, bring the glass-ionomer to a feather-edge at the margin.
- Mix a resin-modified glass-ionomer adhesive, and apply this over the glass-ionomer cement (either cured/set or uncured/setting) and the remaining cavity walls.
- Place a preferred matrix system and wedge as required.
- Insert a small amount of composite resin onto the floor of the proximal box and photo-cure for 10 s (making sure there is an adequate contact of the matrix band with the adjacent tooth).
- Place a further increment of resin-modified glass-ionomer adhesive over the composite resin and cure for 10 s.
- Place the final increment of composite to slightly overfill the remaining cavity space, and photo-cure for a further 10 s.
- Remove the matrix and contour the composite restoration to fit within the occlusal envelope.
- Carry out final contouring and polish the restoration (Figs. 3.23, 3.24 and 3.25).

3.6.5 Silver-Sintered Auto-Cure Glass-Ionomer Cements

Originally looked upon as a means of strengthening auto-cure glass-ionomer cements, silver and gold particles were sintered into the glass particles to form the powder component of the resto-

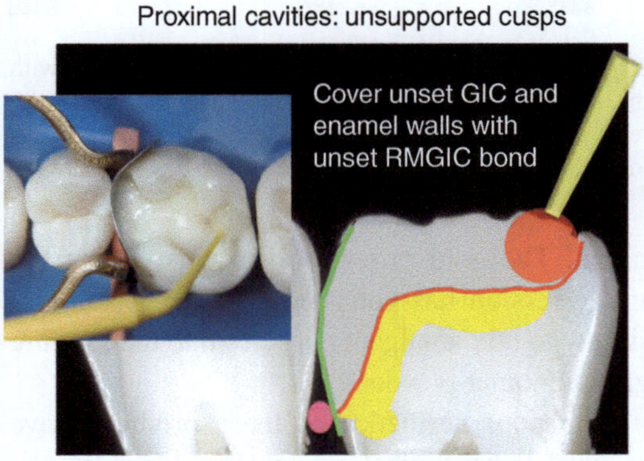

Fig. 3.23 The auto-cure glass-ionomer cement is placed up to the dentino-enamel junction and just short of the margin of the proximal floor. Observe the moat at the dentino-enamel junction margin. Cover the set or unset auto-cure glass-ionomer cement with a thin layer of resin-modified glass-ionomer adhesive (Courtesy of Dr. Geoff Knight)

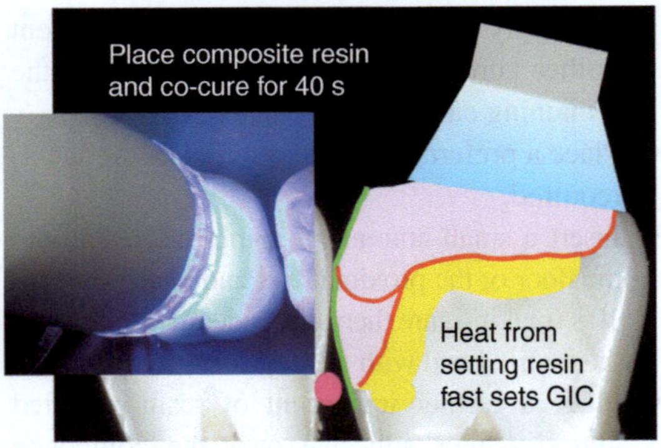

Fig. 3.24 After creating a proximal contact with the composite resin and curing it, fill the remainder of the cavity with composite resin and photo-cure. If the auto-cure glass-ionomer cement has not yet set, curing for 40 s combined with the exothermic setting reaction of the composite will cause a cascade setting reaction within the glass-ionomer, saving valuable clinical time (Courtesy of Dr. Geoff Knight)

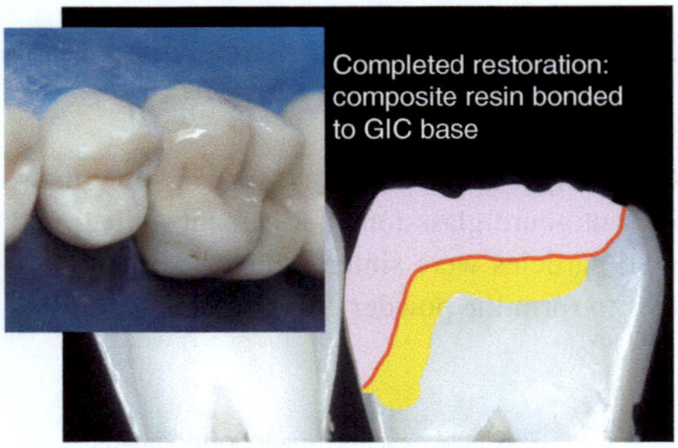

Fig. 3.25 Completed closed-sandwich restoration with the auto-cure glass-ionomer cement and the composite resin chemically bonded with resin-modified glass-ionomer adhesive (Courtesy of Dr. Geoff Knight)

ration. The gold proved too expensive, but the silver version has persisted. Another version is simply to mix amalgam particles into the existing glass-ionomer powder.

The poor aesthetics of these products have reduced their clinical acceptance; however, the high radiopacity makes them suitable for cores, and when used as long-term intermediate restorations, they seem to stay in the cavity well beyond the predicted life expectancy, possibly due to the silver particles acting as a surface lubricant and minimizing the traumatic effects of occlusion.

3.6.6 Managing Endodontically Treated Teeth in a Collapsing Dentition

Many older patients experience collapse of their dentitions as endodontically restored teeth decoronate and leave exposed roots at the gingival margins. The extraction of these teeth adds unnecessary trauma to a frail individual, and they can be managed either by being covered by a denture or left exposed within the dentition by covering the root stumps with auto-cure glass-ionomer cement.

The release of fluoride from the glass-ionomer inhibits caries formation, and minimal cavity preparation is required to produce a smooth surface restoration that prevents tongue lacerations from a jagged cavity margin.

3.6.6.1 Technique

- Minimally prepare the root surface to gain some undercuts if possible.
- Etch for 5 s, wash and dry thoroughly.
- Isolate the cavity with cotton rolls.
- Apply a layer of resin-modified dental adhesive and photo-cure.
- Apply a second layer, but do not photo-cure.
- Apply an increment of auto-cure glass-ionomer cement to slightly overfill the preparation.
- Contour the glass-ionomer with the applicator brush used for the adhesive.
- Photo-cure the auto-cure glass-ionomer and the adhesive for 40 s.

The resin-modified adhesive will triple the bond strength of the glass-ionomer cement, and the energy from the curing light will reduce the normal curing time of the auto-cure glass-ionomer cement (Fig. 3.26).

3.6.7 Resin-Modified Glass-Ionomer Cements

3.6.7.1 Resin-Modified Glass-Ionomer Cement as a Restorative Material

Resin-modified glass-ionomer cements are well suited as luting cements and tooth adhesives

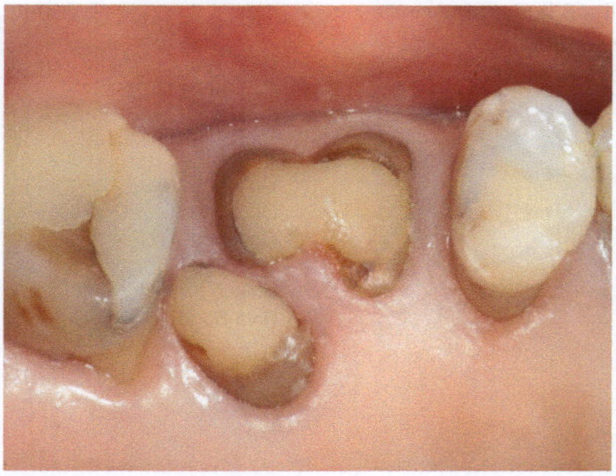

Fig. 3.26 Salvaging a decoronated tooth that has been root-filled with an auto-cure glass-ionomer cement restoration preserves the alveolar ridge and can be incorporated under a denture or left to protect the gingiva from hard food particles (Courtesy of Dr. Geoff Knight)

where thin layers can be photo-cured to polymerize the HEMA present within the cement. In deep cavities, the possibility of unpolymerized HEMA at the floor of the cavity can result in absorption of fluid from the tooth into the restoration or permeation of free HEMA into the dentine and pulp where postoperative sensitivity may develop (Watson 1997).

The clinical use of resin-modified glass-ionomer cements as a restorative material should be limited to shallow cervical restorations where high aesthetics are required and core build-ups in nonvital teeth where there is adequate remaining tooth structure. Resin-modified glass-ionomer cements are well suited as dental adhesives, thin cavity lining materials and luting of translucent ceramic restorations.

3.6.7.2 Cavity Liners

Resin-modified glass-ionomer cements have been successfully used as cavity liners for many years. In thin layers, the free HEMA is mostly polymerized to create an adhesive, bactericidal (Duque et al. 2009), thermally protective and radiopaque liner for use under composite resin or amalgam restorations.

3.6.8 Dental Adhesives

3.6.8.1 Bonding Composite Resin to Tooth Structure

When resin-modified glass-ionomer cements are used as dental adhesives, they are able to eliminate the polymerization shrinkage stress found at the restorative interface between composite resin and tooth structure. Polyacrylic acid is a highly elastic molecule capable of absorbing moisture from the environment and expanding to compensate for the polymerization shrinkage stress generated by the photo-initiation of the composite resin (Naoum et al. 2014). Resin-modified glass-ionomer cements also provide (Forsten et al. 1994) enhanced marginal protection from caries compared to resin adhesives. Capsulated resin-modified glass-ionomer cement adhesives have been shown to resist marginal staining equally well as resin-based adhesives (Tantbirojn et al. 2009) (Figs. 3.27 and 3.28).

3.6.9 Co-curing: Bonding Auto-Cure Glass-Ionomer Cements to Composite Resin

The sandwich technique as described by McLean (1992) required adhering the freshly set glass-ionomer cement to composite resin by first etching the glass-ionomer cement with 37 % phosphoric acid, washing and drying the surface, before applying a layer of unfilled resin as a bonding agent between the resin and composite. The bond strength generated by this technique was about 2 MPa.

Resin-modified glass-ionomer cements will chemically bond either freshly cured or uncured glass-ionomer cements to composite resin (Knight 1994). The resin component in the adhesive bonds to the composite, and the glass-ionomer cement component bonds to the auto-cure glass-ionomer. The bond strength of these bonds exceeds 7 MPa which is the cohesive failure strength of the auto-cure glass-ionomer (Knight et al. 2006) (Figs. 3.29, 3.30 and 3.31).

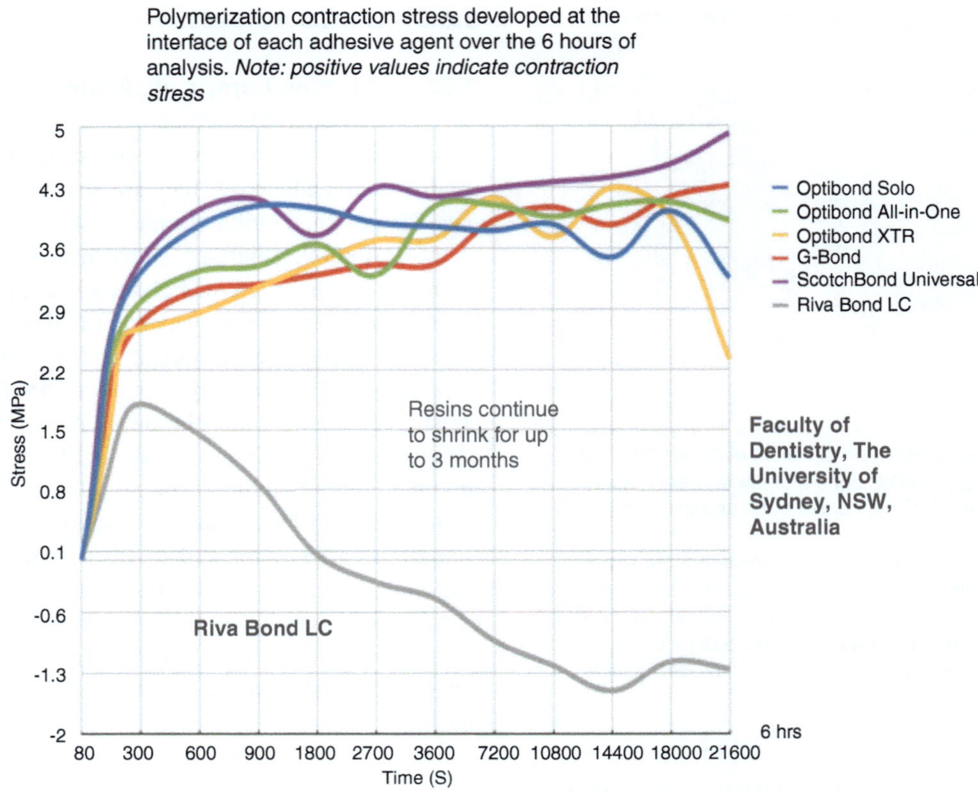

Fig. 3.27 Chart showing the reduction in polymerization shrinkage stress over 6 h at the margins of a composite resin restoration when a resin-modified glass-ionomer adhesive (Riva Bond LC) is used compared to resin-based adhesives (Reprinted from Naoum et al. (2014), with permission from John Wiley & Sons)

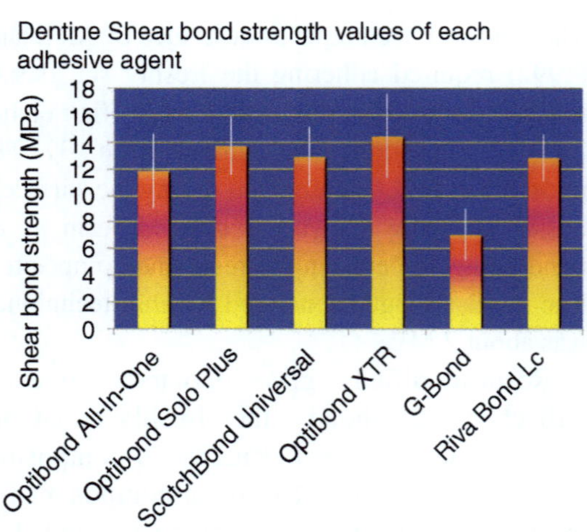

Fig. 3.28 Chart showing the comparisons of the shear bond strength to dentine of various dental adhesives (Reprinted from Naoum et al. (2014), with permission from John Wiley & Sons [Faculty of Dentistry, The University of Sydney, NSW, Australia])

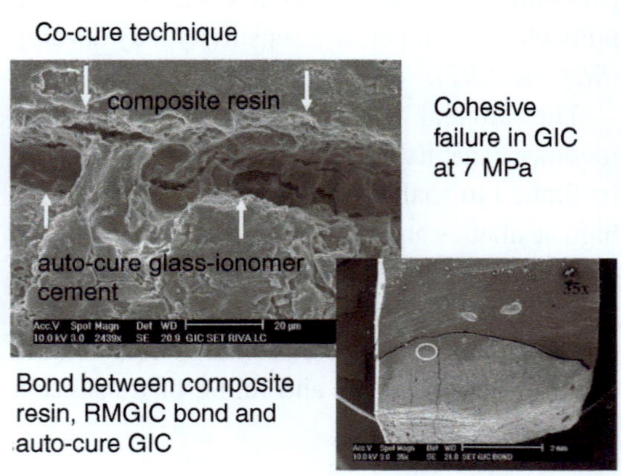

Fig. 3.29 Scanning electron micrograph showing the bond interface between set auto-cure glass-ionomer cement and composite resin using a resin-modified glass-ionomer adhesive at the interface (area indicated in the lower magnification micrograph). Note cohesive failure occurred within the auto-cure glass-ionomer (Courtesy of Dr. Geoff Knight)

3.6.10 Bonding Auto-Cure Glass-Ionomers to Tooth Structure

Resin-modified glass-ionomer bonding agents are capable of increasing the bond strength of auto-cure glass-ionomer cements to dental enamel and dentine. An uncured layer of resin-modified bonding agent is applied over a photo-cured layer followed by the auto-cure glass-ionomer and photo-curing of the combined materials for 40 s. The resin-modified glass-ionomer will photo-cure at the margins and dark-cure beneath the glass-ionomer cement. The bond strength exceeds the cohesive failure of the auto-cure glass-ionomer cement (7 MPa). Increasing the curing time to 40 s transfers heat from the curing light into the auto-cure glass-ionomer, encouraging the setting reaction (Knight et al. 2006) (Figs. 3.32, 3.33 and 3.34).

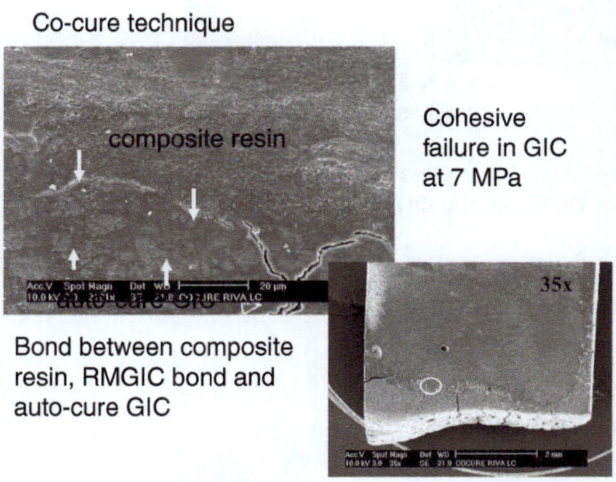

Fig. 3.30 Scanning electron micrograph showing the bond interface between unset (co-cured) auto-cure glass-ionomer cement and composite resin using a resin-modified glass-ionomer adhesive at the interface (area indicated in the lower magnification micrograph). Note how the glass-ionomer and composite resin interface has merged almost undetectably with the resin-based glass-ionomer cement adhesive and that cohesive failure occurred within the auto-cure glass-ionomer (Courtesy of Dr. Geoff Knight)

3.6.11 Resin-Modified Glass-Ionomer Bonding Agents Used as a Carrier for Medicaments Under Restorations

As resin-modified adhesives are water-soluble resin-based materials, they can be used as vehicles to apply medicaments at the base of a restoration. Metallic oxides such as zinc can be

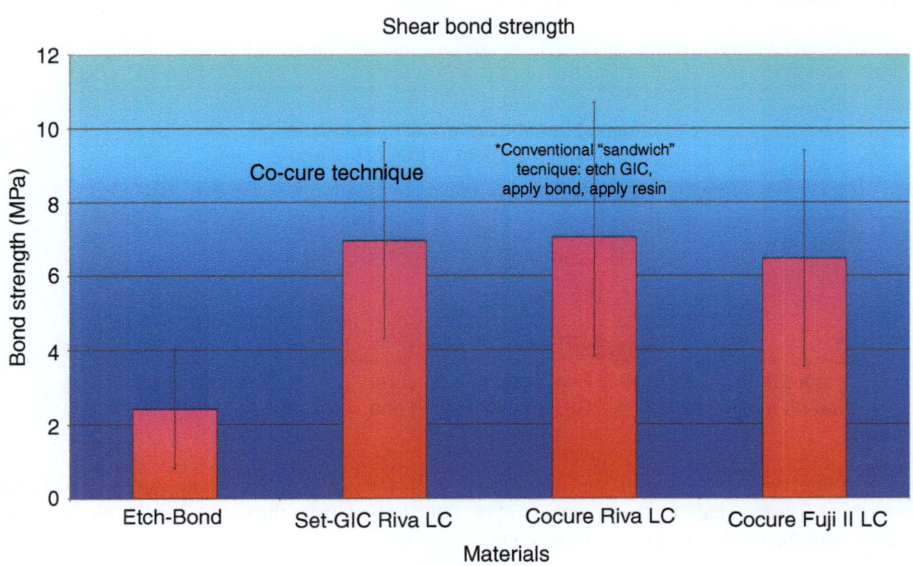

Fig. 3.31 Chart showing the bond strengths of various adhesive techniques between auto-cure glass-ionomer cement and composite resin. There is no statistical difference in the strengths between set and unset (co-cured) glass-ionomer cements as all samples failed cohesively within the glass-ionomer (Courtesy of Dr. Geoff Knight)

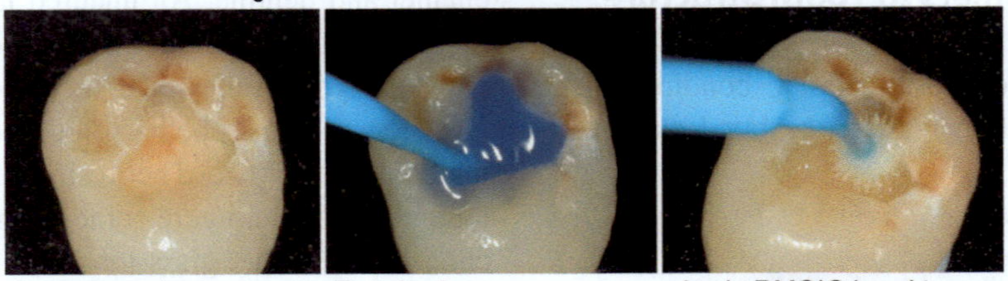

Fig. 3.32 Improving the bond strength between auto-cure glass-ionomer cement and tooth structure. This figure shows the preparation of the cavity and first layer of resin-modified glass-ionomer cement adhesive (Courtesy of Dr. Geoff Knight)

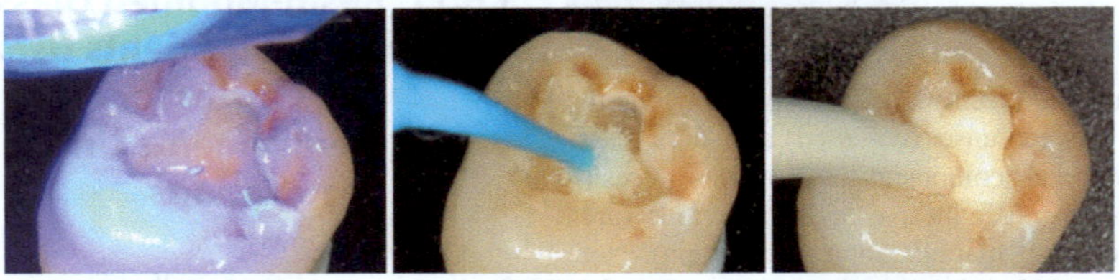

Fig. 3.33 Improving the bond strength between auto-cure glass-ionomer cement and tooth structure. This figure shows photo-curing the first layer and applying the second layer of adhesive followed by the auto-cure glass-ionomer cement (Courtesy of Dr. Geoff Knight)

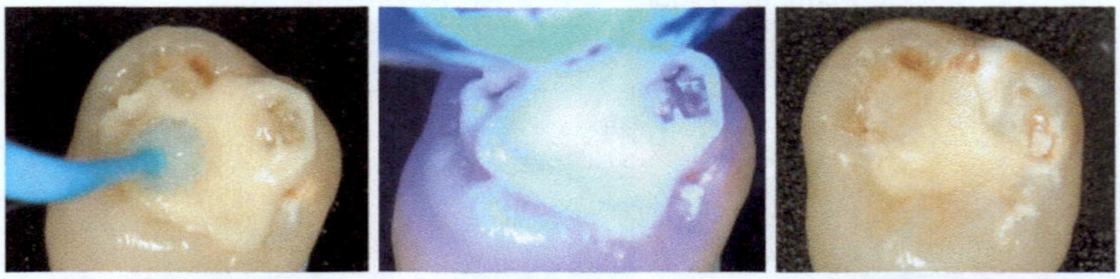

Fig. 3.34 Improving the bond strength between auto-cure glass-ionomer cement and tooth structure. This shows the photo-curing of the adhesive and auto-cure glass-ionomer cement for 40 s to speed the setting time due to heat from the curing light (Courtesy of Dr. Geoff Knight)

incorporated to act as a disinfectant, and small amounts of Ledermix® (Haupt Pharma GmbH, *Wolfratshausen*, Germany) powder can be mixed into the unset bond to create a light-cured version of the liquid/powder combination that has been used for many years as an anti-inflammatory lining beneath deep restorations (Figs. 3.35, 3.36, 3.37 and 3.38).

3.6.12 Bonding Amalgam to Enamel and Dentine

Resin-modified adhesives can be used under dental amalgams to create a chemical bond between the tooth and amalgam. Furthermore, this seals the amalgam and helps protect margins from recurrent caries.

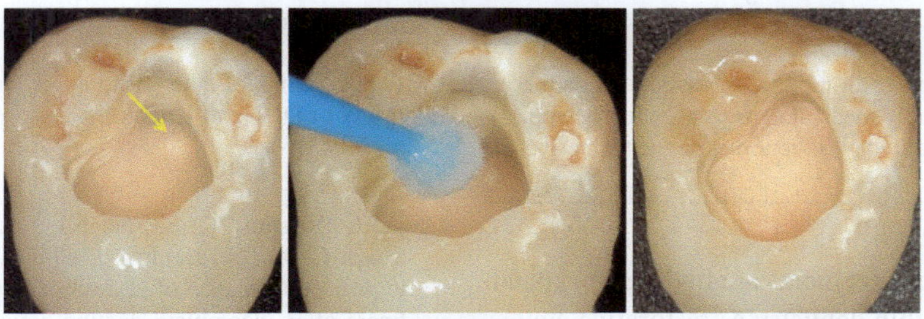

Fig. 3.35 Using a resin-modified glass-ionomer adhesive as a vehicle to apply medicaments to a tooth. This figure shows identification of a small exposure and applying TCA to manage any bleeding (Courtesy of Dr. Geoff Knight)

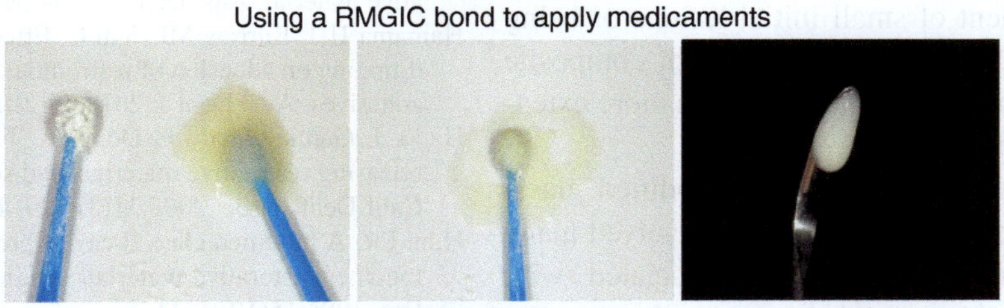

Fig. 3.36 Using a resin-modified glass-ionomer adhesive as a vehicle to apply medicaments to a tooth. This shows the technique for incorporating the medicament into the resin-modified glass-ionomer adhesive (Courtesy of Dr. Geoff Knight)

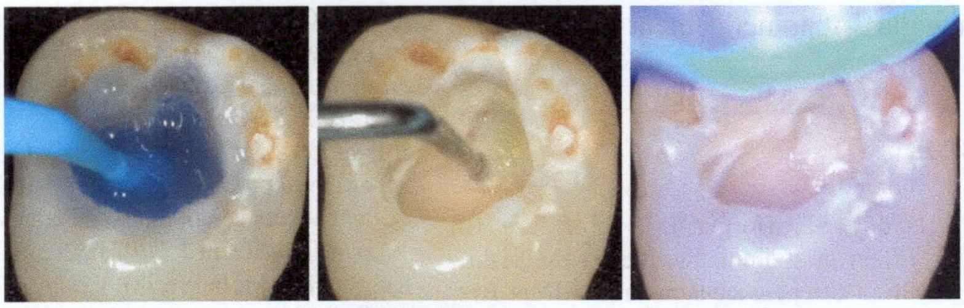

Fig. 3.37 Using a resin-modified glass-ionomer adhesive as a vehicle to apply medicaments to a tooth. This figure shows medicament application to the tooth (Courtesy of Dr. Geoff Knight)

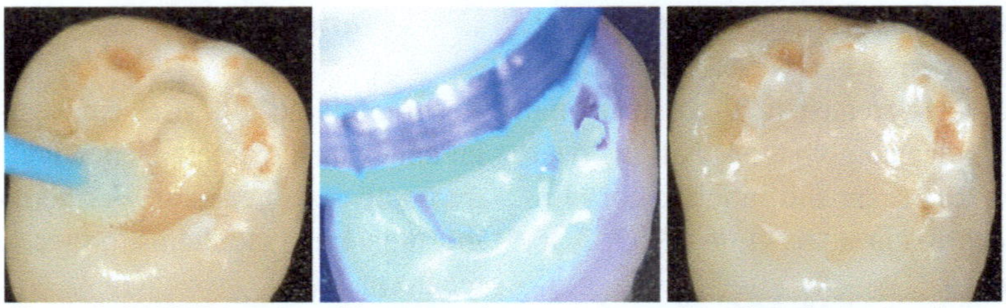
Using a RMGIC bond to apply medicaments
Reapply RMGIC bond over remaining preparation
Photo-cure for a further 10 s
Complete the restoration: either GIC or co-cure sandwich

Fig. 3.38 Using a resin-modified glass-ionomer adhesive as a vehicle to apply medicaments to a tooth. The application of resin-modified glass-ionomer cement adhesive and final placement of the restoration are shown here (Courtesy of Dr. Geoff Knight)

Conclusion

Glass-ionomer cements are finding an expanding role within dentistry as restorative agents, lining materials, luting cements and dental adhesives.

The biomimetic properties of all glass-ionomer cements enable far more conservative cavity preparations either in the management of small initial lesions or being incorporated in combination with composite resin in the management of much more extensive restorations.

The introduction of resin-modified glass-ionomer cement adhesives has resolved many of the inherent problems associated with polymerization shrinkage stress of composite resins and has further enabled the improvement of the bond of auto-cure glass-ionomer cement to tooth structure.

As the dental industry strives for a biomimetic, aesthetic and structurally robust replacement for dental amalgam, it would seem that the answer will certainly incorporate some glass-ionomer cement technology.

References

Brown LR, Handler SF, Horton IM, Streckfuss JL, Dreizen S. Effect of sodium fluoride on the viability and growth of Streptococcus mutans. J Dent Res. 1980;59(2):159–67.

Chow LC, Vogel GL. Enhancing remineralization. Oper Dent. 2001;Suppl 6:27–38.

Duque C, Negrini TC, Sacono NT, Spolidorio DM, de Souza Costa CA, Hebling J. Clinical and microbiological performance of resin-modified glass-ionomer liners after incomplete dentine caries removal. Clin Oral Investig. 2009;13(4):465–71.

Forsten L. Fluoride release and uptake by glass-ionomers and related materials and its clinical effect. Biomaterials. 1998;19(6):503–8.

Forsten L, Mount GJ, Knight GM. Observations in Australia of the use of glass ionomer cement restorative material. Aust Dent J. 1994;39(6):339–43.

Hamama HH, Burrow MF, Yiu C. Effect of dentine conditioning on adhesion of resin-modified glass ionomer adhesives. Aust Dent J. 2014;59(2):193–200.

Hicks J, Garcia-Godoy F, Donly K, Flaitz C. Fluoride-releasing restorative materials and secondary caries. J Calif Dent Assoc. 2003;31(3):229–45.

Hunt PR. A modified class II cavity preparation for glass ionomer restorative materials. Quintessence Int Dent Dig. 1984;15(10):1011–8.

Knight GM. The use of adhesive materials in the conservative restoration of selected posterior teeth. Aust Dent J. 1984;29(5):324–31.

Knight GM. The tunnel restoration – nine years of clinical experience using encapsulated glass ionomer cements. Case report. Aust Dent J. 1992;37(4):245–51.

Knight GM. The co-cured, light-activated glass-ionomer cement – composite resin restoration. Quintessence Int. 1994;25(2):97–100.

Knight GM, McIntyre JM, Mulyani. Bond strengths between composite resin and auto cure glass ionomer cement using the co-cure technique. Aust Dent J. 2006;51(2):175–9.

Knight GM, McIntyre JM, Craig GG, Mulyani. Electron probe microanalysis of ion exchange of selected elements between dentine and adhesive restorative materials. Aust Dent J. 2007a;52(2):128–32.

Knight GM, McIntyre JM, Craig GG, Mulyani, Zilm PS, Gully NJ. An in vitro investigation of marginal dentine caries abutting composite resin and glass ionomer cement restorations. Aust Dent J. 2007b;52(3):187–92.

Lazaridou D, Belli R, Krämer N, Petschelt A, Lohbauer U. Dental materials for primary dentition: are they suitable for occlusal restorations? A two-body wear study. Eur Arch Paediatr Dent. 2015;16(2):165–72.

Lenzi TL, Bonifácio CC, Bönecker M, Amerongen WE, Nogueira FN, Raggio DP. Flowable glass ionomer cement layer bonding to sound and carious primary dentin. J Dent Child (Chic). 2013;80(1):20–4.

Matos AB, Oliveira DC, Vieira SN, Netto NG, Powers JM. Influence of oil contamination on in vitro bond strength of bonding agents to dental substrates. Am J Dent. 2008;21(2):101–4.

McComb D, Erickson RL, Maxymiw WG, Wood RE. A clinical comparison of glass ionomer, resin-modified glass ionomer and resin composite restorations in the treatment of cervical caries in xerostomic head and neck radiation patients. Oper Dent. 2002;27(5):430–7.

McLean JW. Clinical applications of glass-ionomer cements. Oper Dent. 1992;Suppl 5:184–90.

Morand JM, Jonas P. Resin-modified glass-ionomer cement restoration of posterior teeth with proximal carious lesions. Quintessence Int. 1995;26(6): 389–94.

Naoum SJ, Mutzelburg PR, Shumack TG, Thode DJG, Martin FE, Ellakwa A. Reducing composite restoration polymerization shrinkage stress through resin modified glass ionomer based adhesives. Aust Dent J. 2014. doi:10.1111/adj.12265 [Epub ahead of print].

Ngo HC, Mount G, McIntyre J, Tuisuva J, Von Doussa RJ. Chemical exchange between glass-ionomer restorations and residual carious dentine in permanent molars: an in vivo study. J Dent. 2006;34(8):608–13.

Nicholson JW, Aggarwal A, Czarnecka B, Limanowska-Shaw H. The rate of change of pH of lactic acid exposed to glass-ionomer dental cements. Biomaterials. 2000;21(19):1989–93.

Tantbirojn D, Rusin RP, Mitra SB. Inhibition of dentin demineralization adjacent to a glass-ionomer/composite sandwich restoration. Quintessence Int. 2009;40(4):287–94.

Tyas MJ. Placement and replacement of restorations by selected practitioners. Aust Dent J. 2005;50(2):81–9; quiz 127.

Van Meerbeek B, De Munck J, Yoshida Y, Inoue S, Vargas M, Vijay P, Van Landuyt K, Lambrechts P, Vanherle G. Buonocore memorial lecture. Adhesion to enamel and dentin: current status and future challenges. Oper Dent. 2003;28(3):215–35.

Watson TF. Fact and artefact in confocal microscopy. Adv Dent Res. 1997;11(4):433–41.

Welbury RR, Murray JJ. A clinical trial of the glass-ionomer cement-composite resin "sandwich" technique in Class II cavities in permanent premolar and molar teeth. Quintessence Int. 1990;21(6):507–12.

Wilson AD, McLean JW. Glass-ionomer cement. London: Quintessence Publishing; 1988.

The Role of Glass-Ionomer Cements in Minimum Intervention (MI) Caries Management

4

Avijit Banerjee

Abstract

This chapter aims to discuss the evidence available to date from various laboratory and clinical studies about the use of glass-ionomer cements (GICs) in the management of deep caries. The contemporary minimally invasive approach to the operative management of cavitated deep lesions approaching the pulp relies on the selective removal of infected and/or affected dentine close to the pulp, followed by the use of a suitable adhesive restorative material to seal and bond to the underlying peripheral cavity margins/walls. In order to optimize the clinical outcome, an appreciation is required as to how this physico-chemical interaction occurs between GIC and sound as well as caries-affected substrates. The ionic transfer between GIC and tooth structure is described and discussed, with a particular emphasis on its anti-caries and remineralizing potential and also any effects, deleterious or otherwise, on the dental pulp when placed in close proximity to it. The clinical techniques available to restore teeth using high-viscosity GICs are outlined, including Atraumatic Restorative Treatment (ART) and the layered/laminate/sandwich restoration with resin composite. The findings of studies assessing the clinical longevity of such restorations in comparison to other direct plastic restorative materials are analyzed, both in the primary and secondary dentition. From the evidence presented, it is clear that GIC and its derivatives, whilst not perfect, have a major role to play in the minimally invasive restorative management of deep caries lesions.

4.1 Introduction: What is Minimum Intervention Dentistry?

Minimum intervention dentistry (MID) is a term that is used in contemporary dental practice. Its meaning, however, is often misconstrued and

A. Banerjee, BDS, MSc, PhD
Conservative & MI Dentistry,
King's College London Dental Institute
at Guy's Hospital, King's Health Partners,
Guy's Dental Hospital, London, UK
e-mail: avijit.banerjee@kcl.ac.uk

S.K. Sidhu (ed.), *Glass-Ionomers in Dentistry*, DOI 10.1007/978-3-319-22626-2_4

misunderstood, therefore misused and often maligned.

'MID' has two distinct but inter-related definitions:

4.1.1 Minimum Intervention Care (Fig. 4.1)

This describes the overall patient-centred oral and dental healthcare delivery framework where the oral healthcare team (dentist, dental therapist, hygienist, oral health educator, nurse, practice manager and technician) collectively advises patients and offers treatment that promotes health and prevents disease. Included in this framework are disease detection and diagnosis, its non-operative (non-invasive) prevention and control, operative management where necessary, all packaged together with suitably frequent recall consultations. At these vital recall appointments (often undersold to patients by the profession using the valueless term 'check-ups'), the patient's motivation, behaviour and adherence to the preventive lifestyle change advised are reassessed and reinforced. This is within the context of an outcome review of the treatment provided in the previous care episode(s) (restoration status, evidence of disease progression, changes in bacterial/ionic oral balance, etc). The periodicity of these consultations must be tailored to the individual patient's need and ongoing disease risk/susceptibility assessment.

4.1.2 Minimally Invasive (MI) Dentistry

Traditional operative caries management relies upon complete excavation of carious tissue followed by modification of the resulting cavity in terms of its surface finish and overall internal shape to aid restoration retention. The extent of this modification is dictated by the nature of the direct, plastic restorative material used to fill the cavity. Classically, for many years, non-adhesive dental amalgam has been the material of choice for most clinicians, so much so that predetermined cavity shapes are associated erroneously with GV Black's caries classification, classes 1–5, by many dental professionals.

With improved knowledge and understanding of the patho-physiology of the caries process and the subsequent defence reactions of the dentine-pulp complex, scientific and clinical evidence now shows clearly that not all carious tissue requires excavation during interventive operative surgical procedures (Banerjee and Watson 2015). The peripheral seal of restorations with healthy enamel and dentine close to the enamel-dentine junction

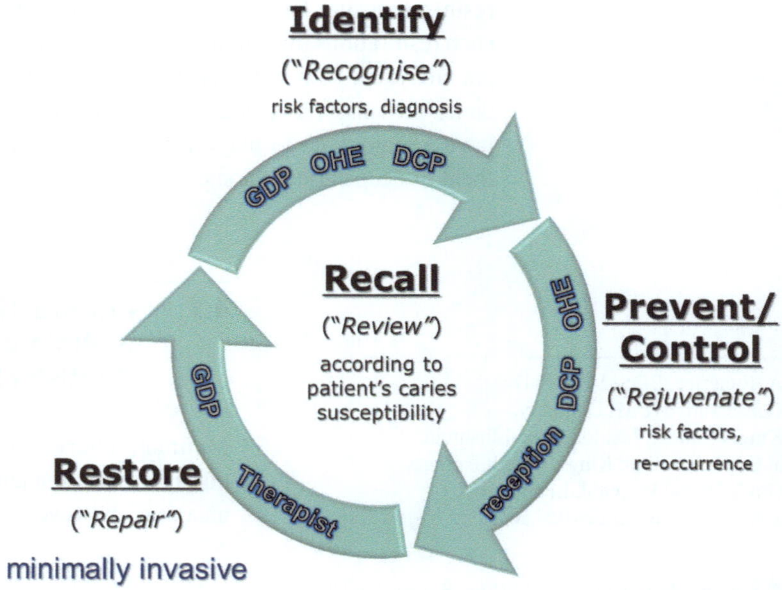

Fig. 4.1 The Minimum Intervention care plan framework for individualised, oral healthcare team-delivered, oral disease management (*GDP* general dental practitioner, *OHE* oral health educator, *DCP* dental care professional (therapist/hygienist))

(EDJ) is of paramount importance to ensure the tooth-restoration complex survives (Banerjee and Watson 2015). This is in conjunction with primary preventive methods instigated by the patient to disturb and/or remove the plaque biofilm, so preventing it from stagnating and becoming cariogenic in nature. Maximum tissue preservation along with maintaining pulp vitality (sensibility) is the tenet of minimally invasive dentistry, and the development of adhesive dentistry has promoted the MI philosophy into mainstream operative care.

Glass-ionomer cements (GICs) are an important part of the contemporary restorative armamentarium for MI operative dentistry. Since their introduction by Wilson and Kent (1971), glass-ionomer cements have had a wide range of clinical uses due to their naturally adhesive, tooth-coloured nature and fluoride-leaching properties, their low coefficient of thermal expansion and ultimate biocompatibility with mineralised tissues (Burke and Lynch 1994; Olivia et al. 2000). Clinically, they have proven to be useful in restorative, lining, luting and sealing applications.

4.2 GIC Adhesion to Tooth Structure

4.2.1 Enamel

Glass-ionomer cements (GICs) bind chemically to calcium ions in hydroxyapatite (HAP), the main constituent of dental enamel. Enamel surface pre-treatment with conditioners including polyacrylic acid (PAA) improves the bond strength between enamel and GIC, based on the exchange of calcium and phosphate ions versus carboxyl ions at the enamel surface. Es-Souni et al. (1999) indicated that the improved adhesion of the GIC on polished and conditioned surfaces resulted from the combined beneficial effects of superficial surface cleanliness, better wettability and surface chemistry. They concluded that PAA conditioning of the enamel prior to GIC bonding led to the formation of a fine polymeric film on the surface. This film may act as a primer and be involved directly in the cement-building reactions, so creating a 'stronger' interfacial layer on the GIC aspect of the bond.

4.2.2 Fluoride and Mineralized Tissues

Bezerra et al. (2012) examined the levels of the fluoride, calcium and phosphate in the enamel and dentine alongside glass-ionomer-based restorations in vivo over time using a high-viscosity GIC (Fuji IX GP, GC Corp, Tokyo, Japan) and a resin-modified GIC (Vitremer, 3M ESPE, St Paul, MN, USA). They described a substantial increase in the fluoride ion concentration adjacent to the glass-ionomer-based restorations attributable to large differences in the ionic gradients and subsequent diffusion patterns (Ngo et al. 2006). This finding raises an important question: does the increase in fluoride ion concentrations in enamel and dentine contribute substantially to an increase in the acid resistance of these two substrates? In-vitro studies had shown an increase in the resistance to demineralization of enamel (Hatibovic-Kofman et al. 1997; Attar and Önen 2002) and dentine (Jang et al. 2001), which was attributed to the release of fluoride ions from the GIC-based restorations. Qvist et al. (2004) reported a reduction in carious lesion progression in enamel surfaces adjacent to glass-ionomer restorations in primary teeth as compared with amalgam restorations over a period of 8 years. This evidence certainly seems to indicate that the fluoride release from glass-ionomer-based materials can play a role in disease arrest in enamel and dentine that is in contact with these materials. When high-viscosity and resin-modified glass-ionomer restorations are used to restore carious lesions in primary molars using the atraumatic restorative treatment (ART) technique, fluoride ions are released into the adjacent enamel and, in particular, into the demineralized, caries-affected dentine.

4.2.3 Sound Dentine

The development of a minimally invasive adhesive approach to conservative dentistry has brought many advantages, such as preservation of tooth tissue, reinforcement/infiltration of weakened remaining tooth structure, reduced marginal leakage and the reduced potential for pulp sensitivity and maintenance of pulp vitality. Adhesive restorative materials should have a close affinity mechanically, physically and chemically to tooth tissue in a way that minimizes the risk of further ingress of bacteria and arrests disease activity. They should also have the ability to bond to a variety of overlying protective restorative materials including resin composite, metals and ceramics. One of the most attractive features of GICs is their ability to bond directly to dentine. Polyacrylate ions either react with apatite by displacing calcium and phosphate ions or bond directly to the calcium within the apatite via hydrogen bonds with the collagen and ionic bonds to the apatite within the dentine (Van Noort 2013).

There have been many studies published reporting varying bond strengths between dentine and GIC. Yip et al. (2001) measured the micro-tensile bond strength (μTBS) of three highly viscous glass-ionomer cements to sound coronal dentine; they found bond strengths in the range of 12–15 MPa, with interfacial (adhesive) and mixed modes of failure. However, previous studies (Cattani-Lorente et al. 1993; Burke and Lynch 1994; Berry and Powers 1994) suggested that bond strengths >5 MPa were seldom achieved using tensile or shear tests *in vitro*, with more cohesive failures occurring within the GIC (Nakajima et al. 1995). It was clear that much of the difference could be explained by variations in the experimental testing technique used, the inconsistencies in sample preparation and the varying specimen sizes as well as their geometry and configuration.

Both scanning and transmission electron microscopy (SEM/TEM) analysis has shown the presence of an intermediate layer between 0.5 and 1.5 mm thick (Ngo et al. 1997a, b; Yip et al. 2001). Depending on the type of GIC, the TEM observations ranged from surface interaction zones consisting of nanometer-sized plate-like structures of calcium and phosphate salt precipitates dispersed among denatured smear layer remnants to plate-like structures being present within the inter-fibrillar spaces of intact, banded collagen fibrils. The inclusion of either smear layer remnants or banded collagen fibrils within the surface intermediate layer may be explained by the aggressiveness of different conditioning protocols used to remove the smear layer and demineralizing the underlying intact dentine. This is associated with the concentration of the polyacrylic acid employed as well as the application time that is recommended by each manufacturer. When the dentine was conditioned with 10 % polyacrylic acid for 10 s (a conventional, clinically recommended protocol), the presence of smear layer remnants within the surface intermediate layer indicated the smear layer was not completely removed. Chemical bonding of polyacrylic acid or polyacrylic acid/maleic acid to the residual hydroxyapatite from the smear layer may result in the retention of these polyelectrolytes on the dentine surface instead of being rinsed off (Yoshida et al. 2000). This could help produce the gel-like, glass-free layer that facilitates subsequent chemical exchange between the leached ions from the setting glass-ionomer matrix and the calcium and phosphate ions from the partially demineralized smear layer. Such a surface intermediate layer that incorporates smear layer remnants was often retained on the dentine surface in specimens that exhibited interfacial or mixed interfacial failures (Yoshida et al. 2000). When a more aggressive conditioning protocol of treating the smear layer-covered dentine with 25 % polyacrylic acid for 25 s was employed, the dentine tubule orifices were rendered patent, and this encouraged the formation of micromechanical dentine tubule tags. Moreover, the smear layer was removed completely and the underlying dentine demineralized to a depth of about 0.5 mm.

Hosoya and Garcia-Godoy (1998) reported an absence of cement tags or a hybrid layer when using a highly viscous GIC (Ketac-Molar, 3MESPE, St Paul, MN, USA). Rinsing off the conditioner probably resulted in a collagen-rich zone that contained retained polyelectrolytes. Subsequent ion exchange between the setting GIC and the partially demineralized collagen fibrils could have resulted in the formation of a surface intermediate layer where the inter-fibrillar spaces were not infiltrated completely by the polyelectrolytes. This could have accounted for the lower bond strength observed when 25 % polyacrylic acid was used as the conditioner in that study. It is further speculated that the clinical situation may be worsened when conditioned and rinsed dentine is then desiccated by the operator before the application of the GIC, as collapse of the collagen network during air-drying will further limit polyelectrolyte diffusion (Gwinnett 1994). It could be concluded that complete removal of the smear layer with more aggressive conditioning protocols that effectively 'etch' into sound dentine does not enhance the dentine-GIC bond strength. The observation of short cement tags that pulled out of the dentine tubules further suggests that they have a limited micro-mechanical contribution to the ultimate retention of GICs.

4.2.4 Caries-Affected Dentine

The MI operative approach to cavitated carious lesion management aims to minimize the excavation of carious dental tissues and instead encourages their preservation, recovery and repair. Dentine caries results from a bacteriogenic demineralizing acid attack from the cariogenic, stagnating biofilm at the tooth surface followed by further enzymatic destruction of the organic, primarily collagenous, matrix in dentine, if the process is unopposed and uninterrupted for a period of time. This ongoing process causes a histo-pathological wave of tissue destruction, divided descriptively into caries-infected and caries-affected dentine zones based on the bacterial load, extent and reparability of the tissue damage sustained (Banerjee and Watson 2015). In the necrotic, caries-infected dentine zone in the heart of the dentine lesion just subjacent to the enamel-dentine junction (EDJ), the mineral and collagenous organic matrices are irreversibly damaged and the bacterial load high. The deeper caries-affected dentine is hypomineralized but with a partially sound collagenous fibrillar structure, which could be repaired and remineralized by the ongoing reparative biological activity of the dentine-pulp complex. The relatively slow progression of the caries process often allows a reparative biochemical reaction which can help restore the mineralized architecture of this zone, especially after having removed the soft, wet, highly infected layer using a minimally invasive operative approach. The interaction between GIC and wet dentine is in the form of an ion exchange where aluminium, fluoride and calcium/strontium leach out of the cement as the glass is dissolved by the polyacid; at the same time, calcium and phosphate ions also move from the underlying dentine as a result of the initial self-etching effect of the acid-base chemical reaction of the setting cement (Watson 1999; Yiu et al. 2004). The release of fluoride and calcium/strontium ions provides GICs with the potential for remineralization of carious tissues (Ngo et al. 2006), where ion exchange could replenish the demineralized tissues' lost ions, thus tipping the balance in favour of mineral deposition/precipitation.

There is little evidence published about the immediate bond/sealing effectiveness or the long-term durability of the bonded interfaces produced by GIC to caries-affected dentine (Czarnecka et al. 2007; Alves et al. 2013). It is still unknown if the type of GIC has an effect on its clinical performance, as there is little published evidence to date regarding the bond strength of high-viscosity or resin-modified GICs (RMGICs) to caries-affected dentine. Some studies have evaluated bond strength degradation of GIC when bonded to sound dentine (De Munck et al. 2004; Fagundes et al. 2009). Bissoto Calvo et al. (2014) examined the in vitro bond strength of different GICs (a high-viscosity GIC and RM GICs with and without nano-particle fillers) to sound and caries-affected primary dentine immediately and after 2 years storage *in vitro*. No statistically significant differences in the immediate bond strength values between the tested materials to either sound or caries-affected dentine were reported. After 2 years, only the RMGIC without nano-particles showed stable bond strength values to both primary sound and caries-affected dentine. Previous to this, Marquezan et al. (2010) reported that a resin-modified GIC showed more resistance to degradation at the bonded interface with caries-affected primary dentine after pH- and load-cycling *in vitro*, compared to an adhesively bonded resin composite. Conventional GIC adheres primarily chemically to dentine, through the interaction of hydroxyapatite and polycarboxylate functional groups. On the other hand, in RMGICs both chemical and micro-mechanical adhesion are involved, which may contribute to the higher immediate and prolonged bond strength values measured.

Although the presence of nano-particles in the formulation of RMGIC potentially reinforces the material's strength, the interfacial area between the nano-particles and the organic matrix is hydrolytically unstable and may favour water sorption and degradation over time. Additionally, the chemical bond of the nano-particulate RMGIC to dentine may be weaker than that produced by a conventional GIC or a conventional RMGIC. This may be due to the reduction in the polycarboxylate content, as a result of nano-particle inclusion, reducing the available functional groups to interact with hydroxyapatite.

The type of the substrate (sound or caries-affected dentine) did not appear to affect the bond strength of GICs, regardless of type or storage time in several studies (Way et al. 1996; Czarnecka et al. 2007; Marquezan et al. 2010). This can be attributed to the hydrophilic properties of GICs. Also, the type of adhesion is chemical and not purely micro-mechanical. In contrast, Cehreli et al. (2013) observed differences between the bond strength values of GICs to sound and simulated caries-affected dentine after 18 months; unfortunately, the immediate bond strength was not recorded, making it impossible to conclude if any bond strength degradation had occurred. Moreover, the authors used caries-affected dentine created artificially using acetic acid as a demineralizing solution. This method results in complete demineralization (Marquezan et al. 2009), which is different to that of the pH-cycling process of de-and remineralization employed in many other studies. This final point is a critical one: 'artificial' data can be produced when using an artificial substrate, and thus clinical extrapolation of such results must be made with considerable caution. The ideal substrate to use is natural caries-affected tissue which needs to be exposed carefully from naturally carious teeth either *in situ* or *in vitro*.

4.3 GIC and Remineralization

Remineralization of demineralized carious dentine using various types of GICs has been demonstrated in several laboratory and clinical studies (Creanor et al. 1998; Ngo 2002a, b). Remineralization can be defined as the deposition of mineral in demineralized defects at a molecular level (Arends and ten Bosch 1986). It has been suggested that the mineral deposited should be apatitic in nature and should not be different from the mineral structure of natural, sound enamel and dentine. Ngo et al. (2006) studied the chemical interaction between a highly viscous GIC and demineralized dentine *in vivo* to determine the level of ion exchange between them. The material they used was Fuji IX GP (GC Corp, Tokyo, Japan), which includes a strontium-containing glass as opposed to the more conventional calcium-based glass in other GICs. They found that a substantial amount of both strontium and fluoride ions crossed the interface into the partially demineralized caries-affected dentine subjacent to the GIC. As the freshly mixed material is placed against the cavity wall, there is a release of ions from the enamel and dentine also leading to the exchange of ions, termed 'ion exchange adhesion'. It is suggested that the same ion exchange can occur in the presence of the partially demineralized carious dentine (Ngo et al. 2006). The ions released from both the GIC and the tooth structure will combine to buffer the low initial pH until such time that it rises to a level where ion activity ceases. During this period of activity there will be both fluoride and strontium ions available to promote mineral deposition in areas of demineralized dentine where the calcium ion levels are low, with strontium ions substituting them. It was suggested that this occurs through a diffusion process driven partly by the concentration gradient which exists between the GIC and the dentine with respect to these two elements. As both strontium and fluoride are apatite-forming elements, they react with the demineralized dentine. If the process is controlled purely by diffusion then one would expect to see the level of ionic strontium and fluoride to be highest at the GIC-dentine interface and lowest deeper towards the sound dentine. The above clinical findings support the laboratory evidence that glass-ionomer can contribute directly to the remineralization of carious dentine. However, there are two important requirements for this to happen: firstly, the restoration has to provide a total seal against the external environment, and secondly, there must be intimate contact between the glass-ionomer and the partly demineralized dentine.

4.4 Clinical Studies of GIC Use in the MI Management of Deep Caries

The treatment of deep carious lesions approaching a vital pulp presents a significant challenge to the practitioner. The traditional management of carious lesions dictates the removal of all infected and affected dentine to prevent further caries progress and to provide a sound base of dentine to support the overlying definitive restoration. In order to prevent, or at least minimize, the serious complications of complete excavation of carious dentine close to the pulp (the dreaded pulp exposure), the minimally invasive, tooth-preserving operative 'stepwise' excavation approach was developed. This involves initially excavating the more superficial soft, wet, necrotic infected dentine, followed by sealing the lesion with calcium hydroxide and a GIC provisional restoration. Some months later the clinician would revisit the lesion and finally remove all or most of the underlying arrested, dry and often darkly stained dentine. The rationale for this is that by this point, any residual bacteria will not have survived, the residual affected dentine will have remineralized and tertiary, reparative dentine will have been deposited. This will make it easier for the dentist to remove any remaining carious tissue without the risk of exposing the vital pulp (Thompson et al. 2008; Banerjee and Watson 2015). As it became increasingly clear that it is the effective peripheral seal of the restoration that is important in preventing the caries process from continuing within an existing cavitated lesion, a fully minimally invasive or ultraconservative approach was developed; this is also referred to as 'partial/selective caries removal'. In this method, all of the infected dentine is removed, the peripheral enamel and dentine are prepared to optimize adhesion and the cavity is sealed (with or without indirect pulp protection) with the definitive adhesive restoration. The 'trade-off' for avoiding pulp exposure, which more often clinically leads to pulp death (Bjørndal et al. 2010), is retaining a layer of potentially radiolucent, affected dentine beneath the definitive restoration (see Fig. 4.2e). This can be defended by citing the substantial evidence that exists in the literature showing that cariogenic bacteria isolated from their source of nutrition by a restoration of sufficient integrity either die or remain quiescent and thus, given a vital pulp, pose no risk to the health of the dentition (Ricketts et al. 2013). Foley et al. (2004) compared the cariostatic effectiveness of alternative restorative materials in both selective and complete removal of carious tissue. They used a split-mouth design in 44 patients (aged 3.7–9.5 years) who had at least one pair of previously unrestored primary molars that had no pulp involvement. One tooth of each pair underwent complete caries removal, and the other had incomplete, selective caries removal followed by restoration using copper phosphate cement, GIC or a material 'of the operator''s choice' (such as amalgam). At 24 months post treatment, teeth that had undergone selective caries removal followed by restoration with copper phosphate cement exhibited greater abscess or sinus formation than did teeth that had undergone other treatments. Teeth treated with GIC alone after selective caries removal exhibited a durability and effectiveness comparable with those placed in teeth that had undergone complete caries removal.

Marchi et al. (2006) studied the effectiveness of two materials as indirect protective pulp liners, a setting calcium hydroxide and a RMGIC, in the treatment of 27 primary molars with deep caries. Four years post treatment, the success rate using the former was 88.8 % and using the GIC was

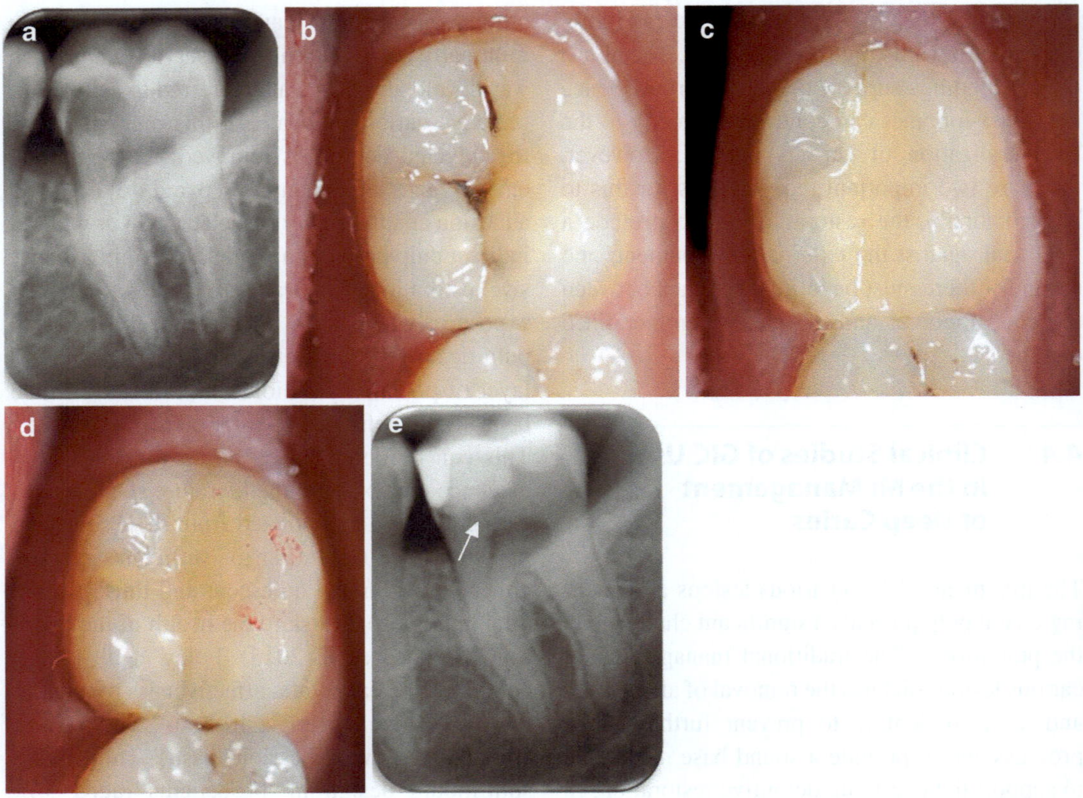

Fig. 4.2 (**a**) Pre-operative periapical radiograph of LL6 and LL7 showing early caries on the distal aspect of LL6 and a large mesio-occlusal carious radiolucency associated with LL7. The LL7 exhibited symptoms of acute pulpitis and positive pulp sensibility tests and showed no loss of lamina dura/widening of the periodontal ligament space around the root apices in the pre-operative radiograph. (**b**) An occlusal clinical image of LL7 showing the underlying shadowing of the lesion mesially and cavitation in the midline fissure. (**c**) After minimally invasive selective caries removal, a GIC was placed as a provisional restoration. (**d**) At the 1-month review, the GIC was cut back and a resin composite restoration veneered onto its surface as a closed sandwich technique. (N.B: The *red marks* show the occlusal articulation at the 1-year review stage). (**e**) The 1-year post-op periapical radiograph: the differences in radiopacities of the GIC and overlying resin composite can be observed. The tooth-restoration complex was sound and the pulp remained vital. The slight radiolucency (*arrowed*) at the dentine border adjacent to the GIC is the retained caries-affected dentine, and is inactive (Hashem et al. 2015)

93 %. The investigators defined 'success' essentially as the absence of any 'clinical or radiographic signs or symptoms of irreversible pulp pathologies or necrosis'. The authors concluded that 'indirect pulp capping in primary teeth arrests the progression of the underlying caries, regardless of the material used as a liner'. In order to provide evidence that the caries process was arrested in the sealed lesions, they sampled teeth for bacterial culture at periods ranging from 1 week to 2 years; at the latter stage, they found a substantial decrease in the number of cultivable micro-organisms in sealed lesions when compared with the unsealed control teeth. Interestingly, they found the greatest amount of bacterial reduction within 2 weeks after treatment. In another microbiological study of dentine samples taken from 40 carious lesions before and after undergoing atraumatic restorative treatment (ART), Bonecker et al. (2003) found significant reductions in the frequency and proportions of the total viable mutans streptococci (but not lactobacilli) in restorations sealed with GIC.

A more recent randomized clinical trial has compared the use of GIC and a calcium silicate cement to restore deep carious cavities in patients

(Hashem et al. 2015). The affected teeth were symptomatic with acute pulpitis. Baseline periapical radiographs, CBCT (cone beam CT) and a full clinical examination were carried out before minimally invasive selective caries removal was performed using burs and hand instruments, assisted with Carisolv™ gel. No pulp exposures occurring at this stage of treatment were included in the study. These deep cavities were restored either with a high-viscosity GIC, Fuji IX (GC Corp, Tokyo, Japan), or a setting calcium silicate cement, Biodentine™ (Septodont, Saint-Maur-des-Fossés, France). They were reviewed after 1 month, and assuming the clinical signs and symptoms indicated healing, these provisional restorations were veneered with a resin composite (a layered definitive restoration – see Fig. 4.2). At the 1 year review, it was clear that both materials had a similar 83 % success rate in maintaining tooth structure as well as pulp vitality and the layered restorations were faring well. Thus, on the basis of the evidence cited, it can be reasonably concluded that the removal of all infected dentine in deep carious lesions is not required for successful caries treatment, provided that the restoration can seal the lesion from the oral environment effectively.

4.5 GIC and Atraumatic Restorative Treatment (ART)

A number of countries have already banned or are considering banning the use of dental amalgam, partly in response to the Minamata Treaty agreed by the United Nations Environment Programme (UNEP 2013). Since then, both the International Dental Federation (FDI) and the World Health Organization (WHO) have called for alternatives to amalgam to be developed for use to operatively manage carious lesions. One alternative is to use currently available glass-ionomer cements. Its high-viscosity variant has become the material of choice for atraumatic restorative treatment (ART). This minimally invasive caries management approach, involving the use of hand instruments only and the placement of a high-viscosity glass-ionomer cement (HVGIC), is considered an alternative to the more traditional maximally invasive restorative treatments (Raggio et al. 2013; Holmgren et al. 2013). In terms of restoration survival, a systematic review concluded that ART/HVGIC and amalgam restorations of the same size, type of dentition and follow-up period are equally successful clinically. However, because of the limited number of suitable data sets for the analysis, the authors of the review suggested that further studies should be carried out to confirm these findings (Mickenautsch et al. 2010).

A weak inherent feature of conventional GIC is its low fracture toughness. By increasing the powder-to-liquid ratio, the fracture toughness can be increased (Peez and Frank 2006), and it was suggested that by using this improved GIC with ART, the survival of ART restorations may be increased, especially in multiple-surface restorations. Hilgert et al. (2014) assessed and compared the cumulative survival rate of amalgam and ART using HVGIC restorations in primary molars over 3 years for single- and multiple-surface restorations. The survival rates over 3 years for all, single- and multiple-surface, amalgam restorations were not significantly different from those of comparable ART/HVGIC restorations. Single-surface restorations had higher survival rates than multiple-surface restorations for both procedures. A higher proportion of restorations failed due to mechanical reasons (94.8 %) than due to caries associated with restorations/sealants (CARS), i.e. secondary caries (5.2 %). The HVGIC used in conjunction with ART is a viable option for restoring carious dentine lesions in single surfaces in vital primary molars. However, the performance of proximal ART restorations using HVGIC is still far from ideal (Ersin et al. 2006; De Amorim et al. 2012). This may be attributed to the highly viscous consistency of the GIC which increases the difficulties with its handling and placement (Frencken and Holmgren 1999). These characteristics can lead to poor adaptation of the material to the cavity base resulting in gaps and leakage, lack of retention and ultimate loss of the restoration (Roeleveld et al. 2006; Bonifácio et al. 2009). More recent laboratory studies showed the insertion of a thin flowable GIC layer at the base of deep proximal cavities prior to the insertion of the regular HVGIC layer (two-layer technique) can improve the material's adaptation to the cavity, so increasing the bond strength to sound tissues (Bonifácio et al. 2010; Lenzi et al. 2013). The success of ART restorations can be influenced by many factors, the most often reported being the operator-induced effect (Frencken et al. 2004; Kemoli et al. 2009). This includes the proper use of hand instruments, cavity pre-conditioning, correct mixing/manipulation of the HVGIC and, in cases of multi-surface restorations, factors such as correct matrix band application, moisture control and sufficient material obturation/adaptation (Kemoli et al. 2009). These differences in individual operative skills are always to be expected (Van Gemert-Schriks et al. 2007; Frencken and Leal 2010).

Bonifácio et al. (2013) investigated the use of a two-layer flowable technique for the insertion of GIC in proximal cavities and assessed the influence of the operator in the survival rate of proximal ART restorations in primary molars. Despite the small sample size, short evaluation period (12 months) and the lack of a control group for comparison, the results showed an acceptable survival rate and no detrimental operator effect over the time period investigated. The retention rate was similar to those previously reported in the literature (Carvalho et al. 2010; da Franca et al. 2011). A 1-year survival rate of 74 % is in agreement with that presented in the literature. In general, the 12-month survival rate of proximal ART restorations in primary posterior teeth ranges between 12 and 88 %, for studies conducted in schools (Ersin et al. 2006; van Gemert-Schriks et al. 2007; Deepa and Shobha 2010). High-viscosity GICs are difficult to handle and can lead to inadequate adaptation to the cavity walls and cervical gaps (Lenzi et al. 2013), both of which contribute to restoration failure (Roeleveld et al. 2006; Mhaville et al. 2006). Bonifácio et al. (2013) concluded that using a flowable layer of the GIC prior to the insertion of a conventional layer leads to an improvement in GIC adaptation and a reduction in the occurrence of the secondary caries (CARS, see earlier). The main reason for failure was bulk fracture or total loss of the restoration, which is in accordance with the published literature (Eden et al. 2006; Van Gemert-Schriks et al. 2007; Topaloglu-Ak et al. 2009; da Franca et al. 2011).

Bulk fractures are related generally to the mechanical properties of the GIC; the use of a flowable layer as a liner may contribute towards reducing the mechanical strength as the final material created has fewer glass particles/unit volume. However, Fonseca et al. (2010) reported that there is no difference in the diametral tensile strength of conventional GIC when the powder/liquid ratio was reduced by 50 %. A disadvantage of the two-layer technique may be that the second layer does not adhere properly to the first, so contributing to bulk fractures. To confirm the potential improvements delivered by the two-layer technique of applying GIC in ART proximal cavities, further studies in the form of controlled clinical trials as well as investigations of the mechanical and adhesive properties of this two-layered GIC should be conducted.

4.6 The Longevity of GIC Restorations

The ultimate success or failure of a restorative material is measured by its longevity in the oral environment whilst maintaining tooth tissue integrity and pulp vitality. As initial laboratory tests of new materials do not always reveal their full limitations or assets, clinical data is essential to provide empirical evidence. Unfortunately, at the present time, there is no consensus on the desired or ideal length of time of a clinical study to accurately predict the performance or clinical life expectancy of restorative dental materials. Differences between study variables, including the sample size, material and restoration type, method of assessment, operator and patient factors, often make data comparisons difficult. Nevertheless, information gleaned from longitudinal assessments is important in the hope that cumulatively, this information adds to the body of evidence to help make informed clinical decisions regarding treatment options. As a 'major undertaking for general dental practitioners is the provision and assessment of dental restorations', observations in clinical practice offer valuable evidence if interpreted appropriately (Sidhu 2010).

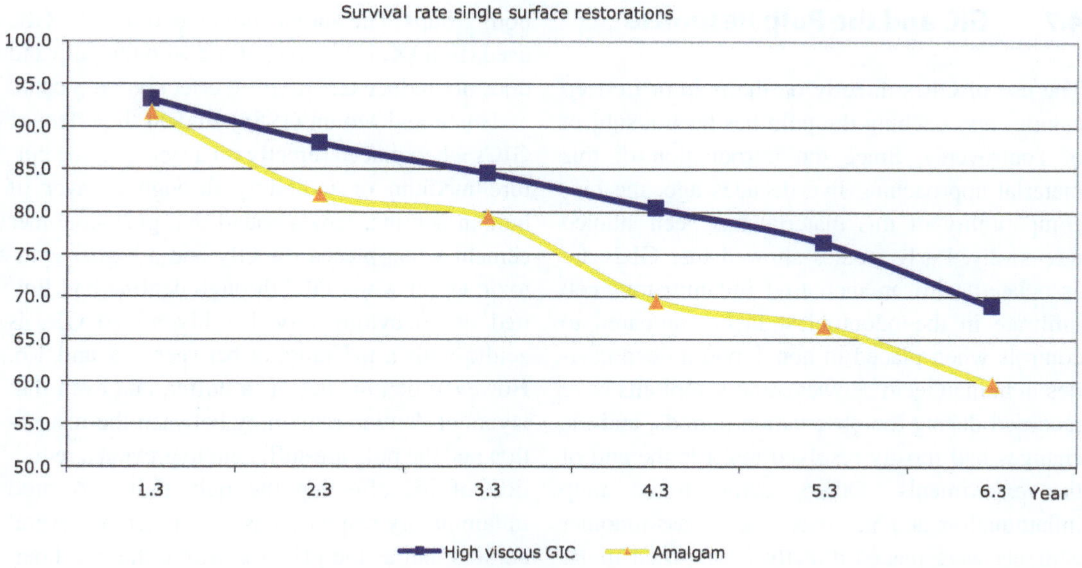

Fig. 4.3 In the permanent dentition, longevity of ART restorations is ≥equivalent amalgam restorations up to 6.3 years, site-dependent. No difference is observed in primary teeth (Frencken et al 2006)

Clinical trials investigating the longevity of GICs in primary molars are mostly short-term studies of less than 3 years. The longest measured survival rates for GICs are in low stress-bearing areas including Class III and Class V restorations (Mount 1993). Vlietstra et al. (1978) reported that 75 % of the conventional glass-ionomer restorations in primary molars were intact after 1 year, and the marginal adaptation, contour and surface finish were all satisfactory. Others (Cho and Cheng 1999) reported that GICs in primary molars showed no significant differences with amalgam restorations in overall failure rates after 2 years. However, a previous 5-year follow-up of restorations showed that GICs had a significantly inferior survival time to amalgam (Welbury et al. 1991). Ostlund et al. (1992) compared Class II restorations of amalgam, resin composite and glass-ionomer cement in primary molars and reported a high failure rate for the glass-ionomer cement of 60 % after 2 years. In contrast, the failure rates for amalgam and resin composite restorations were 8 and 16 % respectively. It is worthwhile noting that these studies were carried out over two decades ago, and much has changed in the chemistry and application of GIC materials since then.

More recently, Fuks et al. (2000) compared the clinical performance of a GIC with amalgam in Class II restorations in primary molars. Only 9 of 101 glass-ionomer restorations met all the quality criteria after 1 year, whereas 90 % of the amalgam restorations met all the evaluation criteria after 3 years. Hickel et al. (2005) investigated the mean survival time of different types of restorations in primary molars and found that the mean survival time for glass-ionomer restorations was only 12 months compared to more than 5 years for stainless-steel crowns and amalgam restorations. The results of these and other studies indicate that conventional GIC is not an appropriate alternative to amalgam in the restoration of primary molars unless the teeth are expected to exfoliate in 1 or 2 years. Indeed, RMGICs may prove to have the highest success rates in terms of longevity in the primary dentition (Toh and Messer 2007).

With regard to the adult dentition, conclusive clinical evidence remains elusive to date. A systematic review of the literature up to 2010 indicated that the longevity of HVGIC restorations is site dependent but in buccal cervical restorations can last successfully over 6 years in clinical service (Frencken et al. 2006; Mickenautsch et al. 2010; see Fig. 4.3).

4.7 GIC and the Pulp Response

The use of GICs directly on the pulp or in deep cavities approaching the pulp has been a subject of controversy. Since the introduction of this material approaching five decades ago, the biocompatibility of this material has been studied intensively. Early studies showed that GICs are associated with an increased inflammatory cell infiltrate in the odontoblast layer compared to controls when placed in non-exposed deep cavities in human teeth. However, no symptoms were recorded during the observation periods, and the changes had mostly resolved towards the end of the experiments. Others demonstrated pulp inflammation and necrosis when glass-ionomer cements were placed directly on exposed molar rat teeth. This finding was corroborated by another in-vitro study assessing the cytotoxicity of eight different GICs by means of pulp cell culture. The authors found that some GICs are more cytotoxic than others and concluded that they should not be placed directly on or near pulps (Müller et al. 1990). However, great caution should be employed when extrapolating results from in-vitro studies to the clinical situation, as the natural protective effect of dentine is ignored and the individual defence and repair mechanisms, which increase tolerance to such materials, are not present.

Indeed, contrary to the above, animal studies have reported no adverse pulp reactions to GIC when placed in non-exposed deep cavities and observed over different time periods (Felton et al. 1991). These results are corroborated by more recent studies using improved GICs, which have shown minimal cytotoxic effects on the pulp. In a study by Six et al. (2000), a HVGIC (Fuji IX, GC Corp, Tokyo, Japan) was placed in deep non-exposed cavities of rat teeth and compared to unfilled cavities as a control. Observation after 8 days revealed few inflammatory cells in both groups, disruption of the odontoblast layer and dilatation of the blood vessels. The inflammatory reaction in the glass-ionomer group was slightly higher than in the control group. After 30 days, complete recovery of the pulp tissue was observed with no disruption of the odontoblast layer. A thick layer of reparative dentine had formed in both groups. The authors concluded that the GIC used (Fuji IX) is biocompatible with the pulp and does not induce any harmful effect on pulp cells.

Hume and Mount (1988) studied the effect of GICs when placed directly on a sterile tissue culture medium or indirectly through a layer of human dentine. It was found that glass-ionomer cement when placed directly had a higher cytotoxic effect while GIC through dentine had limited or no cytotoxicity. Freshly mixed GIC is acidic with a pH ranging between 0.9 and 1.6. However, dentine acts as a buffer, and even thin layers of dentine remaining between the restoration and the pulp are sufficient to prevent a reduction of pH affecting the pulp tissue. A mild inflammatory response has been noted by several authors, but as the pH rises within the first hour, the inflammatory cellular response is transient, resolving within 10–20 days. To a certain extent, the pulp irritation may be accounted for by the high buffering capacity of the hydroxyapatite itself. Also, the low mobility and chelating capacity of the large polyalkenoic acid molecules may be significant in this regard.

It can be concluded from these studies that GICs are not suitable when placed directly on the pulp. However, using them as indirect pulp protection/capping agents or as a dentine replacement material in deep cavities is widely accepted (Sidhu 2011).

4.8 Adhesion Between GIC and Resin Composite

Glass-ionomer cements have many different clinical applications including indirect pulp protection/capping. They consist of a calcium fluoro-alumino-silicate glass powder and an aqueous solution of a poly (acrylic acid—itaconic acid) copolymer containing tartaric acid (Smith 1998). The setting reaction involves the acid-base reaction of the polyacrylic acid and the glass particles and ions (Al^{3+}, Ca^{2+}) located in the glass network (Mount and Hume 1998). Modifications in both components have been made in various commercial brands for both patent and practical reasons (Smith 1998). GICs have been reported to demonstrate excellent sealing properties and good biocompatibility when placed in close proximity with, but not directly on, the pulp (Hilton 2009). In addition, they have the ability to adhere chemically to moist dentine through ionic exchange at the interface leading to the formation of a new intermediate dentine-GIC layer approximately 300 μm thick (Zoergiebel and Ilie 2013). This ionic exchange is triggered at the interface through a diffusion process. This process is partly driven by the concentration gradient which exists between the glass-ionomer and the dentine, with strontium, calcium and fluoride ions undertaking apatitic activity in relation to areas in dentine where the calcium ion levels are low (Ngo et al. 2006).

Drawbacks of GIC include its physical properties as it is susceptible to acid erosion and wear, therefore its successful use lies mainly in the field of dentine replacement in laminate/layered/'sandwich' restorations (Davidson 2006). GICs have been used in both open and closed sandwich restorations with a higher success rate reported for closed sandwich restorations (van Dijken 1994). This is because in open sandwich restorations, GIC is associated with an increased risk of dissolution due to its susceptibility to early moisture contamination. In addition, the proximal area is exposed to longer acid clearance times, which increases the erosion rate at the surface. If a GIC lining cement is used, the cement will be stressed continuously by masticatory forces transferred via the overlying restoration, resulting potentially in crack formation at the cement-restorative interface followed by fracture of the cement. This is due to the lack of strength of the thin cement layer (van Dijken 1994). This problem can be overcome by using a restorative version of the cement which is cut back rather than using a liner variety, resulting in a more robust restoration with better mechanical properties (Cattani-Lorente et al. 1993). This also has an advantage if an overlying resin composite restoration is used as the increased thickness of the GIC reduces the thickness of the resin composite leading to a reduction in the polymerization shrinkage (Woolford 1993).

An interaction between GIC and the overlying resin composite restoration was suggested where GIC reduced the hardness of the surface of resin composite adjacent to it up to a distance of 1 mm into the thickness of the resin composite. This detrimental interaction was observed when resin composite was placed on fresh GIC; therefore, it is recommended to leave the cement to mature as much as possible before the application of the resin composite – a two-visit clinical procedure (Woolford 1993).

Conclusions

This chapter has aimed to discuss the potential attributes of glass-ionomer cements and their use in the contemporary minimally invasive operative management of deep caries lesions. Indeed, low-viscosity GICs have been advocated for use as fissure sealant restorations in clinical cases of primary and tertiary minimally (non)invasive caries prevention. Even though resin composite sealants exhibit better durability and retention clinically, in scenarios with compromised moisture control, GIC sealants still have a part to play, especially in the primary dentition.

Glass-ionomer cements are not necessarily the strongest or toughest direct plastic restorative material available clinically to withstand the occlusal forces and the changing environment generated in the oral cavity. However, their ability to chemically bond to and seal enamel and dentine substrate without the need for a separate chemical adhesive, to leach ions that can aid mineralization, including fluoride, all help to encourage resistance and repair of caries-affected tissues and also the dentine-pulp complex. Clinically, modern GIC derivatives exhibit improved handling characteristics, aesthetics and strength/durability. With the potential global reduction in use of dental amalgam to restore teeth with carious cavities, GICs form an invaluable member of the remaining restorative armamentarium to the clinician treating dental caries in their patients.

References

Alves FBT, Hesse D, Lenzi TL, et al. The bonding of glass ionomer cements to caries-affected primary dentin. Pediatr Dent. 2013;35(4):320–4.

Arends J, ten Bosch JJ. In vivo de- and remineralization of dental enamel. In: Leach SA, editor. Factors relating to demineralization and remineralization of the teeth. Oxford: IRL Press; 1986. p. 1–11.
Attar N, Önen A. Artificial formed caries-like lesions around esthetic restorative materials. J Clin Pediatr Dent. 2002;26:289–96.
Banerjee A, Watson TF. Pickard's guide to minimally invasive operative dentistry. 10th ed. London: Oxford University Press; 2015.
Berry EA, Powers JM. Bond strength of glass ionomers to coronal and radicular dentin. Oper Dent. 1994;19:122–6.
Bezerra AC, Novaes RC, Faber J, et al. Ion concentration adjacent to glass-ionomer restorations in primary molars. Dent Mater. 2012;28:e259–63.
Bissoto Calvo AF, Alves FBT, Lenzi TL, et al. Glass ionomer cements bond stability in caries-affected primary dentin. Int J Adhes Adhes. 2014;48:183–7.
Bjørndal L, Reit C, Bruun G, et al. Treatment of deep caries lesions in adults: randomised clinical trials comparing stepwise vs. direct complete excavation, and direct pulp capping vs. partial pulpotomy. Eur J Oral Sci. 2010;118(3):290–7.
Bonecker M, Toi C, Cleaton-Jones P. Mutans streptococci and lactobacilli in carious dentine before and after atraumatic restorative treatment. J Dent. 2003;31(6):423–8.
Bonifácio CC, Kleverlaan CJ, Raggio DP, et al. Physical-mechanical properties of glass ionomer cements indicated for atraumatic restorative treatment. Aust Dent J. 2009;54:233–7.
Bonifácio CC, van Amerongen WE, Meschini TG, et al. Flowable glass ionomer cement as a liner: improving marginal adaptation of atraumatic restorative treatment restorations. J Dent Child. 2010;77:12–6.
Bonifácio CC, Hesse D, Bönecker M, et al. A preliminary clinical trial using flowable glass-ionomer cement as a liner in proximal-ART restorations: the operator effect. Med Oral Patol Oral Cir Bucal. 2013;18(3):e529–32.
Burke F, Lynch E. Glass polyalkenoate bond strength to dentine after chemo-mechanical caries removal. J Dent. 1994;22:283–91.
Carvalho TS, Sampaio FC, Diniz A, et al. Two years survival rate of Class II ART restorations in primary molars using two ways to avoid saliva contamination. Int J Paediatr Dent. 2010;20:419–25.
Cattani-Lorente MA, Godin C, Meyer JM. Early strength of glass ionomer cements. Dent Mater. 1993;9:57–62.
Cehreli ZC, Akca T, Altay N. Comparison of bonding ability of single-step self- etching adhesives with different etching aggressiveness to root dentin. Am J Dent. 2013;16:47A–50.
Cho S, Cheng AC. A review of glass ionomer restorations in the primary dentition. J Can Dent Assoc. 1999;65:491–5.
Creanor SL, Awawdeh LA, Saunders WP, et al. The effect of a resin-modified glass ionomer restorative material on artificially demineralized dentine caries in vitro. J Dent. 1998;26(5–6):527–31.
Czarnecka B, Deregowska-Nosowicz P, Limanowska-Shaw H, et al. Shear bond strengths of glass-ionomer cements to sound and to prepared carious dentine. J Mater Sci. 2007;18(5):845–9.
Da Franca C, Colares V, Van Amerongen E. Two-year evaluation of the atraumatic restorative treatment approach in primary molars class I and II restorations. Int J Paediatr Dent. 2011;21:249–53.
Davidson CL. Advances in glass-ionomer cements. J Applied Oral Sci. 2006;14:3–9.
De Amorim RG, Leal SC, Frencken JE. Survival of atraumatic restorative treatment (ART) sealants and restorations: a meta-analysis. Clin Oral Investig. 2012;16:429–41.
De Munck J, Inoue S, Suzuki K, et al. Four-year water degradation of a resin-modified glass-ionomer adhesive bonded to dentin. Eur J Oral Sci. 2004;112(1):73–83.
Deepa G, Shobha T. A clinical evaluation of two glass ionomer cements in primary molars using a traumatic restorative treatment technique in India: 1 year follow up. Int J Paediatr Dent. 2010;20:410–8.
Eden E, Topaloglu-Ak A, Frencken JE, et al. Survival of self-etch adhesive Class II composite restorations using ART and conventional cavity preparations in primary molars. Am J Dent. 2006;19:359–63.
Ersin NK, Candan U, Aykut A, et al. A clinical evaluation of resin-based composite and glass ionomer cement restorations placed in primary teeth using the ART approach: results at 24 months. J Am Dent Assoc. 2006;137:1529–36.
Es-Souni M, Zimehl R, Fischer-Brandies H. Microscopic and electron spectroscopic characterization of dental enamel surfaces. Colloid Polym Sci. 1999;277:382–7.
Fagundes TC, Toledano M, Navarro MF, et al. Resistance to degradation of resin-modified glass-ionomer cements dentine bonds. J Dent. 2009;37(5):342–7.
Felton DA, Cox CF, Odom M, et al. Pulpal response to chemically cured and experimental light-cured glass ionomer cavity liners. J Prosthet Dent. 1991;65:704–12.
Foley J, Evans D, Blackwell A. Partial caries removal and cariostatic materials in carious primary molar teeth: a randomised controlled clinical trial. Br Dent J. 2004;197(11):697–701.
Fonseca RB, Branco CA, Quagliatto PS, et al. Influence of powder/liquid ratio on the radiodensity and diametral tensile strength of glass ionomer cements. J Appl Oral Sci. 2010;18:577–84.
Frencken JE, Holmgren CJ. How effective is ART in the management of dental caries? Community Dent Oral Epidemiol. 1999;27:423–30.
Frencken JE, Leal SC. The correct use of the ART approach. J Appl Oral Sci. 2010;18:1–4.
Frencken JE, Van't Hof MA, Van Amerongen WE, et al. Effectiveness of single-surface ART restorations in the permanent dentition: a meta-analysis. J Dent Res. 2004;83:120–3.

Frencken JE, Taifour D, Van't Hof MA. Survival of ART and amalgam restorations in permanent teeth of children after 6.3 years. J Dent Res. 2006;85:622–6.

Fuks AB, Araujo FB, Osorio LB, et al. Clinical and radiographic assessment of Class II aesthetic restorations in primary molars. Pediatr Dent. 2000;22(6):479–85.

Gwinnett AJ. Chemically conditioned dentin: a comparison of conventional and environmental scanning electron microscopy findings. Dent Mater. 1994;10:150–5.

Hashem D, Mannocci F, Patel S, et al. Efficacy of calcium silicate indirect pulp capping; a randomized controlled clinical trial. J Dent Res. 2015;94(4):562–8.

Hatibovic-Kofman S, Suljak JP, Koch G. Remineralization of natural carious lesions with a glass ionomer cement. Swed Dent J. 1997;21:11–7.

Hickel R, Kaaden CH, Paschos E, et al. Longevity of occlusally-stressed restorations in posterior primary teeth. Am J Dent. 2005;18(3):198–211.

Hilgert LA, de Amorim RG, Leal SC, et al. Is high-viscosity glass-ionomer-cement a successor to amalgam for treating primary molars? Dent Mater. 2014;30:1172–8.

Hilton TJ. Keys to clinical success with pulp capping: a review of the literature. Oper Dent. 2009;34:615–25.

Holmgren CJ, Roux D, Doméjean S. Minimal intervention dentistry: part 5. Atraumatic restorative treatment (ART) – a minimum intervention and minimally invasive approach for the management of dental caries. Br Dent J. 2013;214:11–8.

Hosoya Y, Garcia-Godoy F. Bonding mechanism of Ketac-Molar Applicap and Fuji IX GP to enamel and dentin. Am J Dent. 1998;11:235–9.

Hume WR, Mount GJ. In vitro studies on the potential for pulpal cytotoxicity of glass-ionomer cements. J Dent Res. 1988;67:915–8.

Jang KT, Garcia-Godoy F, Donly KJ, et al. Remineralizing effects of the glass ionomer restorations on adjacent interproximal caries. ASDC J Dent Child. 2001;68:125–8.

Kemoli AM, van Amerongen WE, Opinya G. Influence of the experience of operator and assistant on the survival rate of proximal ART restorations: two-year results. Eur Arch Paediatr Dent. 2009;10:227–32.

Lenzi TL, Bonifácio CC, Bönecker M, et al. Flowable glass ionomer cement layer bonding to sound and caries affected primary dentin. J Dent Child (Chic). 2013;80:20–4.

Marchi JJ, de Araujo FB, Froner AM, et al. Indirect pulp capping in the primary dentition: a 4 year follow-up study. J Clin Pediatr Dent. 2006;31(2):68–71.

Marquezan M, Corrêa FN, Sanabe ME, et al. Artificial methods of dentine caries induction: a hardness and morphological comparative study. Arch Oral Biol. 2009;54(12):1111–7.

Marquezan M, Osório Ciamponi AL, Toledano M. Resistance to degradation of bonded restorations to simulated caries-affected primary dentin. Am J Dent. 2010;23(1):47–52.

Mhaville RJ, van Amerongen WE, Mandari GJ. Residual caries and marginal integrity in relation to Class II glass ionomer restorations in primary molars. Eur Arch Paediatr Dent. 2006;7:81–4.

Mickenautsch S, Yengopal V, Banerjee A. Atraumatic restorative treatment versus amalgam restoration longevity: a systematic review. Clin Oral Invest. 2010;14:233–40.

Mount GJ. Clinical placement of modern glass ionomer cements. Quintessence Int. 1993;24:99–107.

Mount GJ, Hume WR. Preservation and restoration of tooth structure, chapter 8. St Louis: Mosby; 1998. p. 80–2.

Müller J, Bruckner G, Kraft E, et al. Reaction of cultured pulp cells to eight different cements based on glass ionomers. Dent Mater. 1990;6:172–7.

Nakajima M, San H, Burrow MF, et al. Tensile bond strength and SEM evaluation of caries-affected dentin using dentin adhesive. J Dent Res. 1995;74:1679–88.

Ngo H. Remineralization of artificial carious dentine exposed to two glass ionomers. J Dent Res. 2002a; 81(Special Issue):386.

Ngo HC. Biological potential of glass-ionomer. In: Mount GJ, editor. An atlas of glass-ionomer cements. London: Martin Dunitz; 2002b. p. 43–55.

Ngo HC, Mount GJ, Peters MC. A study of glass-ionomer cement and its interface with enamel and dentin using a low-temperature, high resolution scanning electron microscopic technique. Quintessence Int. 1997a;28:63–9.

Ngo HC, Ruben J, Arends J, et al. Electron probe microanalysis and transverse microradiography studies of artificial lesions in enamel and dentin: a comparative study. Adv Dent Res. 1997b;11:426–32.

Ngo HC, Mount G, McIntyre J, et al. Chemical exchange between glass-ionomer restorations and residual carious dentine in permanent molars: an in vivo study. J Dent. 2006;34(8):608–13.

Olivia A, Della Ragione F, Salerno A. Biocompatibility studies on glass ionomer cements by primary cultures of human osteoblasts. Biomaterials. 2000;17:1351–6.

Ostlund J, Möller K, Koch G. Amalgam, composite resin and glass ionomer cement in Class II restorations in primary molars – a three year clinical evaluation. Swed Dent J. 1992;16(3):81–6.

Peez R, Frank S. The physical–mechanical performance of the new Ketac Molar Easymix compared to commercially available glass ionomer restoratives. J Dent. 2006;34:582–7.

Qvist V, Laurberg L, Poulsen A, et al. Eight-year study on conventional glass ionomer and amalgam restorations in primary teeth. Acta Odontol Scand. 2004;62:37–45.

Raggio DP, Hesse D, Lenzi TL, et al. Is atraumatic restorative treatment an option for restoring occluso-proximal caries lesions in primary teeth? A systematic review and meta-analysis. Int J Paediatr Dent. 2013; 23:435–43.

Ricketts DNJ, Lamont T, Innes P et al (2013) Operative caries management in adults and children. Cochrane Database Syst Rev (3):CD003808

Roeleveld AC, van Amerongen WE, Mandari GJ. Influence of residual caries and cervical gaps on

the survival rate of Class II glass ionomer restorations. Eur Arch Paediatr Dent. 2006;7:85–91.
Sidhu SK. Clinical evaluations of resin-modified glass-ionomer restorations. Dent Mater. 2010;2:7–12.
Sidhu SK. Glass-ionomer cement restorative materials: a sticky subject? Aust Dent J. 2011;56 Suppl 1:23–30.
Six N, Lasfargues JJ, Goldberg M. *In vivo* study of the pulp reaction to Fuji IX, a glass ionomer cement. J Dent. 2000;28:413–22.
Smith DC. Development of glass-ionomer cement systems. Biomaterials. 1998;19:467–78.
Thompson V, Craig RG, Curro FA, et al. Treatment of deep carious lesions by complete excavation or partial removal: a critical review. J Am Dent Assoc. 2008; 139(6):705–12.
Toh SL, Messer LB. Evidence-based assessment of tooth-colored restorations in proximal lesions of primary molars. Pediatr Dent. 2007;29(1):8–15.
Topaloglu-Ak A, Eden E, Frencken JE, et al. Two year survival rate of class II composite resin restorations prepared by ART with and without a chemomechanical caries removal gel in primary molars. Clin Oral Investig. 2009;13:325–32.
United Nations Environment Programme (2013) Minamata Convention on Mercury UNEP(DTIE)/Hg/CONF/3
Van Dijken JW. A 6-year evaluation of a direct composite resin inlay/onlay system and glass ionomer cement-composite resin sandwich restorations. Acta Odontol. 1994;52:368–76.
Van Gemert-Schriks MC, van Amerongen WE, ten Cate JM, et al. Three-year survival of single- and two-surface ART restorations in a high-caries child population. Clin Oral Investig. 2007;11:337–43.
Van Noort R. Introduction to dental materials. 4th ed. Edinburgh/New York: Mosby Elsevier; 2013. p. 113.
Vlietstra JR, Plant CG, Shovelton DS, et al. The use of glass ionomer cement in deciduous teeth. Br Dent J. 1978;145:164–6.
Watson TF. Bonding glass-ionomer cements to tooth structure. In: Davidson CL, Mjör IA, editors. Advances in glass-ionomer cements. Germany: Quintessence Publishing Co Inc.; 1999.
Way JL, Caputo AA, Jedrychowski JR. Bond strength of light-cured glass ionomers to carious primary dentin. ASDC J Dent Child. 1996;63(4):261–4.
Welbury RR, Walls AW, Murray JJ, McCabe JF. The 5-year results of a clinical trial comparing a glass polyalkenoate (ionomer) cement restoration with an amalgam restoration. Br Dent J. 1991;170:177–81.
Wilson AD, Kent BE. The glass ionomer cement. A new translucent dental filling material. J Appl Chem Biotechnol. 1971;21:313.
Woolford M. Composite resin attached to glass polyalkenoate (ionomer) cement—the laminate technique. J Dent. 1993;21:31–8.
Yip HK, Tay FR, Ngo HC, et al. Bonding of contemporary glass ionomer cements to dentin. Dent Mater. 2001; 17(5):456–70.
Yiu CK, Tay FR, King NM, et al. Interaction of glass-ionomer cements with moist dentin. J Dent Res. 2004;83(4):283–9.
Yoshida Y, Van Meerbeek B, Nakayama Y, et al. Evidence of chemical bonding at biomaterial-hard tissue interfaces. J Dent Res. 2000;79(2):709–14.
Zoergiebel J, Ilie N. An in vitro study on the maturation of conventional glass ionomer cements and their interface to dentin. Acta Biomater. 2013;9:9529–37.

Glass-Ionomers in Contemporary Endodontics

5

Josette Camilleri

Abstract

Glass-ionomer cements have a wide range of applications in dentistry and are also used in endodontics. Their main desirable properties include adhesion to tooth structure, fluoride release, biocompatibility and antimicrobial properties. Due to these properties, glass-ionomer cements have been indicated for use in endodontics in both nonsurgical (e.g. as temporary interim dressings during root canal therapy, intra-orifice barriers and root canal sealers) and surgical situations (e.g. as root-end filling materials). Glass-ionomers used in endodontics have been extensively researched and have been in clinical use for a number of years.

5.1 Introduction

Glass-ionomer cements are composed of an acid-reactive glass powder which is mixed with polyacrylic acid, resulting in a material which has particular properties. These properties lead to the use of glass-ionomer cements for a variety of applications in dentistry, one of which is its use in endodontics. In the current chapter, only the conventional glass-ionomer cement (the powder/liquid) formulations will be discussed.

The most desirable properties of glass-ionomer cement which make it suitable for use in endodontics include its adhesive properties in the form of a bond to dentine (Wilson and McLean 1988), fluoride release (Cattani-Lorente et al. 1994; Mitra and Kedrowski 1994) and biocompatibility (Sidhu and Schmalz 2001). Furthermore, glass-ionomers have exhibited antibacterial properties against a number of bacterial strains (Meiers and Miller 1996; DeSchepper et al. 1989; Vermeersch et al. 2005).

5.2 Properties Relevant to Endodontics

5.2.1 Adhesive Properties

Glass-ionomers bond to dental hard tissues chemically (Lin et al. 1992). Although bonding is reported for glass-ionomers as restorative materials, this bond seems not to be optimal within the

J. Camilleri, BChD, MPhil, PhD
Department of Restorative Dentistry,
Faculty of Dental Surgery, Medical School,
Mater Dei Hospital, University of Malta,
Msida, Malta
e-mail: josette.camilleri@um.edu.mt

S.K. Sidhu (ed.), *Glass-Ionomers in Dentistry*, DOI 10.1007/978-3-319-22626-2_5

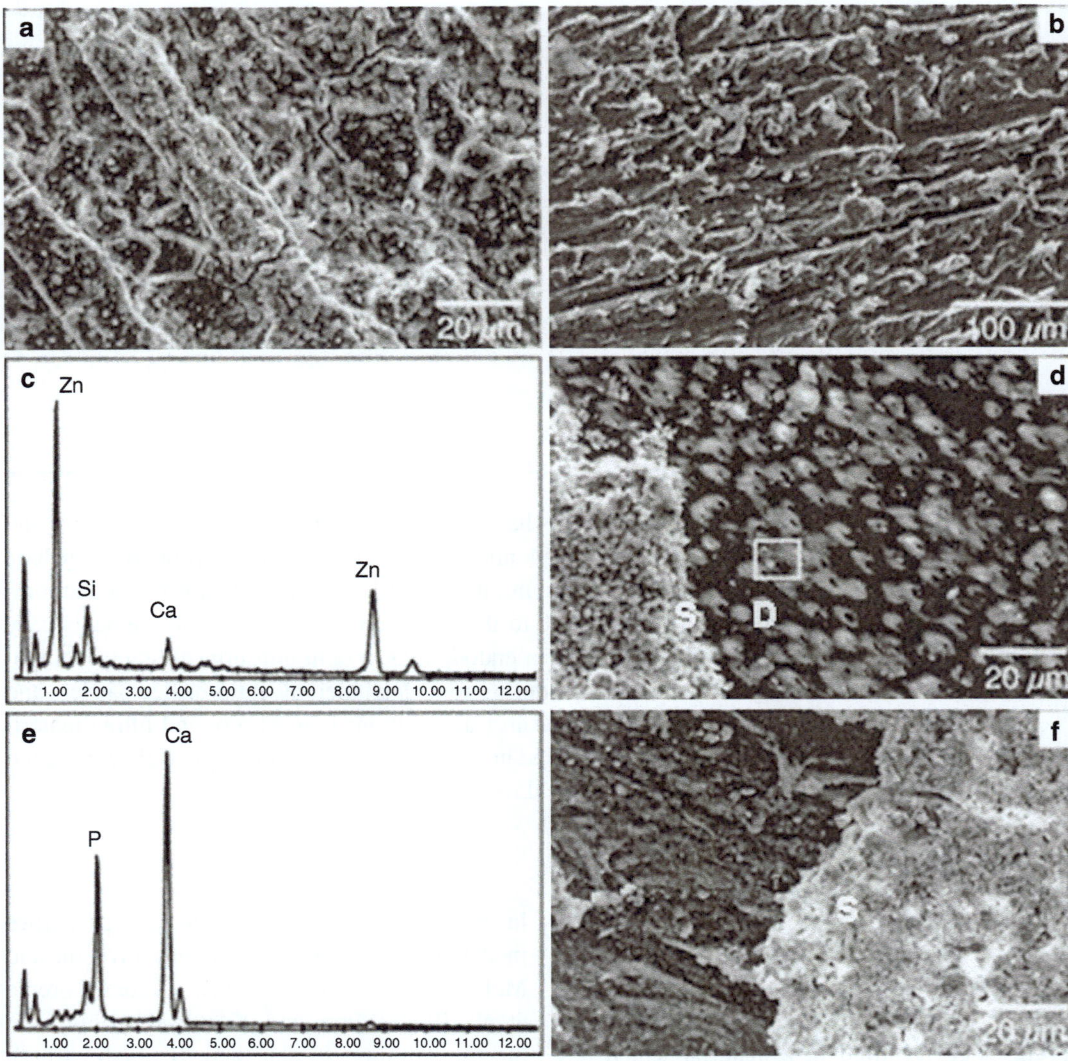

Fig. 5.1 Root dentine surface of debonded specimens with different dentine pretreatments, in which Ketac Endo sealer had been used. (**a**) Scanning electron micrograph (SEM) (×800) of dentine surface completely covered with sealer (citric acid pretreatment). (**b**) SEM (×200) of gutta-percha surface (citric acid pretreatment). (**c**) EDS analysis of gutta-percha surface revealing traces of sealer. Gutta-percha is mostly organic with zinc making up most of its inorganic component. The calcium and silicon in the EDS analysis are derived from the sealer. (**d**) SEM (×800) of dentine surface partly covered with sealer (*S*). Open dentinal tubules (*D*) with no sealer tags are seen in most of the figure elsewhere (EDTA pretreatment). (**e**) EDS analysis of the area indicated within the *white square* in (**d**), showing that this area appears to be clear dentine, i.e. without any remnants of sealer. Dentine is composed of calcium and phosphorus as seen in the EDS analysis. (**f**) SEM (×800) of gutta-percha surface partly covered with sealer (*S*) (EDTA pretreatment) (Reprinted from Saleh et al. (2003). With permission from Elsevier)

root canal when the material is used as a root canal sealer (Chung et al. 2001; Timpawat et al. 2001; Tagger et al. 2002; Najar et al. 2003).

Investigation of the shear bond strength of a glass-ionomer sealer showed bond strengths higher than calcium hydroxide-based sealers and lower bond strengths when compared to methacrylate sealers (Lalh et al. 1999a; Gogos et al. 2004). The failure was mostly cohesive (Lalh et al. 1999a; Gogos et al. 2004) with a layer of glass-ionomer evident on the wall of the root canal after failure occurred, regardless of the lack of sealer penetration in dentinal tubules (Fig. 5.1; Saleh et al. 2003). When compared to an epoxy resin-based sealer (Sealer 26, Dentsply, DeTrey, Konstanz, Germany), the glass-ionomer sealer (Ketac Endo, 3M ESPE, St Paul, MN, USA) exhibited very low bond strengths, which were similar to that of a zinc oxide-eugenol-based sealer (Grossman's sealer). The push-out bond strength of glass-ionomers in general appears to be inferior to epoxy resin-based sealers (Nagas et al. 2009; Tagger et al. 2002). The use of glass-ionomer cements as root canal sealers is not as widespread as other categories of sealers.

The removal of the smear layer with ethylenediaminetetracetic acid (EDTA) did not appear to have any effect on the bond strength of a glass-ionomer sealer (Ketac Endo) (Najar et al. 2003). In fact, when EDTA was used to remove the smear layer from root canal walls, no penetration of glass-ionomer sealer was shown inside the dentinal tubules as indicated in Fig. 5.1 (Saleh et al. 2003). Ketac Endo exhibited continuous penetration when phosphoric acid and citric acid were used to pretreat the dentine (Saleh et al. 2003). The bond strengths of a glass-ionomer sealer to gutta-percha were weaker than other test sealers (Saleh et al. 2002). The bond strength of glass-ionomer to gutta-percha was also shown to be low when compared to other classes of sealer cements (Lee et al. 2002). It has been suggested that pretreatment with phosphoric acid or citric acid should be done in association with glass-ionomer root canal sealer to achieve the most effective removal of the smear layer and to provide better adhesion (Timpawat et al. 2001; Saleh et al. 2003). On the other hand, the use of 2.6 % sodium hypochlorite solution used as a dentine conditioner improved the sealer adhesion, and the presence of a hybrid layer was noted (Lalh et al. 1999b). The adhesion of glass-ionomer sealers to root canal walls is also affected by the presence of calcium hydroxide and formocresol medicaments used in the root canal during root canal treatment (Chung et al. 2001). Although bonding of glass-ionomer cement to dentine walls can potentially minimize microleakage, no correlation between microleakage and adhesive properties was found when four commonly used sealers including glass-ionomer cement were evaluated (Pommel et al. 2003).

Testing for adhesive properties has been mostly conducted by performing a shear bond strength test (Lalh et al. 1999a, b; Chung et al. 2001; Gogos et al. 2004) and tensile testing (Tagger et al. 2002; Lee et al. 2002; Saleh et al. 2002, 2003). The push-out bond strength test has also been used to test the sealing ability and bonding using different sealers including a glass-ionomer sealer (Nagas et al. 2009). Push-out bond strength testing is currently the most popular test to assess adhesive properties of materials used within the root canal.

5.2.2 Fluoride Release

Fluoride ion release is one of the properties of glass-ionomer cements. The action of polyacrylic acid on the glass particle results in ion dissolution over time. In the early stages, calcium and aluminium ions are preferentially released in solution, while sodium and fluorine are leached in the long term. While the fluoride ion release has been shown to result in remineralization of tooth tissue (Arends et al. 1990; Almqvist and Lagerlöf 1993), this property has not been extensively researched for glass-ionomer cements used for endodontic applications. There is no literature on the effect of fluoride released from glass-ionomers used for endodontic applications and its effect on root dentine remineralization.

The acidic environs of glass-ionomer-based materials are not known to promote bioactivity and remineralization when compared to the local bioactivity of the tricalcium silicate-based materials like mineral trioxide aggregate (MTA) and Biodentine (Septodont, Saint-Maur-des-Fossés, France). Materials based on tricalcium silicate release calcium hydroxide on hydration; this in turn results in an alkalinizing medium that has been shown to produce mineralization within the adjacent dentine substrate, extending deep within the tissues. This suggests that the local ion-rich alkaline environment may be more favourable to mineral repair and reconstruction (Tay and Pashley 2008; Dong et al. 2011), compared with glass-ionomers (Watson et al. 2014). To this effect, a remineralization medium consisting of a Portland cement/phosphate-containing fluid that included polyacrylic acid and polyvinylphosphonic acid biomimetic analogues resulted in both interfibrillar and intrafibrillar apatites becoming readily discernible within the hybrid layers after 2–4 months (Tay and Pashley 2009). Thus, the calcium ion release from the tricalcium silicates may have a significant effect on remineralization of dentine.

Root canals are often irrigated with solutions such as EDTA and citric acid that remove the smear layer. The best combination for effective removal of a smear layer has been found to be alternate use of sodium hypochlorite (NaOCI) and EDTA (Baumgartner and Mader 1987; Fig. 5.2). Removal of the smear layer allows the sealers to enter some of the dentinal tubules. The use of a fluoride-containing sealer potentially may enhance dentine remineralization. The concentration of fluoride in the dentine in the coronal part of the root canal was found to be increased after obturation with gutta-percha and a glass-ionomer sealer (Saunders et al. 1992). In another study assessing a silver-reinforced glass-ionomer cement used as a root-end filling material, fluoride ion release was also reported, but its effect on dentine was not assessed; the corrosion potential of the silver was however investigated (Roth 1991). It was shown that there was no difference in dye leakage of the different glass-ionomers investigated when using vertically condensed gutta-percha. It was thus concluded that glass-ionomer cement is possibly a clinical alternative for the sealing of retrograde cavities. The silver-reinforced materials, however, may cause tissue irritation from release of silver ions and their corrosion products (Roth 1991).

Fluoride-releasing glass-ionomer cement seems to be an appropriate material to seal the root canals of overdenture abutments, because it has an inhibiting effect on demineralization at the cavity wall in vitro (Ikebe et al. 2001). When glass-ionomer was used over carious root surfaces in one study, fluoride concentrations varied markedly along the outer edge of both normal and carious root tissues (Shu et al. 1998). However, fluoride increase at the edge of the lesion was found to be a result of remineralization events during caries (Shu et al. 1998). A sealer composed of pre-reacted glass-ionomer filler particles leaching aluminium, boron, fluoride, sodium, silicon, strontium and zinc showed that the incorporation of fluoride, strontium, silicon and boron along the outermost dentine of the sealer-dentine interface and the incorporation depth increased with prolonged immersion (Han and Okiji 2011). This provides evidence that fluoride causes remineralization of root dentine and hence, glass-ionomer cements may offer some potential benefits in this regard.

5.2.3 Biocompatibility

The biocompatibility of glass-ionomer materials is an important property when the materials are used as root-end fillers and to a certain extent when used as sealers which come into contact with the tissues at the apex. The biocompatibility of glass-ionomer cements has been assessed mostly at the cellular level, with osteosarcoma cells (Peltola et al. 1992; Lee et al. 2012) and gingival fibroblasts (Peltola et al. 1992; Koulaouzidou et al. 2005; Vajrabhaya et al. 2006; Al-Hiyasat et al. 2012; Subbarao et al. 2012) being the preferred cell lines. Animal models have also been used (Kolokuris et al. 1996; Tassery et al. 1999; Ogasawara et al. 2003) with intraosseous implantation in rabbit mandible being more reliable than implantation in femurs (Tassery et al. 1999). Subcutaneous implantation was also used for assessment of biocompatibility of glass-ionomers (Kolokuris et al. 1996). Mild inflammatory reaction was observed with Ketac Endo on the 5th day (Fig. 5.3a); the connective tissue was infiltrated with plasma cells as well as lymphocytes and macrophages were observed. The intensity of the reaction diminished by the 15th day (Fig. 5.3b), and this reduction continued progressively through the 60th and 120th days (Fig. 5.3c). The control material, a zinc oxide-eugenol-based sealer, remained irritating even after long-term implantation periods (Kolokuris et al. 1996).

The biocompatibility of glass-ionomer cement used as a root-end filling material was previously compared to zinc oxide-eugenol cement, where in every assessment, the glass-ionomer

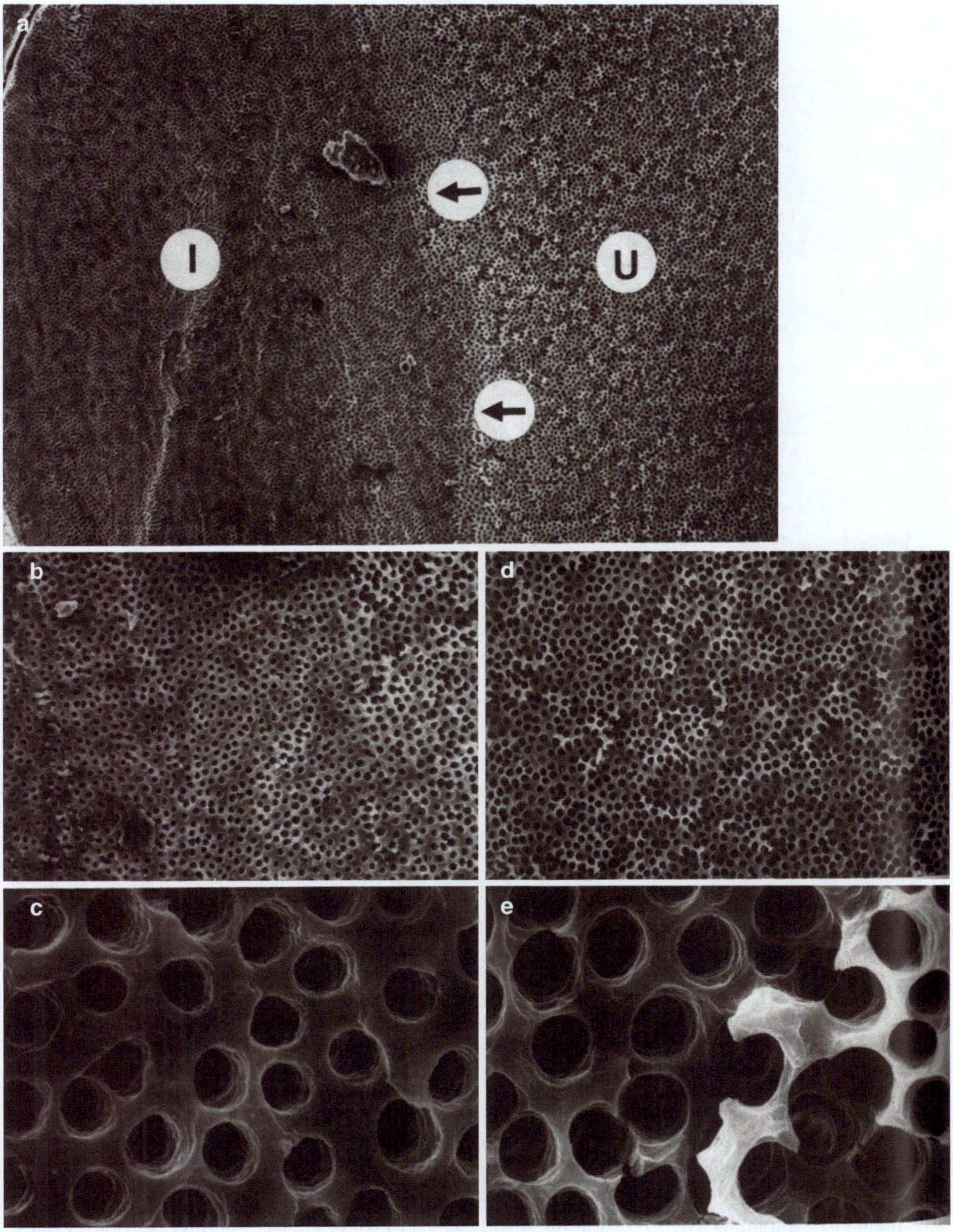

Fig. 5.2 SEMs of the root canal wall showing the effects of removal of the smear layer by using a regimen of NaOCl and EDTA alternately. (**a**) SEM (×148) of the junction (*arrowed*) between the instrumented (*I*) and un-instrumented (*U*) halves of the canal wall. (**b**) SEM of the instrumented half of the canal wall at a lower magnification (×504) and (**c**) at higher magnification (×4,040). Note the clean, smoothly planed appearance of the canal wall and the sharply defined orifices of the dentinal tubules. (**d**) Lower magnification (×506) and higher magnification (**e**) (×4,000) micrographs of the un-instrumented half of the canal wall. Note the erosion of the globular surface of the calcospherites and enlargement of the orifices of the dentinal tubules (Reprinted from Baumgartner and Mader (1987). With permission from Elsevier)

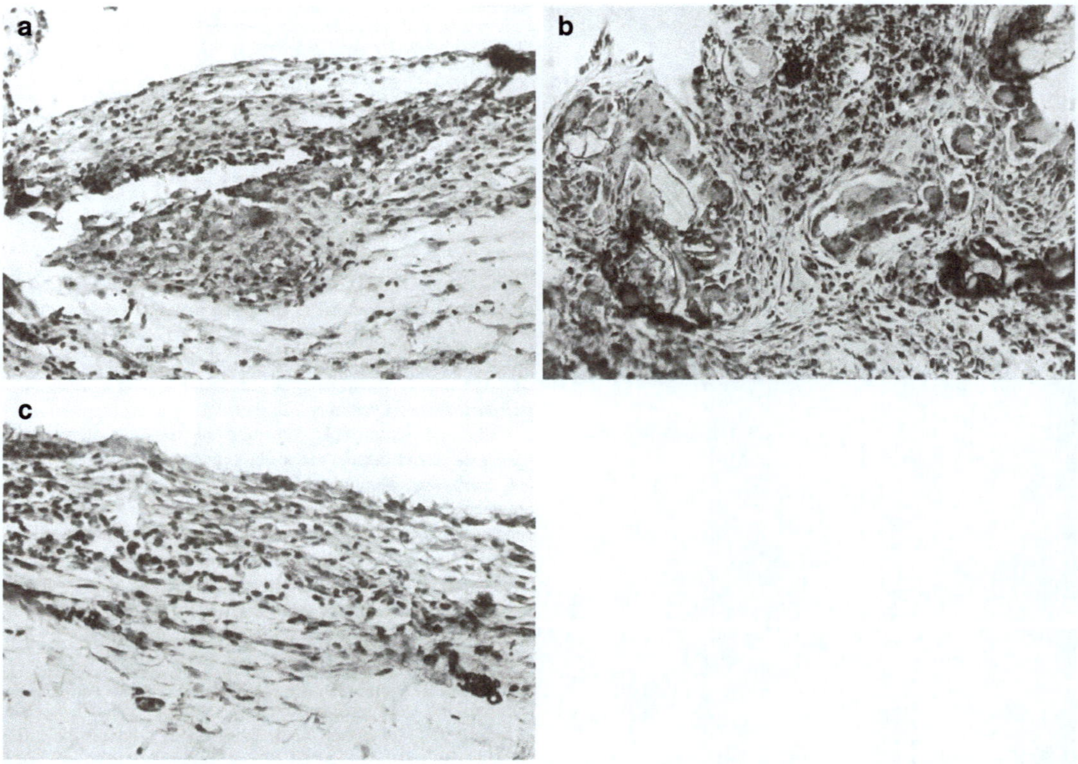

Fig. 5.3 Histological assessment of tissue biocompatibility of Ketac Endo sealer in rat connective tissue showing microscopic appearance on the (**a**) 5th day: mild inflammation with the presence of mononuclear cells. (**b**) 15th day: presence of giant cells and macrophages. Note also the presence of connective tissue. (H ×215). (**c**) 60th day: presence of a few mononuclear cells. (H ×325) (Reprinted from Kolokuris et al. (1996). With permission from Elsevier)

outperformed the zinc oxide. It was found that the zinc oxide-eugenol sealer was largely absorbed and surrounded by fibrous tissue with many macrophages. The disintegrated material was completely engulfed by macrophages, whereas the glass-ionomer cement remained in the bone cavity with no inflammatory reaction (Ogasawara et al. 2003). The short-term biocompatibility of glass-ionomer cement was similar to zinc oxide-eugenol, but after 12 weeks, the former had better performance when assessed by intraosseous implantation (Tassery et al. 1999). Subcutaneous implantation of glass-ionomer cement (Fig. 5.3) and zinc oxide-eugenol showed connective tissue infiltration with plasma cells for glass-ionomers, while necrosis was evident with zinc oxide-eugenol (Kolokuris et al. 1996). Thus, glass-ionomer cement appears to have at least similar but probably better biocompatibility than zinc oxide-eugenol.

Further studies on glass-ionomer biocompatibility were performed to compare glass-ionomers to MTA. Glass-ionomer cements were comparable to MTA in one study (Lee et al. 2012), but the biocompatibility of glass-ionomers was generally lower than that of MTA in several other reports (Koulaouzidou et al. 2005; Vajrabhaya et al. 2006; Al-Hiyasat et al. 2012). The surface of a glass-ionomer restorative material (Ketac Fil, 3M ESPE, St Paul, MN, USA) showed very sparse cellular growth, with cells of round shape, and a rough surface due to the

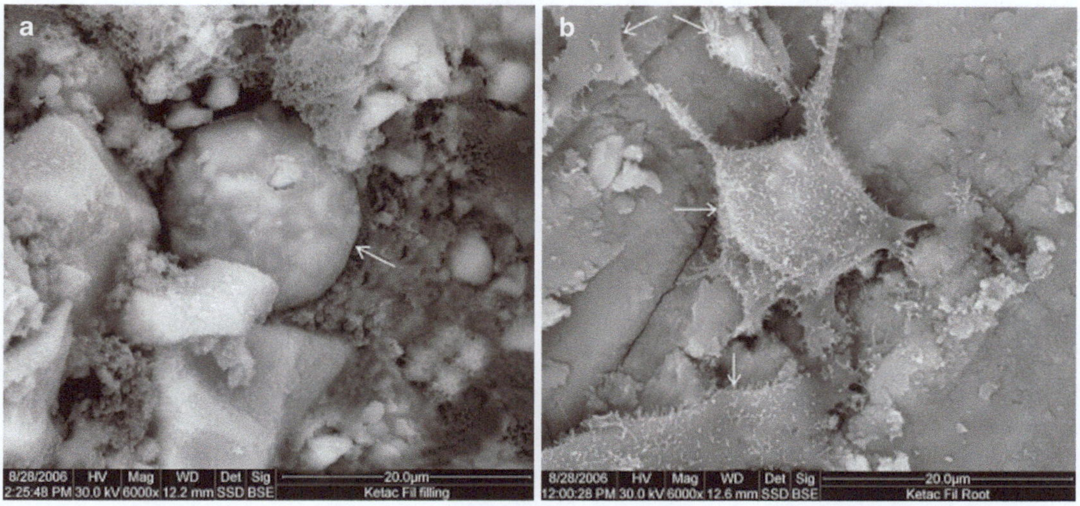

Fig. 5.4 Scanning electron micrograph of Ketac Fil: (**a**) material surface (×6,000) showing limited cell attachment. (**b**) Root surface (×6,000) showing very good cell attachment. (*Arrows* indicate cells.) (Reprinted from Al-Hiyasat et al. (2012). With permission from *Journal of Applied Oral Sciences (JAOS)*)

extending processes, namely, microvilli. While on the root surface, cells demonstrated excellent attachment features including a spindle shape, lamellipodia, filopodia and microvilli (Fig. 5.4). This was in contrast to MTA where cell attachment to the material was similar to the attachment on the dentine surface (Al-Hiyasat et al. 2012). Glass-ionomer was less biocompatible than composite resin, titanium and amalgam (Peltola et al. 1992). The biocompatibility of glass-ionomer cement to fibroblasts appeared to be improved by the addition of bioactive glass than by the addition of collagen. The glass-ionomer and modified glass-ionomer still exhibited reduced biocompatibility when compared to MTA (Subbarao et al. 2012).

5.2.4 Antibacterial Properties

The antibacterial effect of glass-ionomer cement is related to its acidity (Vermeersch et al. 2005); adjustment of the liquid to pH 5 results in a loss of antibacterial activity (DeSchepper et al. 1989). Furthermore, the fluoride concentration has been linked with the antimicrobial activity, with no antimicrobial activity reported when the fluoride release is lowered (DeSchepper et al. 1989). The effect of fluoride does not have a great impact on glass-ionomers used as sealers, root-end filling materials and materials used in perforation repair sites as fluoride recharge is necessary for sustained fluoride release by glass-ionomers, and these sites are relatively inaccessible for recharge. In fact, the antibacterial activity of glass-ionomers is increased with topical applications of fluoride toothpaste and gels (Seppä et al. 1993).

Glass-ionomer sealers exhibit antibacterial activity initially, but this effect reduces drastically after 7 days according to some studies (Shalhav et al. 1997; Anumula et al. 2012). In other reports, it exhibits no antimicrobial activity at all (Heling and Chandler 1996). However, the technique used to test antibacterial activity, time of incubation and the ingredients of the materials tested can affect the results of the microbiological studies (Cobankara et al. 2004). This should be taken into consideration when reviewing conflicting results which prevent firm conclusions to be drawn.

5.3 Uses of Glass-Ionomer Cements in Endodontics

Glass-ionomers are used in endodontics for the following:

- Nonsurgical applications: for temporary inter-appointment restoration during root canal treatment, as intra-orifice barrier materials, as root canal sealers and for nonsurgical perforation repair
- Surgical applications: as root-end filling materials and for surgical perforation repair

There are no specifications for root-end filling and perforation repair materials although root canal sealer properties have to comply with ANSI/ADA Specification 57 (2000) and ISO 6876 (2012).

5.3.1 Root Canal Sealers

Root canal sealer properties have to comply with ANSI/ADA Specification 57 (2000) and ISO 6876 (2012). Regardless of the extensive use of glass-ionomers as root canal sealers, there is very limited research on the material properties and compliance to the specifications for root canal sealers. Only the compliance of glass-ionomer materials for radiopacity (Shah et al. 1996; Tanomaru-Filho et al. 2008) has been reported. Unfortunately, glass-ionomer sealers have also shown high solubility and disintegration (Carvalho-Júnior et al. 2003), which is not in compliance with the ADA specifications for root canal sealers (ADA Specifications No. 57, 2000).

The main scope of a root canal sealer is to bind the gutta-percha to the dentine walls. Thus, the ideal sealer should adhere to both the gutta-percha and also to the dentine. Glass-ionomer sealers have shown poor adhesive properties to both root dentine and gutta-percha. This lack of adhesion would imply a potential for increased microleakage if glass-ionomer is used as a sealer.

Studies evaluating microleakage of glass-ionomer sealers show that they consistently perform worse than epoxy-based resin sealers and were comparable or even worse than zinc oxide-based root canal sealers. These evaluations were performed using dye leakage with methylene blue (Smith and Steiman 1994; Rohde et al. 1996; Oliver and Abbott 1998; Kumar and Shruthi 2012), India ink (Goldberg et al. 1995; Leonard et al. 1996), dye leakage with three-dimensional reconstruction (Lyroudia et al. 2000), salivary bacterial leakage (Malone and Donnelly 1997) and the fluid transport model (Cobankara et al. 2002; Miletić et al. 2002; Economides et al. 2005).

Glass-ionomer sealer provided adequate sealing of the root canal and was comparable to a number of commercial sealers (Miletić et al. 1999). The apical seal exhibited by glass-ionomer cement was not significantly different from that provided by zinc oxide-eugenol cement regardless of the presence or absence of a smear layer (Timpawat and Sripanaratanakul 1998), but inferior to that of a resin-based sealer used in conjunction with a dentine bonding agent (Leonard et al. 1996) and a polydimethylsiloxane-based root canal sealer (Cobankara et al. 2002). Epoxy resin-based sealers invariably exhibited a better seal than glass-ionomer sealers (De Almeida et al. 2000). In a previous study, both a glass-ionomer sealer (Ketac Endo) and a zinc oxide-eugenol-based sealer prevented coronal microleakage in the absence of a coronal restoration (Malone and Donnelly 1997). In the Oliver and Abbott (1998) study, interestingly enough, coronal gutta-percha was removed and the coronal 3 mm filled with Ketac Endo only but not in the AH 26 (Dentsply, DeTrey, Konstanz, Germany) group which served as the control. The study found comparable coronal leakage of Ketac Endo specimens to the control group (AH 26), regardless of the different methodologies used to obturate the root canals (Oliver and Abbott 1998). In another study, the area of adhesive failure was 88 % for the glass-ionomer sealer compared to 15 % for the epoxy resin-based root

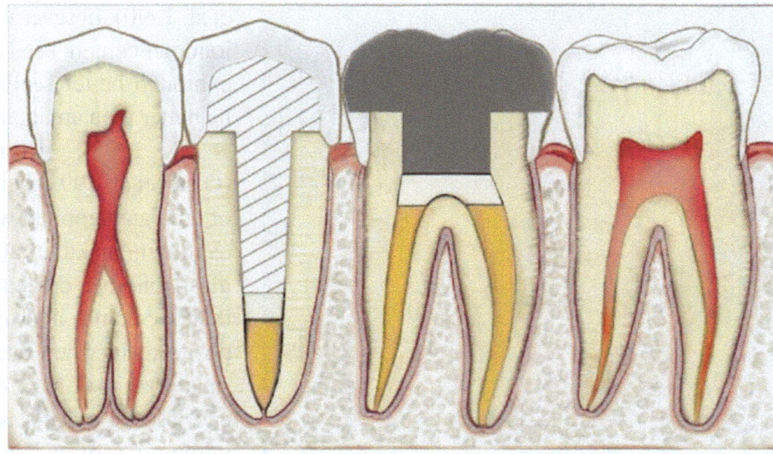

Fig. 5.5 Intra-canal glass-ionomer barrier illustrated under the post in the second premolar. Intra-orifice glass-ionomer barriers over the canals and over the pulpal floor are illustrated in the first molar (Reprinted from Mavec et al. (2006). With permission from Elsevier)

canal sealer (De Gee et al. 1994). In general, the thickness of the sealer and sealer type has been shown to affect the adequacy of the obturation and subsequent microleakage (Georgopoulou et al. 1995). Glass-ionomer sealer exhibited a better seal when used in very thin sections than other sealer types but did not perform as well when thicker amounts of materials were used (Wu et al. 1994, 1997).

Regardless of the poor outcomes of the results of leakage studies, it is now widely believed that there is little value in using in vitro models as they are not totally adept at quantifying the seal of root canals. In addition, the major limitations of in vitro leakage studies are their lack of reproducibility, relatively small sample size and inadequate statistical power, lack of standardization as well as lack of correlation among different leakage models (Wu and Wesselink 1993; Schuurs et al. 1993; Lucena et al. 2013). The clinical implications for experimental laboratory-based sealability models are unclear. The ideal assessment of endodontic treatment outcome is still clinical evaluation.

5.3.2 Intra-orifice Barrier and Restorative Material

The use of glass-ionomer cement as an intra-orifice barrier material and as an interim dressing relies on the material's sealing ability, antimicrobial properties and adhesion. The use of glass-ionomer cements to block the root canal orifice used in conjunction with gutta-percha obturations is shown diagrammatically in Fig. 5.5. Glass-ionomer significantly reduced coronal microleakage compared to a previously available thermoplastic synthetic polymer-based root canal filling, Resilon (resin-based solid cones) (Epiphany, Pentron Clinical Technologies, Wallingford, CT, USA), used without sealer and the glass-ionomer intra-orifice barrier (Jack and Goodell 2008). When used as a coronal barrier in cases of nonvital bleaching, glass-ionomer provided adequate seal comparable to that of white MTA (Vosoughhosseini et al. 2011). However, another research has shown a high degree of leakage when glass-ionomer was used as an intra-canal orifice barrier during tooth bleaching with sodium perborate and peroxide gel (Canoglu et al. 2012).

Glass-ionomer used as a restorative material after root canal treatment is not affected by the presence of other endodontic materials used for temporary filling or sealers present on dentine which are left from previous endodontic visits. The bond strength of dentine with and without the presence of other endodontic materials was the same (Capurro et al. 1993). A clinical picture of glass-ionomer used as a temporary dressing is shown in Fig. 5.6.

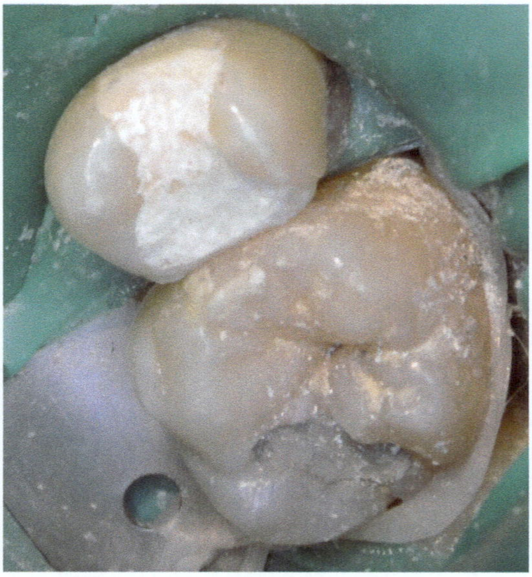

Fig. 5.6 Glass-ionomer cement used as a temporary filling material (Courtesy of Ms. Chiara Brincat and Dr. Matthew Cachia, University Dental Clinic, Faculty of Dental Surgery, University of Malta, Malta)

When glass-ionomer cement is used over MTA, as in cases of pulpotomy, the glass-ionomer appeared to exhibit a high degree of microcracking and some porosity in the interfacial region with MTA (Camilleri 2011). In addition, strontium from the glass-ionomer was detected at 200 μm within the MTA (Camilleri 2011). Hence, it appears that the pH disparity between MTA and glass-ionomer cement affects the properties of both materials and their interaction.

5.3.3 Root-End Filling Material

Root-end (retrograde) filling materials should exhibit an adequate seal and also encourage cell growth and differentiation particularly with periodontal ligament cells. The sealing ability of glass-ionomer root-end filling materials was reported to be comparable to that of amalgam, and it was preferable to use a root-end filling material rather than leave the tooth unfilled at the root-end (Olson et al. 1990). In several studies, conventional glass-ionomer cement used as a root-end filling material exhibited better sealing ability; it was shown to be better than amalgam (Chong et al. 1991; Ozata et al. 1993), silver-reinforced glass-ionomer (Ozata et al. 1993), amalgam applied with varnish or amalgam applied with a dentine bonding agent (Sutimuntanakul et al. 2000). Both amalgam and glass-ionomer cement leaked significantly more than a calcium hydroxide-based sealer and composite resin when used as root-end filling materials (Danin et al. 1992). Glass-ionomer cement can also be placed as a root-end filling material without a root-end cavity preparation. The resin-modified version of glass-ionomer materials exhibits particularly good adaptation to the root canal walls (Chong et al. 1993).

In more recent studies, glass-ionomer root-end filling materials exhibited high levels of marginal gaps when compared to Biodentine and MTA, which are both tricalcium silicate-based materials (Xavier et al. 2005; Ravichandra et al. 2014). In contrast, good marginal adaptation was observed with glass-ionomer cements when measured directly and on resin replicas (Costa et al. 2009) and using capillary flow porometry (De Bruyne et al. 2005). No correlation was observed between marginal adaptation and apical sealing ability (Xavier et al. 2005; Costa et al. 2008).

Glass-ionomers were shown to be biocompatible as cells seeded on the materials were dense and confluent; the biocompatibility was similar to that of calcium silicate-based materials (Lee et al. 2012). In contrast, in another study, poor cellular attachment was demonstrated in contrast to that of MTA (Al-Hiyasat et al. 2012), with cellular apoptosis of periodontal ligament cells (Lin et al. 2004).

5.3.4 Perforation Repair

Glass-ionomer cement has also been suggested for use as a perforation repair material. It is not

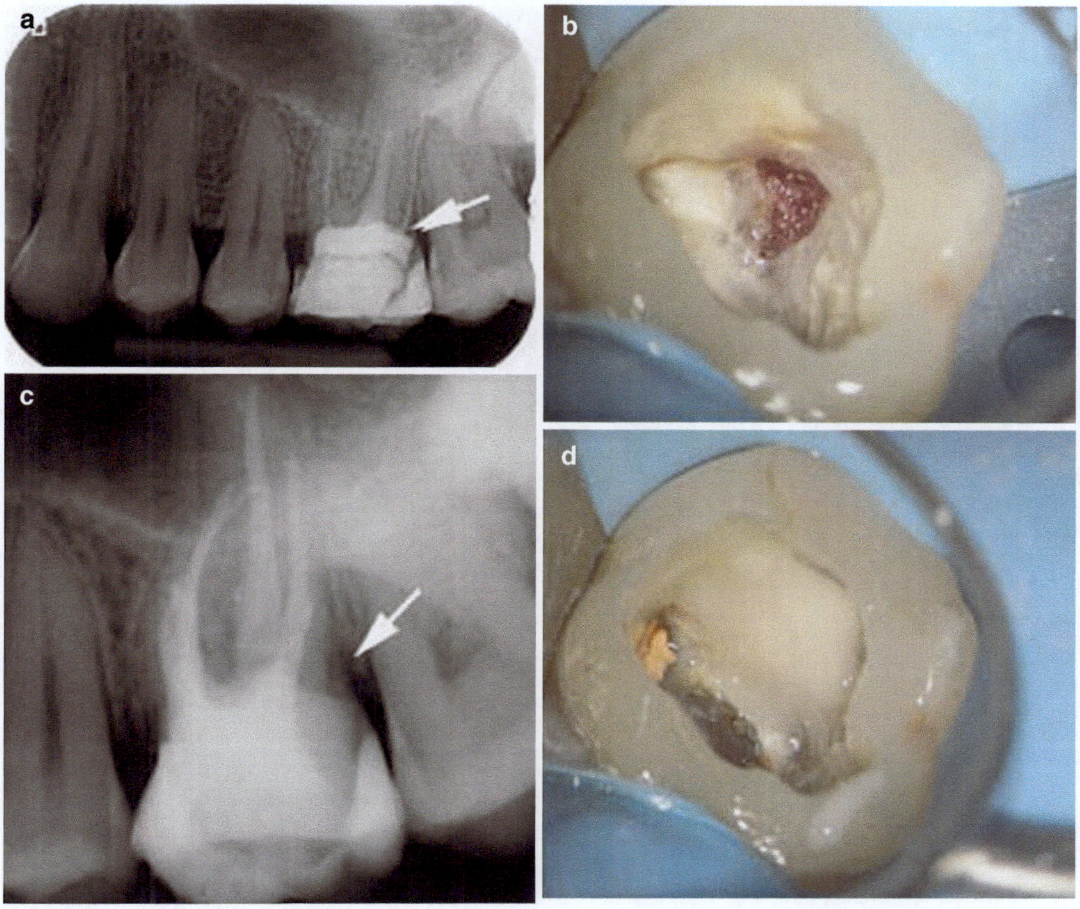

Fig. 5.7 Nonsurgical repair of root perforation in a maxillary molar tooth. (**a**) Preoperative radiograph showing supra-crestal perforation in Tooth 26 (*arrowed*). (**b**) Clinical picture of perforation prior to repair. (**c**) Periapical radiograph of perforation repaired (*arrowed*) with glass-ionomer cement. The root canal treatment was also redone. (**d**) Clinical appearance after placement of glass-ionomer cement (Courtesy of Dr. Roberto Critescu, Private Practice Limited to Endodontics, Amsterdam, the Netherlands)

the ideal material for perforation repair as it does not preserve the integrity of the periodontal tissues (Vanni et al. 2011). In fact, glass-ionomer cement suppressed the growth of human periodontal ligament fibroblast cells (Vajrabhaya et al. 2006), and its extracts were worse than Super EBA, amalgam and MTA in inhibiting cell proliferation (Souza et al. 2006). However, it was better than composite resin (Tai and Chang 2000) and leaked significantly less (Lodiene et al. 2011) but is not as effective as MTA for perforation repair (Bellam et al. 2009). A clinical case showing the use of glass-ionomer cement to repair a lateral root perforation nonsurgically is shown in Fig. 5.7, and a case of surgical perforation repair is shown in Fig. 5.8.

Although glass-ionomer cements have been used for endodontic applications for a number of years, clinical studies to assess their performance are scarce.

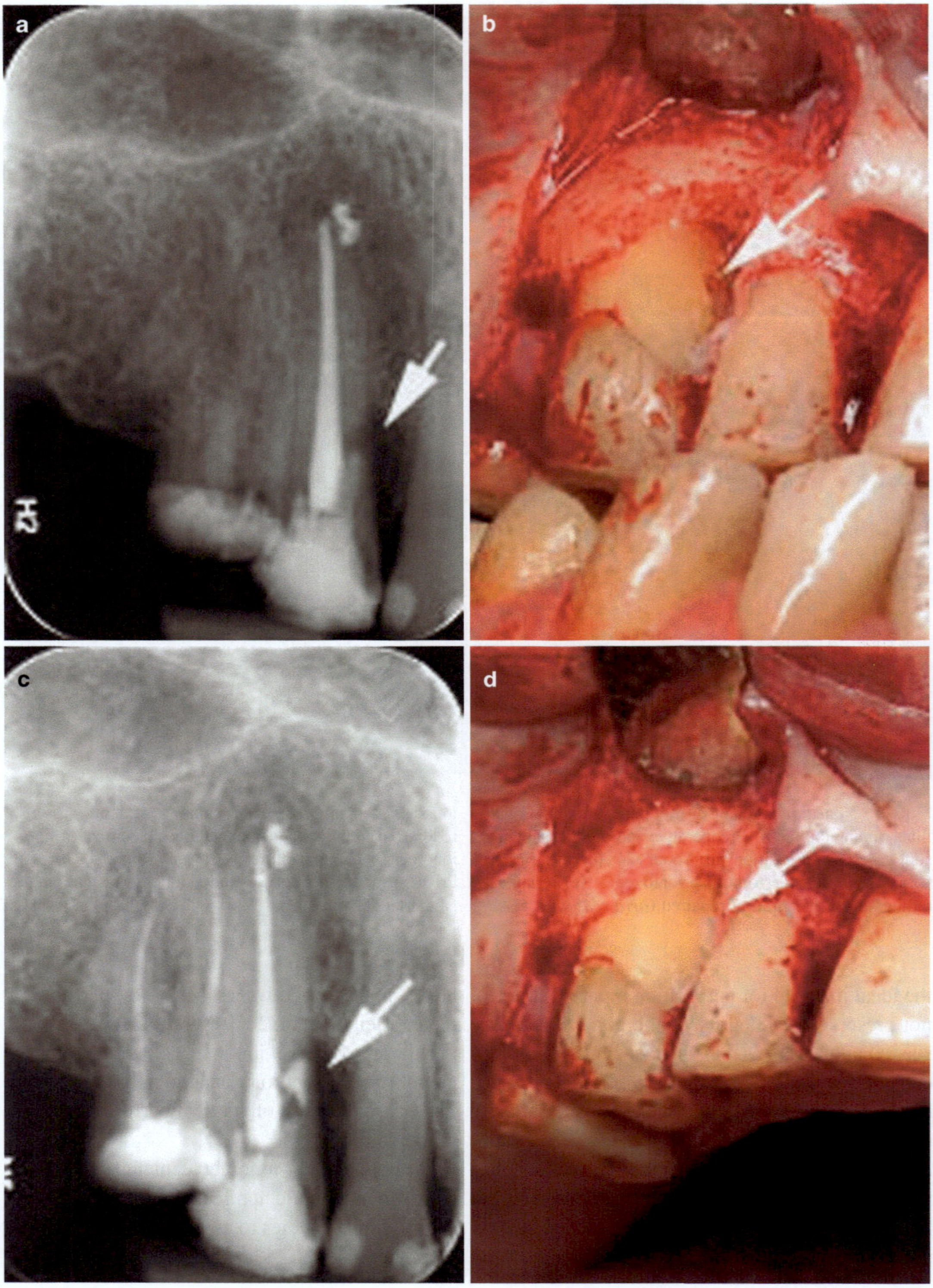

Fig. 5.8 Surgical repair of root perforation in a maxillary premolar tooth. (**a**) Preoperative radiograph showing perforation in Tooth 14 (*arrowed*). (**b**) Clinical picture of perforation (*arrowed*) with muco-periosteal flap raised. (**c**) Periapical radiograph of perforation repaired (*arrowed*) with glass-ionomer cement. (**d**) Clinical appearance after placement of glass-ionomer cement (*arrowed*) (Courtesy of Dr. Carlos Aznar Portoles, Verwijspraktijk voor Endodontologie, Santpoort-Zuid, the Netherlands)

Conclusions

Glass-ionomers are marketed depending on their particular use in dentistry. For root-end filling, perforation repair and interim dressings, the restorative glass-ionomers are usually employed. For this purpose, several brands are available and further material developments have been undertaken to improve the material properties over the years. Root canal sealers should have different material properties; thus, glass-ionomer restorative materials cannot be employed for this purpose. The material properties, namely, adhesion to dental hard structures, fluoride release, antimicrobial properties and biocompatibility, make glass-ionomers suitable for use in endodontics. However, research has indicated that they have been outperformed by other materials that have been in clinical use or have been developed over the years.

References

Al-Hiyasat AS, Al-Sa'Eed OR, Darmani H. Quality of cellular attachment to various root-end filling materials. J Appl Oral Sci. 2012;20(1):82–8.

Almqvist H, Lagerlöf F. Effect of intermittent delivery of fluoride to solution on root hard-tissue de- and remineralization measured by 125I absorptiometry. J Dent Res. 1993;72(12):1593–8.

American National Standards Institute/American Dental Association (2000) Endodontic sealing material. ANSI/ADA Specification No 57

Anumula L, Kumar S, Kumar VS, Sekhar C, Krishna M, Pathapati RM, Venkata Sarath P, Vadaganadam Y, Manne RK, Mudlapudi S. An assessment of antibacterial activity of four endodontic sealers on Enterococcus faecalis by a direct contact test: an in vitro study. ISRN Dent. 2012;2012:989781.

Arends J, Ruben JL, Christoffersen J, Jongebloed WL, Zuidgeest TG. Remineralization of human dentine in vitro. Caries Res. 1990;24(6):432–5.

Baumgartner JC, Mader CL. A scanning electron microscopic evaluation of four root canal irrigation regimens. J Endod. 1987;13(4):147–57.

Bellam KK, Namburi SK, Tripuraneni SC. In vitro evaluation of bacterial leakage through different perforation repair materials of teeth. J Appl Biomater Biomech. 2009;7(3):179–84.

Camilleri J. Scanning electron microscopic evaluation of the material interface of adjacent layers of dental materials. Dent Mater. 2011;27(9):870–8.

Canoglu E, Gulsahi K, Sahin C, Altundasar E, Cehreli ZC. Effect of bleaching agents on sealing properties of different intraorifice barriers and root filling materials. Med Oral Patol Oral Cir Bucal. 2012;17(4):e710–5.

Capurro MA, Herrera CL, Macchi RL. Influence of endodontic materials on the bonding of glass ionomer cement to dentin. Endod Dent Traumatol. 1993;9(2):75–6.

Carvalho-Júnior JR, Guimarães LF, Correr-Sobrinho L, Pécora JD, Sousa-Neto MD. Evaluation of solubility, disintegration, and dimensional alterations of a glass ionomer root canal sealer. Braz Dent J. 2003;14(2):114–8.

Cattani-Lorente MA, Godin C, Meyer JM. Mechanical behavior of glass ionomer cements affected by long-term storage in water. Dent Mater. 1994;10(1):37–44.

Chong BS, Pitt Ford TR, Watson TF. Light-cured glass ionomer cement as a retrograde root seal. Int Endod J. 1993;26(4):218–24.

Chong BS, Pitt Ford TR, Watson TF. The adaptation and sealing ability of light-cured glass ionomer retrograde root fillings. Int Endod J. 1991;24(5):223–32.

Chung HA, Titley K, Torneck CD, Lawrence HP, Friedman S. Adhesion of glass-ionomer cement sealers to bovine dentin conditioned with intracanal medications. J Endod. 2001;27(2):85–8.

Cobankara FK, Adanir N, Belli S, Pashley DH. A quantitative evaluation of apical leakage of four root-canal sealers. Int Endod J. 2002;35(12):979–84.

Cobankara FK, Altinöz HC, Ergani O, Kav K, Belli S. In vitro antibacterial activities of root-canal sealers by using two different methods. J Endod. 2004;30(1):57–60.

Costa AT, Konrath F, Dedavid B, Weber JB, de Oliveira MG. Marginal adaptation of root-end filling materials: an in vitro study with teeth and replicas. J Contemp Dent Pract. 2009;10(2):75–82.

Costa AT, Post LK, Xavier CB, Weber JB, Gerhardt-Oliveira M. Marginal adaptation and microleakage of five root-end filling materials: an in vitro study. Minerva Stomatol. 2008;57(6):295–300.

Danin J, Linder L, Sund ML, Strömberg T, Torstenson B, Zetterqvist L. Quantitative radioactive analysis of microleakage of four different retrograde fillings. Int Endod J. 1992;25(4):183–8.

De Almeida WA, Leonardo MR, Tanomaru Filho M, Silva LA. Evaluation of apical sealing of three endodontic sealers. Int Endod J. 2000;33(1):25–7.

De Bruyne MA, De Bruyne RJ, Rosiers L, De Moor RJ. Longitudinal study on microleakage of three root-end filling materials by the fluid transport method and by capillary flow porometry. Int Endod J. 2005;38(2):129–36.

De Gee AJ, Wu MK, Wesselink PR. Sealing properties of Ketac-Endo glass ionomer cement and AH26 root canal sealers. Int Endod J. 1994;27(5):239–44.

DeSchepper EJ, White RR, von der Lehr W. Antibacterial effects of glass ionomers. Am J Dent. 1989;2(2):51–6.

Dong Z, Chang J, Deng Y, Joiner A. Tricalcium silicate induced mineralization for occlusion of dentinal tubules. Aust Dent J. 2011;56(2):175–80.

Economides N, Panagiotis B, Kolokouris I, Gogos C, Kokorikos I. Comparative study of the sealing ability of a polydimethylsiloxane-based root canal sealer. Braz Dent J. 2005;16(2):145–8.

Georgopoulou MK, Wu MK, Nikolaou A, Wesselink PR. Effect of thickness on the sealing ability of some root canal sealers. Oral Surg Oral Med Oral Pathol Oral Radiol Endod. 1995;80(3):338–44.

Gogos C, Economides N, Stavrianos C, Kolokouris I, Kokorikos I. Adhesion of a new methacrylate resin-based sealer to human dentin. J Endod. 2004;30(4):238–40.

Goldberg F, Artaza LP, De Silvio A. Apical sealing ability of a new glass ionomer root canal sealer. J Endod. 1995;21(10):498–500.

Han L, Okiji T (2011) Evaluation of the ions release / incorporation of the prototype S-PRG filler-containing endodontic sealer. Dent Mater J. 2011;30(6): 898–903.

Heling I, Chandler NP. The antimicrobial effect within dentinal tubules of four root canal sealers. J Endod. 1996;22(5):257–9.

Ikebe K, Ettinger RL, Wefel JS. In vitro evaluation of fluoride-releasing restorative materials for sealing the root canals of overdenture abutments. Int J Prosthodont. 2001;14(6):556–62.

International Standards Organization (2012) Dentistry. Root canal sealing materials. ISO 6876

Jack RM, Goodell GG. In vitro comparison of coronal microleakage between Resilon alone and gutta-percha with a glass-ionomer intraorifice barrier using a fluid filtration model. J Endod. 2008;34(6): 718–20.

Kolokuris I, Beltes P, Economides N, Vlemmas I. Experimental study of the biocompatibility of a new glass-ionomer root canal sealer (Ketac-Endo). J Endod. 1996;22(8):395–8.

Koulaouzidou EA, Papazisis KT, Economides NA, Beltes P, Kortsaris AH. Antiproliferative effect of mineral trioxide aggregate, zinc oxide-eugenol cement, and glass-ionomer cement against three fibroblastic cell lines. J Endod. 2005;31(1):44–6.

Kumar RV, Shruthi C. Evaluation of the sealing ability of resin cement used as a root canal sealer: an in vitro study. J Conserv Dent. 2012;15(3):274–7.

Lalh MS, Titley K, Torneck CD, Friedman S. The shear bond strength of glass ionomer cement sealers to bovine dentine conditioned with common endodontic irrigants. Int Endod J. 1999a;32(6):430–5.

Lalh MS, Titley KC, Torneck CD, Friedman S. Scanning electron microscopic study of the interface of glass ionomer cement sealers and conditioned bovine dentin. J Endod. 1999b;25(11):743–6.

Lee BN, Son HJ, Noh HJ, Koh JT, Chang HS, Hwang IN, Hwang YC, Oh WM. Cytotoxicity of newly developed ortho MTA root-end filling materials. J Endod. 2012;38(12):1627–30.

Lee KW, Williams MC, Camps JJ, Pashley DH. Adhesion of endodontic sealers to dentin and gutta-percha. J Endod. 2002;28(10):684–8.

Leonard JE, Gutmann JL, Guo IY. Apical and coronal seal of roots obturated with a dentine bonding agent and resin. Int Endod J. 1996;29(2):76–83.

Lin A, McIntyre NS, Davidson RD. Studies on the adhesion of glass-ionomer cements to dentin. J Dent Res. 1992;71(11):1836–41.

Lin CP, Chen YJ, Lee YL, Wang JS, Chang MC, Lan WH, Chang HH, Chao WM, Tai TF, Lee MY, Lin BR, Jeng JH. Effects of root-end filling materials and eugenol on mitochondrial dehydrogenase activity and cytotoxicity to human periodontal ligament fibroblasts. J Biomed Mater Res B Appl Biomater. 2004;71(2):429–40.

Lodiene G, Kleivmyr M, Bruzell E, Ørstavik D. Sealing ability of mineral trioxide aggregate, glass ionomer cement and composite resin when repairing large furcal perforations. Br Dent J. 2011;210(5), E7.

Lucena C, Lopez JM, Pulgar R, Abalos C, Valderrama MJ. Potential errors and misuse of statistics in studies on leakage in endodontics. Int Endod J. 2013;46:323–31.

Lyroudia K, Pantelidou O, Mikrogeorgis G, Chatzikallinikidis C, Nikopoulos N, Pitas I. The use of 3D computerized reconstruction for the study of coronal microleakage. Int Endod J. 2000;33(3):243–7.

Malone 3rd KH, Donnelly JC. An in vitro evaluation of coronal microleakage in obturated root canals without coronal restorations. J Endod. 1997;23(1):35–8.

Mavec JC, McClanahan SB, Minah GE, Johnson JD, Blundell Jr RE. Effects of an intracanal glass ionomer barrier on coronal microleakage in teeth with post space. J Endod. 2006;32(2):120–2.

Meiers JC, Miller GA. Antibacterial activity of dentin bonding systems, resin-modified glass ionomers, and polyacid-modified composite resins. Oper Dent. 1996;21(6):257–64.

Miletić I, Anić I, Pezelj-Ribarić S, Jukić S. Leakage of five root canal sealers. Int Endod J. 1999;32(5):415–8.

Miletić I, Ribarić SP, Karlović Z, Jukić S, Bosnjak A, Anić I. Apical leakage of five root canal sealers after one year of storage. J Endod. 2002;28(6):431–2.

Mitra SB, Kedrowski BL. Long-term mechanical properties of glass ionomers. Dent Mater. 1994;10(2):78–82.

Nagas E, Altundasar E, Serper A. The effect of master point taper on bond strength and apical sealing ability of different root canal sealers. Oral Surg Oral Med Oral Pathol Oral Radiol Endod. 2009;107(1):e61–4.

Najar AL, Saquy PC, Vansan LP, Sousa-Neto MD. Adhesion of a glass-ionomer root canal sealer to human dentine. Aust Endod J. 2003;29(1):20–2.

Ogasawara T, Yoshimine Y, Yamamoto M, Akamine A. Biocompatibility of an experimental glass-ionomer cement sealer in rat mandibular bone. Oral Surg Oral Med Oral Pathol Oral Radiol Endod. 2003;96(4):458–65.

Oliver CM, Abbott PV. An in vitro study of apical and coronal microleakage of laterally condensed gutta percha with Ketac-Endo and AH-26. Aust Dent J. 1998;43(4):262–8.

Olson AK, MacPherson MG, Hartwell GR, Weller RN, Kulild JC. An in vitro evaluation of injectable thermoplasticized gutta-percha, glass ionomer, and amalgam when used as retrofilling materials. J Endod. 1990;16(8):361–4.

Ozata F, Erdilek N, Tezel H. A comparative sealability study of different retrofilling materials. Int Endod J. 1993;26(4):241–5.

Ravichandra PV, Vemisetty H, Deepthi K, Reddy SJ, Ramkiran D, Jaya Nagendra Krishna M, Malathi G. Comparative evaluation of marginal adaptation of Biodentine™ and other commonly used root end filling materials-an invitro study. J Clin Diagn Res. 2014;8(3):243–5.

Peltola M, Salo T, Oikarinen K. Toxic effects of various retrograde root filling materials on gingival fibroblasts and rat sarcoma cells. Endod Dent Traumatol. 1992;8(3):120–4.

Pommel L, About I, Pashley D, Camps J. Apical leakage of four endodontic sealers. J Endod. 2003;29(3):208–10.

Rohde TR, Bramwell JD, Hutter JW, Roahen JO. An in vitro evaluation of microleakage of a new root canal sealer. J Endod. 1996;22(7):365–8.

Roth S. A laboratory study of glass ionomer cement as a retrograde root-filling material. Aust Dent J. 1991;36(5):384–90.

Saleh IM, Ruyter IE, Haapasalo M, Ørstavik D. The effects of dentine pretreatment on the adhesion of root-canal sealers. Int Endod J. 2002;35(10):859–66.

Saleh IM, Ruyter IE, Haapasalo MP, Orstavik D. Adhesion of endodontic sealers: scanning electron microscopy and energy dispersive spectroscopy. J Endod. 2003;29(9):595–601.

Saunders WP, Saunders EM, Herd D, Stephens E. The use of glass ionomer as a root canal sealer – a pilot study. Int Endod J. 1992;25(5):238–44.

Schuurs AH, Wu MK, Wesselink PR, Duivenvoorden HJ. Endodontic leakage studies reconsidered. Part II. Statistical aspects. Int Endod J. 1993;26:44–52.

Seppä L, Forss H, Ogaard B. The effect of fluoride application on fluoride release and the antibacterial action of glass ionomers. J Dent Res. 1993;72(9):1310–4.

Shah PM, Chong BS, Sidhu SK, Ford TR. Radiopacity of potential root-end filling materials. Oral Surg Oral Med Oral Pathol Oral Radiol Endod. 1996;81(4):476–9.

Shalhav M, Fuss Z, Weiss EI. In vitro antibacterial activity of a glass ionomer endodontic sealer. J Endod. 1997;23(10):616–9.

Shu M, Pearce EI, Sissons CH, Coote GE, Miller JH. Fluoride distribution in sound and carious root tissues of human teeth. Caries Res. 1998;32(4):239–46.

Sidhu SK, Schmalz G. The biocompatibility of glass-ionomer cement materials. A status report for the American Journal of Dentistry. Am J Dent. 2001;14(6):387–96.

Smith MA, Steiman HR. An in vitro evaluation of microleakage of two new and two old root canal sealers. J Endod. 1994;20(1):18–21.

Souza NJ, Justo GZ, Oliveira CR, Haun M, Bincoletto C. Cytotoxicity of materials used in perforation repair tested using the V79 fibroblast cell line and the granulocyte-macrophage progenitor cells. Int Endod J. 2006;39(1):40–7.

Subbarao C, Neelakantan P, Subbarao CV. In vitro biocompatibility tests of glass ionomer cements impregnated with collagen or bioactive glass to fibroblasts. J Clin Pediatr Dent. 2012;36(3):269–74.

Sutimuntanakul S, Worayoskowit W, Mangkornkarn C. Retrograde seal in ultrasonically prepared canals. J Endod. 2000;26(8):444–6.

Tagger M, Tagger E, Tjan AH, Bakland LK. Measurement of adhesion of endodontic sealers to dentin. J Endod. 2002;28(5):351–4.

Tai KW, Chang YC. Cytotoxicity evaluation of perforation repair materials on human periodontal ligament cells in vitro. J Endod. 2000;26(7):395–7.

Tanomaru-Filho M, Jorge EG, Tanomaru JM, Gonçalves M. Evaluation of the radiopacity of calcium hydroxide- and glass-ionomer-based root canal sealers. Int Endod J. 2008;41(1):50–3.

Tassery H, Pertot WJ, Camps J, Proust JP, Déjou J. Comparison of two implantation sites for testing intraosseous biocompatibility. J Endod. 1999;25(9):615–8.

Tay FR, Pashley DH. Guided tissue remineralisation of partially demineralised human dentine. Biomaterials. 2008;29(8):1127–37.

Tay FR, Pashley DH. Biomimetic remineralization of resin-bonded acid-etched dentin. J Dent Res. 2009;88(8):719–24.

Timpawat S, Harnirattisai C, Senawongs P. Adhesion of a glass-ionomer root canal sealer to the root canal wall. J Endod. 2001;27(3):168–71.

Timpawat S, Sripanaratanakul S. Apical sealing ability of glass ionomer sealer with and without smear layer. J Endod. 1998;24(5):343–5.

Vajrabhaya LO, Korsuwannawong S, Jantarat J, Korre S. Biocompatibility of furcal perforation repair material using cell culture technique: Ketac Molar versus ProRoot MTA. Oral Surg Oral Med Oral Pathol Oral Radiol Endod. 2006;102(6):e48–50.

Vanni JR, Della-Bona A, Figueiredo JA, Pedro G, Voss D, Kopper PM. Radiographic evaluation of furcal perforations sealed with different materials in dogs' teeth. J Appl Oral Sci. 2011;19(4):421–5.

Vermeersch G, Leloup G, Delmée M, Vreven J. Antibacterial activity of glass-ionomer cements, compomers and resin composites: relationship between acidity and material setting phase. J Oral Rehabil. 2005;32(5):368–74.

Vosoughhosseini S, Lotfi M, Shahmoradi K, Saghiri MA, Zand V, Mehdipour M, Ranjkesh B, Mokhtari H, Salemmilani A, Doosti S. Microleakage comparison of glass-ionomer and white mineral trioxide aggregate used as a coronal barrier in nonvital bleaching. Med Oral Patol Oral Cir Bucal. 2011;16(7):e1017–21.

Watson TF, Atmeh AR, Sajini S, Cook RJ, Festy F. Present and future of glass-ionomers and calcium-silicate cements as bioactive materials in dentistry: biophotonics-based interfacial analyses in health and disease. Dent Mater. 2014;30(1):50–61.

Wilson AD, McLean JW. Glass-ionomer cement. Chicago: Quintessence Publishing; 1988.

Wu MK, De Gee AJ, Wesselink PR. Leakage of AH26 and Ketac-Endo used with injected warm gutta-percha. J Endod. 1997;23(5):331–6.

Wu MK, De Gee AJ, Wesselink PR. Leakage of four root canal sealers at different thickness. Int Endod J. 1994;27(6):304–8.

Wu MK, Wesselink PR. Endodontic leakage studies reconsidered. Part I. Methodology, application and relevance. Int Endod J. 1993;26:37–43.

Xavier CB, Weismann R, de Oliveira MG, Demarco FF, Pozza DH. Root-end filling materials: apical microleakage and marginal adaptation. J Endod. 2005;31(7):539–42.

The Role of Glass-ionomers in Paediatric Dentistry

6

David John Manton and Katie Bach

Abstract

Children provide many challenges in clinical dentistry and behaviour management. All dental care provided for a child should consider the characteristics of that individual such as age, behavioural capabilities and 'total treatment load'. Especially in the child at high risk of dental caries, the use of low-viscosity glass-ionomer cements (GICs) in timely protection of 'at-risk' surfaces of molar teeth is of great benefit. The selection of an appropriate restorative material can be influenced by the caries risk, age to exfoliation of the primary tooth, size and position of the carious lesion, pulpal status and other factors such as appearance. GICs are the primary material of choice for the cementation of preformed metal crowns and are also useful in sealing over pulpotomy agents to maintain seal and pulpal health. The use of GIC in orthodontics, especially in those individuals with increased caries risk, is advisable. Whether used as a band or bracket cement, GIC decreases the risk and extent of white spot lesion formation around orthodontic fixtures, and if applied accordingly, bond strengths are high enough to undertake orthodontic care efficiently.

6.1 Introduction

Glass-ionomer cements (GICs) are one of the materials that are highly suited for use in children; however, due to the apparent simplicity of its use and often claimed (but sometimes overstated) widespread suitability for many restorative situations, it is also prone to misuse as well. From pit and fissure sealing to temporisation of a carious lesion to definitive restorative care, GIC can be used widely in the child; however, like all materials, the suitability of GIC should be considered in the context of the individual case.

D.J. Manton, BDSc, MDSc, PhD (✉)
Department of Growth and Development,
University of Melbourne, Melbourne Dental School,
Carlton, VIC, Australia
e-mail: djmanton@unimelb.edu.au

K. Bach, BDS, DCD
Oral Health Unit, Auckland District Health Board,
Auckland, New Zealand

S.K. Sidhu (ed.), *Glass-Ionomers in Dentistry*, DOI 10.1007/978-3-319-22626-2_6

6.2 Prevention of Caries

In the developing child, the occlusal surfaces of the first permanent molars are at high risk for the development of carious lesions due to the inability to clean the pits and fissures effectively, so protection of these surfaces in a child is imperative to reduce the need for restorative care. The risk of occlusal caries can be reduced by the placement of fissure sealants on these surfaces (Beauchamp et al. 2008). Traditionally, the fissure sealant of choice has been resin based; however, for resin sealants to be successful, excellent moisture control must be obtained, and this often relies on the placement of rubber dam (Simonsen and Neal 2011). For many children, it is not possible to achieve adequate moisture control due to inability to place a rubber dam clamp, often due to partial tooth eruption or behavioural issues.

Glass-ionomer cements can provide an effective alternative option for fissure sealing, where moisture control or access may prove difficult (Fig. 6.1). This may be advantageous in young children with partially erupted teeth or in patients with special needs. It must be appreciated that these surface protectants may not have retention rates as successful as traditional resin sealants placed in a carefully controlled environment. However, the important issue to consider is that prevention of caries is the outcome of interest with sealants, and many studies report that caries prevention is similar between resin- and GIC-based sealants. Using an impression technique, Frencken et al. (2007) reported micro-retention of GIC in the base of the fissures in teeth that appeared to have lost their GIC sealant, possibly providing a mechanism and explanation of why complete retention may not be as important for GICs as it is for resin-based sealants (Fig. 6.2). The leaching of fluoride from the sealant is another mechanism that may influence caries prevention, especially with the high fluoride release of low-viscosity products such as Fuji VII/Fuji Triage (GC Corp, Tokyo, Japan).

Whilst resin-based sealants have higher retention rates, this does not necessarily equate to higher rates of caries prevention (Ulusu et al. 2012). Much of the evidence regarding both resin and GIC sealants may be affected by selection and publication bias (Simonsen 1996). The literature does not suggest that there is any difference between the caries-preventive effects of GIC and resin-based fissure sealants (Mickenautsch and Yengopal 2011). When GIC sealants clinically appear partially or totally lost, often the base of the fissures still remains sealed (Mickenautsch et al. 2011). There is evidence to suggest that whilst the bulk of the GIC sealant material placed may be lost within 2–3 years post-placement, newly erupted teeth that are sealed with GIC show a significantly lower dentine caries rate than those that were not sealed (Taifour et al. 2003).

Glass-ionomer sealants have the added benefit that they may be placed outside the traditional 'dental environment', as they can be placed with limited dental instrumentation and infrastructure. This may have added benefits in developing

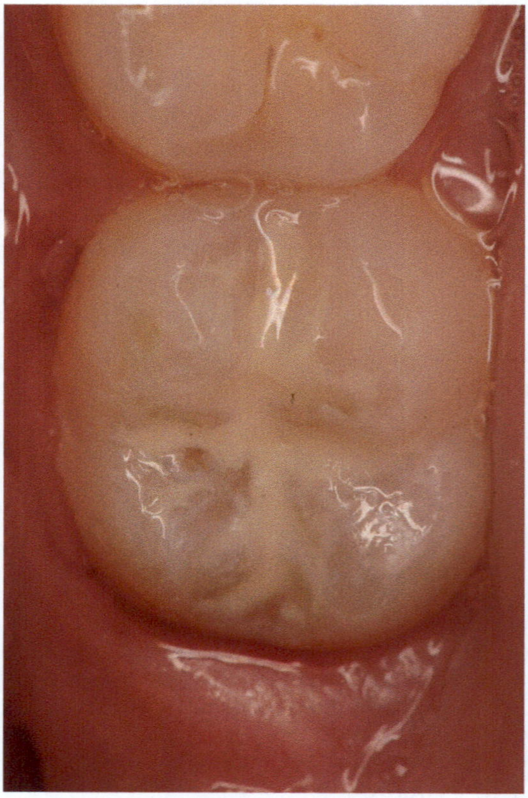

Fig. 6.1 Glass-ionomer sealant (Fuji IX GP Extra, GC Corp, Tokyo, Japan) on first permanent molar (Courtesy of A/Prof J. Lucas)

countries or for school-based sealant programmes, especially as they can be hand mixed, negating the need for electricity for a triturator or suction and a light-curing unit required for resin-based sealants. However, this is not to suggest that GIC sealants can be placed in an environment heavily contaminated by saliva, as this will reduce the sealing capability and retention rate, although nowhere near the effect contamination has on resin-based sealants – environmental

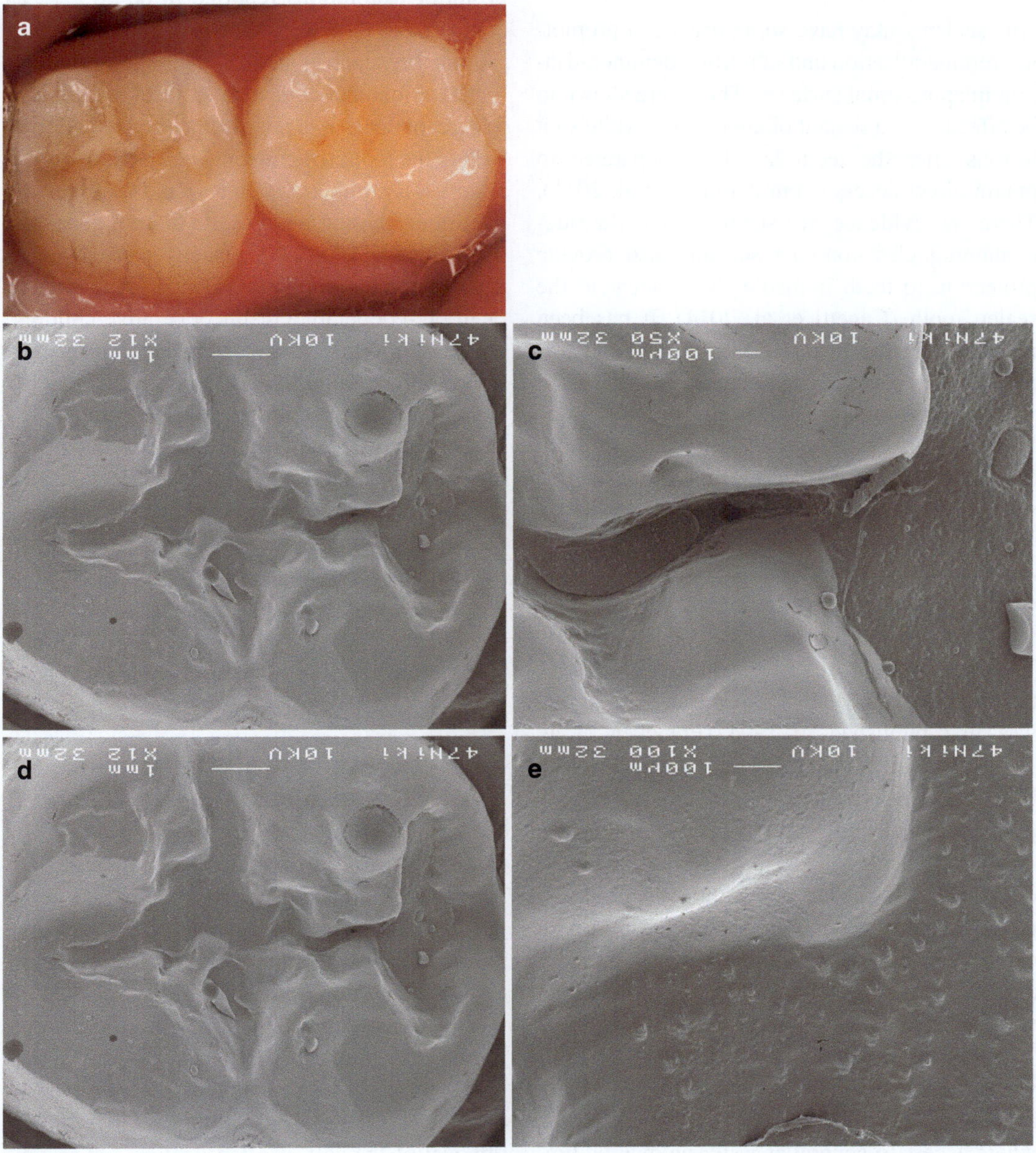

Fig. 6.2 Glass-ionomer cement (Fuji IX, GC Corp) sealant placed on tooth 46 (13 years previously) and tooth 47 (12 years previously). (**a**) Clinical image of GIC sealant. (**b**) SEM of resin replica of remnant GIC in 47 fissure (area highlighted in Fig. 6.2a is highlighted here) (×12). (**c**) SEM of resin replica of remnant GIC in 47 fissure: higher magnification of area outlined in Figs. 6.2a, b (×50). (**d**) SEM of close surface adaptation of GIC in 47 fissure (×12). (**e**) SEM of close surface adaptation of GIC in 47 fissure: higher magnification of area outlined in Fig. 6.2d (×100) (Courtesy of Prof J. Frencken)

control is still important for GIC sealants (Kulczyk et al. 2005; Farmer et al. 2014).

6.3 Effects on Approximal Surfaces

GIC sealants may have some benefit in promoting remineralisation and inhibiting demineralisation in approximal surfaces. They were shown to be effective as a sealant of approximal white spot lesions after the teeth had been separated to obtain direct access (Trairatvorakul et al. 2011). There is evidence to suggest that fluoride-containing glass-ionomer sealants also provide protection to teeth immediately adjacent to the sealed tooth (Cagetti et al. 2014). It has been reported that the distal surfaces of second primary molars next to first permanent molars sealed with a glass-ionomer have significantly lower levels of carious lesion development than those approximating a first permanent molar sealed with a resin-based material (Cagetti et al. 2014).

6.4 Restorative Care

The atraumatic restorative treatment or ART technique, developed by Frencken and Holmgren, was first published in 1994 (Frencken et al. 1994). This technique allows a carious lesion to be prepared using hand instruments for carious tissue removal and restored using an adhesive material such as GIC. This technique is more often than not carried out without local anaesthetic. The ART technique should be used with careful case selection and is not a gold standard alternative to conventional tooth preparation and restoration where this is available.

This technique may be useful in populations where access to conventional dentistry is not available or in young and uncooperative children where access to general anaesthesia may be limited. A definitive diagnosis must be made before considering whether ART is an appropriate treatment; teeth with signs and symptoms of irreversible pulpitis, or those with lesions that extend to the pulp on radiographs, are not appropriate for this mode of treatment. The extent of the lesion must also be assessed as ART has higher success rates in teeth with single surface lesions compared to multiple surfaces (Frencken et al. 2007). The site of the lesion also has some influence, with survival rates after 6.4 years of non-occlusal posterior restorations reported to be 80.2 %, as compared to 64.8 % for occlusal posterior restorations (Frencken et al. 2007).

Glass-ionomer cement is an ideal material for this treatment as it is relatively cheap and adheres well to the tooth structure and can be hand mixed if necessary, although some would consider the quality of capsule-mixed GIC to be higher than hand mixed. As ART is usually carried out in environments with limited dental infrastructure or in pre-cooperative or uncooperative children, obtaining a retentive cavity preparation or ideal moisture control may be difficult; therefore, GIC becomes a more favourable material compared to resin composite and silver amalgam. However, the clinician should not ignore the effect of good moisture control on the success of GIC restorations. In hot and humid areas, care taken over maintaining 'normal' temperatures of the materials should be considered, as setting times and handling characteristics can vary greatly, often to the detriment of the success of the procedure.

6.5 'Contemporary' Carious Tissue Removal

A relatively recent treatment modality in dentistry, which coincides with the increased popularity of ART, is that of a more conservative attitude towards dentine caries removal (Borges et al. 2012). Teeth must be carefully selected for this procedure; clinical and radiographic diagnosis must rule out any signs and symptoms of pulpitis unable to be reversed or the presence of periapical lesions. The technique relies on the removal of the soft infected dentine and recommends leaving a small amount of firmer affected dentine. This serves to preserve tooth structure and to avoid carious or iatrogenic pulp exposure, with improved outcomes in both primary and permanent teeth (Ricketts et al. 2013). The main limitation with this concept is that it is basically impossible to determine what is affected or infected dentine in the clinical situation – and physical features such as hardness or resistance to the excavation instrument should be considered as a primary indicator, although these are also prone to subjective variability. A sound perimeter is required so that a seal can be obtained at the margins, decreasing the chance of leakage and subsequent lesion progression (Fig. 6.3).

For any restorative technique to be successful, there must be arrest of the carious process, hardening (remineralisation) of the dentine on the cavity floor, and the formation of reactionary dentine to provide protection to the pulp. The material placed over the pulp must provide an adequate seal, and antibacterial properties may be of advantage, although the seal is the primary feature the clinician should seek (Duque et al. 2009). Historically, calcium hydroxide cements have been used for both direct and indirect pulp capping. However, they have some disadvantages such as high solubility and low-compression resistance, and they do not bond well to dentine (Duque et al. 2009). There is now evidence indicating that GICs may assist with the remineralisation process of the affected dentine, due to their antibacterial properties, ion exchange capabilities involving strontium and fluoride, and favourable bonding characteristics to dentine (Duque et al. 2009; Watson et al. 2014). Recently a calcium-based remineralising agent, casein phosphopeptide-amorphous calcium phosphate (CPP-ACP), has been added to a low-viscosity GIC material to increase calcium ion release (Fuji VII EP, GC Corp, Tokyo Japan). However, there is limited evidence whether this material increases remineralisation of dentine due to its high concentration of bioavailable calcium and phosphate. The recent introduction and promotion of a calcium silicate cement (Biodentine®, Septodont, Saint-Maur-des-Fossés, France) as a dentine substitute has created another option for coverage of deep lesions. Recent research indicates that Biodentine may produce better outcomes at 12 months compared with glass-ionomer cement in deep lesions at least three-quarters into the dentine when it is used as an indirect pulp capping material. However, further research with longer-term follow-up and increased subject numbers is needed (Hashem et al. 2015).

Glass-ionomer cements may be used as a conventional restorative material in carefully selected cases. There are several factors that should be considered when selecting a restorative material for the primary dentition. The age of the child and caries risk are the first factors that should be considered, in conjunction with the size of the lesion. Caries risk is often thought of as a static factor; however, it can vary throughout life, so consistent assessment is necessary to allow the clinician to make informed decisions regarding the most appropriate preventive and restorative care of the child. The estimated time until tooth exfoliation is another important factor that varies with tooth type. Location of the lesion to be restored with respect to functional load also influences material selection, and the use of GIC in areas of high loading or in poorly supported multi-surface lesions is often inappropriate.

Glass-ionomer cements are a good base material for two-surface resin composite restorations in children. With options of the 'open' or 'closed' sandwich technique, this restoration is comprised of a GIC or resin-modified GIC (RMGIC) base that is sealed with a resin composite restoration. The open technique leaves a layer of GIC material exposed at the gingival margin of the approximal box. It is advisable to avoid having GIC at the contact point, due to possible material wear and subsequent loss of arch space. The success of open sandwich restorations has been reported to be high (Atieh 2008). The closed sandwich uses GIC as a dentine seal with resin composite enclosing the GIC. With this technique, the presence of enamel at the gingival floor of the cavity preparation is an advantage as bond strengths are increased and microleakage decreased compared to a dentine margin.

Cavity design is based around removal of soft demineralised necrotic dentine and establishment of a sound perimeter or margin. Currently, there is a lack of evidence-based definitions that relate to the treatment of carious lesions, such as what is 'hard' dentine, what is necrotic dentine, how does the clinician identify these conditions and

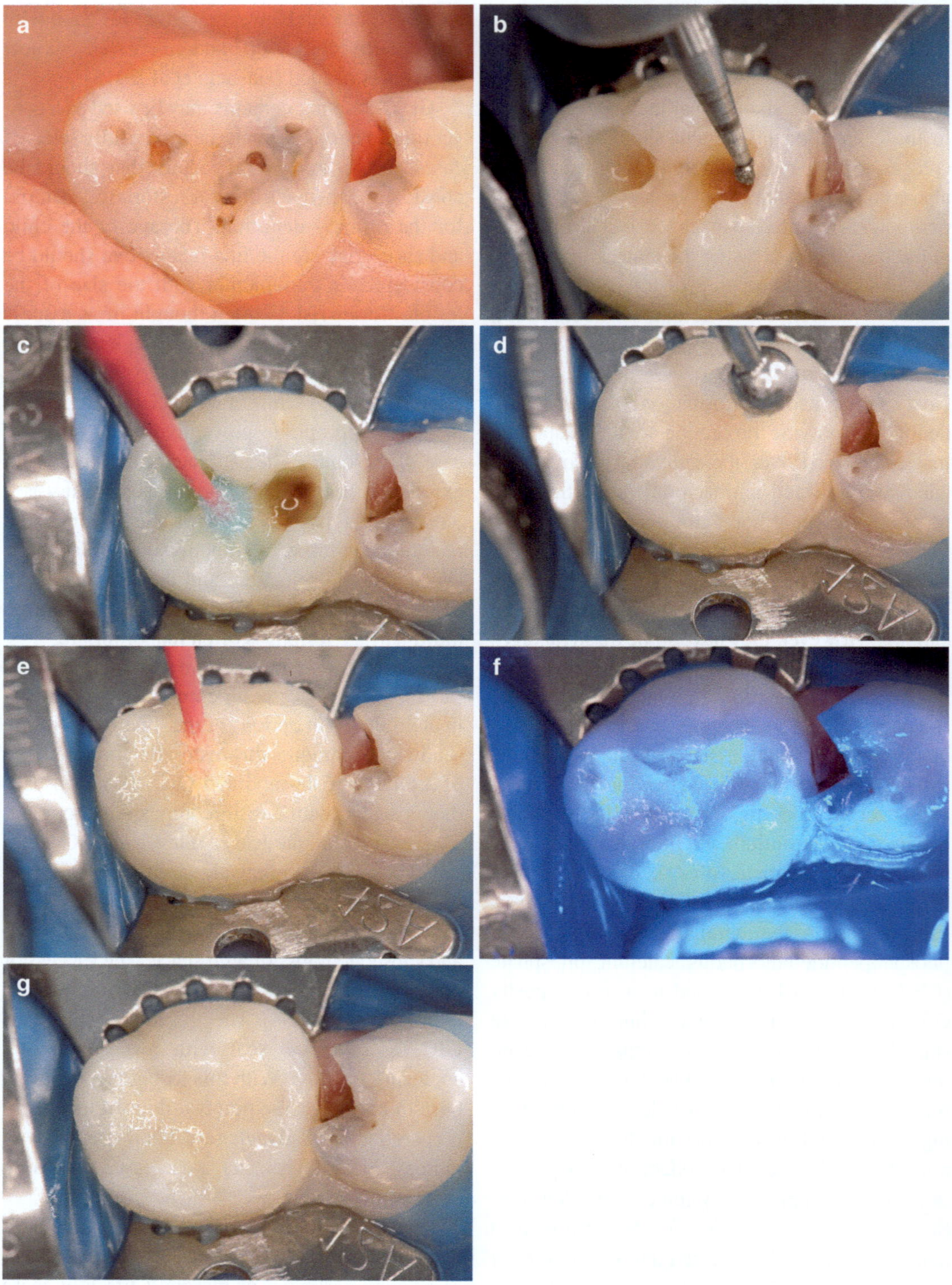

Fig. 6.3 Placement of GIC (Fuji IX) restoration in second primary molar. (**a**) Occlusal (pit and fissure) carious lesions. (**b**) Removal of degraded carious tissue. (**c**) Conditioning of prepared surfaces (note residual hard stained dentine). (**d**) Placement of GIC restorative (Fuji IX Extra, GC Corp). (**e**) Placement of resin laminate coating (G-bond, GC Corp). (**f**) Light-curing of resin laminate coating. (**g**) Final restoration. Note the carious lesion in the first primary molar. This would be suitable for preformed crown placement luted with low-viscosity GIC over GIC core – with pulp therapy if indicated (Courtesy of A/Prof J. Lucas)

also what a sound margin actually is? Fortunately, the recently established International Caries Consensus Collaboration (ICCC) is establishing guidelines for these often subjective definitions.

It is recommended that after a pulpotomy is performed on a primary molar tooth, a preformed metal crown is cemented with GIC. This provides protection of the remaining structure and a high success rate when compared to an intra-coronal tooth-coloured restoration (Kindelan et al. 2008; Hutcheson et al. 2012).

GICs can be effective materials for the cementation of preformed metallic crowns, which rely on high retentive strength and a good marginal seal to ensure that they are a successful restoration (Yilmaz et al. 2004). Poor seal may lead to the development of biofilm at the margins and subsequent microleakage, both of which may result in the development of a new carious lesion or periodontal complications. Another major issue with the lack of patency of a cement seal is the problem with pulpal health, and leakage increases the chances of pulp inflammation and necrosis, whether a pulpotomy has been undertaken or not. Adhesive cements such as glass-ionomer cements have the advantage of providing a mechanical and adhesive bond between the stainless steel crown and the tooth (Memarpour et al. 2011).

Whilst preformed metallic crowns are the most durable restorations we have in paediatric dentistry, they are still prone to wear due to excessive occlusal forces. With significant wear, areas of the occlusal surface of the crown can be perforated, exposing the luting cement and tooth structure below. In cases where the crown is soundly sealed at the gingival margin and displays no movement or signs of symptoms, one option is for the occlusal surface to be repaired, especially if the tooth is within a few years of exfoliation, with the other option being crown replacement. The material that is chosen to repair the crown must display satisfactory sealing ability to both the crown and the tooth surface, as well as create a seal that will prevent microleakage that can lead to failure of the repair or the crown/pulp complex itself. It has been shown that preformed metallic crowns that have been repaired with a GIC display lower levels of microleakage than crowns that were repaired with a resin composite (Yilmaz et al. 2011). Crown repair would usually be appropriate when the tooth is within a year or two of exfoliating; if the child is younger than this, replacement is more appropriate.

Dental care of the paediatric patient involves the consideration of a number of factors, including caries risk, age, behavioural capabilities and compliance of the child and the parents. Following are two cases illustrating differing clinical scenarios.

Clinical examples:

1. A 3-year-old male – the current high caries risk was illustrated by a highly cariogenic diet of processed foods, soft drinks and frequent snacking, poor oral hygiene and intermittent use of fluoridated toothpaste. After discussion of the risk factors with his mother, it was felt that it was unlikely that the caries risk would change in the short term. After examination and bitewing radiography, eight approximal lesions in the first and second primary molars, all cavitated and reaching the inner half of the dentine, were noted. Due to the limited ability to change caries risk, it was suggested that these teeth were restored with preformed (stainless steel) crowns cemented with a low-viscosity GIC, with pulp treatment as appropriate. This is due to the high long-term success rate of preformed crowns and the ability to 'seal off' other surfaces of the tooth at risk of developing carious lesions in the future.
2. An 8-year-old female – with high caries risk during childhood; however, this is decreasing due to a low cariogenic diet and excellent oral hygiene (assisted by her parents), so it can be considered that her caries risk is likely to become low. After examination and bitewing radiography, two approximal lesions on the distal surfaces of the maxillary second primary molars limited to the outer half of the dentine were noted. She is dentally advanced, so therefore the use of GIC or RMGIC is appropriate due to the relatively short survival time before exfoliation and her decrease in

caries risk. Care should be taken in examining the mesial surfaces of the first permanent molars when restoring the teeth, as white spot lesions may be present.

6.6 Endodontic Care

The use of GICs in the endodontic care of children can be widespread. As previously mentioned, maintenance of retention and seal of a preformed metal crown is implicitly associated with pulpal health. Other uses of GICs include orthograde and retrograde canal/apical seal and repair of root resorptive defects and perforations (De Bruyne and De Moor 2004). More recently, the use of calcium silicate cements such as mineral trioxide aggregate (MTA) and Biodentine® has taken the place of GIC in many of these endodontic procedures such as perforation and resorptive defect repair as well as apical sealing (Watson et al. 2014).

6.7 Orthodontic Care

Glass-ionomer cements have many applications in orthodontic practice. GICs can be used to cement orthodontic molar bands. These molar bands may be used as anchorage in full fixed appliances or for orthodontic appliances such as quad helices, band and loop space maintainers or habit-breaking devices. De-cementation is a common reason for failure of these appliances. However, there may be some advantage associated with a weaker bond when compared to resin-based cements, as these appliances will all eventually need to be removed, preferably without damaging any tooth structure. Another advantage is that if more than one cementation point exists, an issue with resin-based cements is that one area of adhesion can fail. However, the strength of the remaining bond allows the appliance to stay in place, with a potential for leakage and subsequent demineralisation of the underlying tooth structure, due to the inability of the patient to clean this surface. On the other hand, when there is cement failure of a bracket to the enamel, the tendency for GIC-based cements is to fail completely and the bracket debonds; this decreases the chance of enamel demineralisation from partial cement failure. The release of fluoride from the GIC-based cement also decreases demineralisation potential under the appliance. More recent RMGIC materials have been reported to have similar bond strengths to resin cements, especially if the enamel surface is pretreated (Cheng et al. 2011).

The downside of using GICs with orthodontic brackets is that they have lower bond strengths than conventional resin cements (Wiltshire 1994). The bond strength of a GIC may be improved by adding resin as in RMGICs. These resin-modified GICs have higher bond strengths and may have an advantage in cementation of brackets (Shimazu et al. 2013).

There is building evidence of the benefits that RMGIC cements may bring for bonding of orthodontic brackets in patients with increased caries risk. In many cases, orthodontic appliances increase an individual's caries risk, with many patients developing white spot lesions adjacent to brackets (Sudjalim et al. 2006; Benson et al. 2013). Apart from the potential of a need for restoration if advanced, these lesions are unsightly and pose a challenge to remineralise with an aesthetic result in an acceptable time period for the patient. Glass-ionomer cements provide the advantage of fluoride release that reduces the progression and extent of carious lesion development (Czochrowska et al. 1998; Benson et al. 2005; Paschos et al. 2015). There are also reported antibacterial effects from a commercially available RMGIC orthodontic lute (Fuji ORTHO LC, GC Corp, Tokyo, Japan) which may have some impact on demineralisation in the local area (Slutzky et al. 2014).

The use of protective coatings around brackets in high-risk patients has been suggested. Materials such as resin-based sealants have been proposed; however, recent in vitro research indicates that low-viscosity high-F-release materials such as GICs may have more of a role in this area, especially due to their long-term fluoride release (Yap et al. 2014).

In some cases, prior or during orthodontic treatment, it may be advantageous to temporarily increase the vertical dimension for occlusal clearance of interferences. Occlusal clearance may be required to correct crossbites or create space to move teeth. This can be achieved with the placement of GIC or RMGIC on the occlusal surfaces of the posterior teeth. This involves no tooth preparation of the teeth and the material is easily removed.

6.8 Parental Concerns

There are growing numbers of parents who have increasing demands with respect to the materials that are used as restorative materials in their children; these are often parents who demand the most aesthetic restoration for their child. Many resin-based sealants and resin composites include in their ingredient list a derivative of bisphenol A (BPA), most often BPA glycidyl dimethacrylate (bis-GMA) (Fleisch et al. 2010). Pure BPA may have some oestrogenic properties and disrupt some endocrine functions, and the evidence suggests that exposure to BPA may have some adverse health effects (Fleisch et al. 2010). Some researchers have suggested that exposure to BPAs may increase the prevalence of hypomineralised enamel defects (Jedeon et al. 2013). The current evidence suggests that exposure to BPA from dental materials is transient and that exposure can be well controlled in the dental surgery as long as the resin cement is cured effectively (Fleisch et al. 2010; Purushothaman et al. 2015). However, in the current climate of 'google medicine' and the ability of parents to find reports from many sources, there can be times where they will be reluctant to consent to some materials being used; unfortunately, these parents may also be those who are reluctant to have fluoride-containing materials placed in their children. Glass-ionomer cements may be useful in these cases provided that the material is clinically indicated and appropriate and that the parent will accept a fluoride-containing restorative material. In these cases, parents must be warned of the limitations of this material over resin composite in certain situations. However, some parents may be concerned about the other constituents of GICs such as aluminium and their putative relationship with neurodegenerative diseases. There is little evidence to support such a relationship; however, clinicians need to be aware of possible concerns of parents and be able to answer their concerns readily.

Conclusions

Glass-ionomer cements can be used in a variety of situations in children from prevention of dental caries to endodontics and orthodontics. The selection of an appropriate restorative material can be influenced by the caries risk, age to exfoliation of the primary tooth, size and position of the carious lesion, pulpal status and other factors such as appearance. GICs may be used as a conventional restorative material in carefully selected cases, as well as in the ART technique, as a base material under resin composite restorations, in the treatment of uncooperative children and those with special needs. They are also useful for the protection of pits/fissures and 'at-risk' surfaces of molar teeth, especially in the child at high risk of dental caries. GICs are the primary material of choice for the cementation of preformed metal crowns and are also useful in sealing over pulpotomy agents to maintain seal and pulpal health. The use of GIC in orthodontics, especially in those individuals with increased caries risk, reduces the risk and extent of white spot lesion formation around orthodontic fixtures. With appropriate treatment planning and consideration of the child's individual needs, the use of GICs can be of great benefit and simplify the treatment for the child and the clinician.

Bibliography

Atieh M. Stainless steel crown versus modified open-sandwich restorations for primary molars: a 2-year randomized clinical trial. Int J Paediatr Dent. 2008;18:325–32.

Beauchamp J, Caufield PW, Crall JJ, Donly K, Feigal R, Gooch B, Ismail A, Kohn W, Siegal M, Simonsen R,

Frantsve-Hawley J. Evidence-based clinical recommendations for the use of pit-and-fissure sealants – a report of the American Dental Association Council on Scientific Affairs. J Am Dent Assoc. 2008;139:257–68.

Benson P, Shah A, Millett D, Dyer F, Parkin N, Vine R. Fluorides, orthodontics and demineralization: a systematic review. J Orthod. 2005;32:102–14.

Benson PE, Parkin N, Dyer F, Millett DT, Furness S, Germain P. Fluorides for the prevention of early tooth decay (demineralised white lesions) during fixed brace treatment. Cochrane Database Syst Rev. 2013;(12):CD003809.

Borges BCD, De Souza Borges J, Braz R, Montes MAJR, De Assunção Pinheiro IV. Arrest of non-cavitated dentinal occlusal caries by sealing pits and fissures: a 36-month, randomised controlled clinical trial. Int Dent J. 2012;62:251–5.

Cagetti M, Carta G, Cocco F, Sale S, Congiu G, Mura A, Strohmenger L, Lingström P, Campus G, Bossù M. Effect of fluoridated sealants on adjacent tooth surfaces a 30-mo randomized clinical trial. J Dent Res. 2014;93:59s–65.

Cheng HY, Chen CH, Li CL, Tsai HH, Chou TH, Wang WN. Bond strength of orthodontic light-cured resin-modified glass ionomer cement. Eur J Orthod. 2011;33:180–4.

Czochrowska E, Ogaard B, Duschner H, Ruben J, Arends J. Cariostatic effect of a light-cured, resin-reinforced glass-ionomer for bonding orthodontic brackets in vivo. J Orofac Orthop. 1998;59:265–73.

De Bruyne MAA, De Moor RJG. The use of glass ionomer cements in both conventional and surgical endodontics. Int Endod J. 2004;37:91–104.

Duque C, De Cássia Negrini T, Sacono NT, Spolidorio DMP, De Souza Costa CA, Hebling J. Clinical and microbiological performance of resin-modified glass-ionomer liners after incomplete dentine caries removal. Clin Oral Investig. 2009;13:465–71.

Farmer SN, Ludlow SW, Donaldson ME, Tantbirojn D, Versluis A. Microleakage of composite and two types of glass ionomer restorations with saliva contamination at different steps. Pediatr Dent. 2014;36:14–7.

Fleisch AF, Sheffield PE, Chinn C, Edelstein BL, Landrigan PJ. Bisphenol A and related compounds in dental materials. Pediatrics. 2010;126:760–8.

Frencken JE, Songpaisan Y, Phantumvanit P, Pilot T. An atraumatic restorative treatment (ART) technique: evaluation after one year. Int Dent J. 1994;44:460–4.

Frencken J, Van't Hof M, Taifour D, Al-Zaher I. Effectiveness of art and traditional amalgam approach in restoring single-surface cavities in posterior teeth of permanent dentitions in school children after 6.3 years. Community Dent Oral Epidemiol. 2007;35:207–14.

Hashem D, Mannocci F, Patel S, Manoharan A, Brown JE, Watson TF, Banerjee A. Clinical and radiographic assessment of the efficacy of calcium silicate indirect pulp capping: a randomized controlled clinical trial. J Dent Res. 2015;94:562–8.

Hutcheson C, Seale NS, Mcwhorter A, Kerins C, Wright J. Multi-surface composite vs stainless steel crown restorations after mineral trioxide aggregate pulpotomy: a randomized controlled trial. Pediatr Dent. 2012;34:460–7.

Jedeon K, De La Dure-Molla M, Brookes SJ, Loiodice S, Marciano C, Kirkham J, Canivenc-Lavier M-C, Boudalia S, Berges R, Harada H, Berdal A, Babajko S. Enamel defects reflect perinatal exposure to bisphenol A. Am J Pathol. 2013;183:108–18.

Kindelan SA, Day P, Nichol R, Willmott N, Fayle SA. UK National Clinical Guidelines in Paediatric Dentistry: stainless steel preformed crowns for primary molars. Int J Paediatr Dent. 2008;18:20–8.

Kulczyk KE, Sidhu SK, Mccabe JF. Salivary contamination and bond strength of glass-ionomers to dentin. Oper Dent. 2005;30:676–83.

Memarpour M, Mesbahi M, Rezvani G, Rahimi M. Microleakage of adhesive and nonadhesive luting cements for stainless steel crowns. Pediatr Dent. 2011;33:501–4.

Mickenautsch S, Yengopal V. Caries-preventive effect of glass ionomer and resin-based fissure sealants on permanent teeth: an update of systematic review evidence. BMC Res Notes. 2011;4:22.

Mickenautsch S, Mount G, Yengopal V. Therapeutic effect of glass-ionomers: an overview of evidence. Aust Dent J. 2011;56:10–5.

Paschos E, Galosi T, Huth K, Rudzki I, Wichelhaus A, Kunzelmann K-H. Do bonding agents protect the bracket-periphery?—Evaluation by consecutive μCT scans and fluorescence measurements. Clin Oral Investig. 2015;19:159–68.

Purushothaman D, Kailasam V, Chitharanjan AB. Bisphenol a release from orthodontic adhesives and its correlation with the degree of conversion. Am J Orthod Dentofacial Orthop. 2015;147:29–36.

Ricketts D, Lamont T, Innes NP, Kidd E, Clarkson JE. Operative caries management in adults and children. Cochrane Database Syst Rev. 2013;(3):CD003808.

Shimazu K, Ogata K, Karibe H. Evaluation of the caries-preventive effect of three orthodontic band cements in terms of fluoride release, retentiveness, and microleakage. Dent Mater J. 2013;32:376–80.

Simonsen RJ. Glass ionomer as fissure sealant—a critical review. J Public Health Dent. 1996;56:146–9.

Simonsen RJ, Neal RC. A review of the clinical application and performance of pit and fissure sealants. Aust Dent J. 2011;56:45–58.

Slutzky H, Feuerstern O, Namuz K, Shpack N, Lewinstein I, Matalon S. The effects of in vitro fluoride mouth rinse on the antibacterial properties of orthodontic cements. Orthod Craniofac Res. 2014;17:150–7.

Sudjalim TR, Woods MG, Manton DJ. Prevention of white spot lesions in orthodontic practice: a contemporary review. Aust Dent J. 2006;51:284–9.

Taifour D, Frencken JE, Beiruti N, Truin GJ. Effects of glass ionomer sealants in newly erupted first molars after 5 years: a pilot study. Community Dent Oral Epidemiol. 2003;31:314–9.

Trairatvorakul C, Itsaraviriyakul S, Wiboonchan W. Effect of glass-ionomer cement on the progression of proximal caries. J Dent Res. 2011;90:99–103.

Ulusu T, Odabaş ME, Tüzüner T, Baygin Ö, Sillelioğlu H, Deveci C, Gökdoğan FG, Altuntaş A. The success rates of a glass ionomer cement and a resin-based fissure sealant placed by fifth-year undergraduate dental students. Eur Arch Paediatr Dent. 2012;13:94–7.

Watson TF, Atmeh AR, Sajini S, Cook RJ, Festy F. Present and future of glass-ionomers and calcium-silicate cements as bioactive materials in dentistry: biophotonics-based interfacial analyses in health and disease. Dent Mater. 2014;30:50–61.

Wiltshire WA. Shear bond strengths of a glass-ionomer for direct bonding in orthodontics. Am J Orthod Dentofacial Orthop. 1994;106:127–30.

Yap J, Walsh LJ, Naser-Ud Din S, Ngo H, Manton DJ. Evaluation of a novel approach in the prevention of white spot lesions around orthodontic brackets. Aust Dent J. 2014;59:70–80.

Yilmaz Y, Dalmis A, Gurbuz T, Simsek S. Retentive force and microleakage of stainless steel crowns cemented with three different luting agents. Dent Mater J. 2004;23:577–84.

Yilmaz Y, Belduz Kara N, Yilmaz A, Sahin H. Wear and repair of stainless steel crowns. Eur J Paediatr Dent. 2011;12:25–30.

7 The Future of Glass-ionomers

Joshua J. Cheetham

Abstract

As the use and acceptance of glass-ionomer cement (GIC) increase, the scientific community will endeavour to improve current limitations due to their relatively low physical properties compared to other materials. This chapter discusses a range of future improvements in glass-ionomer cements which will increase their longevity and allow them to be used in place of other materials such as the widely used amalgam.

To improve their material properties, many paths can be investigated. New glass filler systems, including a variety of additions, modifications and pre-reacted GIC filler particles, and their effect on physical properties are detailed in this chapter. Other categories of filler particles, including spherical particles, glass fibre reinforcement and nanoparticle developments, as well as their effect on improving GIC properties such as fracture toughness, wear and other physical and aesthetic properties are documented.

Technologies utilising GIC materials as controlled-release vehicles for different materials are discussed. The importance of new mechanisms, such as self-healing technologies and self-cleaning glass technology, is documented in efforts to improve the longevity of GICs and their physical properties. Novel polymer networks, developed for improvements in strength and other properties, and technologies related to porosity reduction, methods to improve fracture toughness and improvements in adhesion durability are also be provided. Future delivery systems provide the user with an insight of what could be the new delivery systems of GICs. Important avenues for the improvement of GIC wear properties, and improvements in aesthetic properties are discussed.

J.J. Cheetham, BE, MBA, PhD
Department of Research and Development,
SDI Limited, Bayswater, VIC 3153, Australia
e-mail: joshua.cheetham@sdi.com.au

S.K. Sidhu (ed.), *Glass-Ionomers in Dentistry*, DOI 10.1007/978-3-319-22626-2_7

Other topics focus on the future use of GIC participating in pharmacological approaches to caries reduction and restorative dentistry and include biomineralisation and biopromoting improvements, biofilm alterations, the antimicrobial/bioprotection properties of GICs and the possibility of antibiotic additions.

7.1 Introduction

As permanent restorative materials, glass-ionomer cements (GICs) (both resin-modified and conventional self-cure versions) still have limitations when placed in stress-bearing restorations due to their relatively low fracture strength, toughness and wear properties (Lohbauer 2009). GICs are generally inferior in aesthetics and physical properties compared to composite resin materials.

Although the GIC bond is considered to be one of the most resilient with a lower annual failure rate compared to adhesively bonded composite resins, the bulk material mechanical properties still hinder its wide usage (Peumans et al. 2005). Variants of GICs are now available to restore different classes of cavities; however, amalgam and adhesively bonded composite resins remain the popular choice for restorative materials. A recent study has highlighted the importance of a dental material's ability to preserve existing tooth structure and prevent secondary caries, which places GICs in a good position against other materials (Seemann et al. 2014). It is unlikely that in the short term, GICs will achieve wear, strength or longevity properties seen in amalgam and composite resins, but the focus of future developments may deliver GICs with great improvements in these properties.

7.2 GIC as an Alternative to Amalgam

GICs are specifically used for their dynamic interaction with the tooth structure, compared to the relatively "inert" and static relationship that composite resin and amalgam have with the adjacent tooth structure interface. It is this "dynamic" environment and distinct interface created by GIC materials that has enabled their use to grow.

As more advanced analytical techniques are employed to investigate and critique restorative material interfaces, GICs continue to find an unique position in terms of their technical offering to the clinician. Glass-ionomer cements have gained relevance due to their ability to self-adhere to tooth structure, biomimetic/re-mineralising properties, anti-cariogenic potential and their relative ease of use (Peumans et al. 2005; Benelli et al. 1993). Currently, bulk-fill composite resin restorations are replacing amalgam as an accepted choice for a permanent restoration, and it is this area where new GIC advances are likely to play a role.

Furthermore, as a response to the Minamata Convention on Mercury (Mackey et al. 2014), the use of amalgams is decreasing, and clinicians are now choosing alternative materials. Currently, GIC has been recommended for small, non-load-bearing permanent restorations. Although lacking the strength or wear properties achieved by amalgam, the use of modern GIC materials is similar in many ways to amalgam. For example, both amalgam and GIC placement does not require the use of an adhesive. As GICs contain water in their formulations, they can be placed on moist dentine.

Furthermore, new-generation GICs such as Chemfil™ Rock (Dentsply DeTrey GmbH, Konstanz, Germany), Ketac™ Universal Aplicap™ (3MESPE Dental Products, St. Paul, MN, USA) and Equi Forte (GC Corporation, Itabashi-ku, Tokyo, Japan) do not necessarily require cavity conditioning and can be placed in cavity preparations similar to amalgam. Modern "condensable" high viscosity GIC materials are immediately condensable, and as their setting reaction proceeds, they become even more condensable, which facilitates their "packing" into the cavity in a similar way to amalgam. In addition, resin-modified GICs (RMGICs) have also been shown to place minimum polymerisation stress on cavity walls, which could further explain their durable bonding mechanism (Cheetham et al. 2014a).

In contrast, variables such as adhesive placement, isolation procedures, visible light-curing and polymerisation shrinkage stress make adhesively bonded composites more difficult to use (Gerdolle et al. 2008). Prior to 2012, the majority of GIC manufacturers recommended conditioning the prepared cavity (both enamel and dentine) with some form of acid solution (Zhang et al. 2013; Altunsoy et al. 2014; Powis et al. 1982).

Recently, a high viscosity, nonsticky, packable GIC was released that did not require cavity conditioning, i.e. placement is directly into the cavity as in the case of amalgam (Giray et al. 2014; Huo et al. 2011). This represented the first attempt to provide a viable encapsulated high viscosity GIC alternative to amalgam for certain cavity classes.

7.3 Improvements in Glass Filler Systems

The current filler present in glass-ionomer materials typically consists of ground glass particles. Their composition is based on silica and alumina as well as calcium, strontium and zinc oxide as well as other components. Fluorine, phosphate and sodium are also incorporated into multicomponent glass structures (Lohbauer 2009; Moshaverinia et al. 2011). Additions and modifications to powder systems have been described previously, but few have been incorporated into commercial GICs (Moshaverinia et al. 2011). The fillers vary in size depending on the manufacturer and are typically produced by some form of attrition (grinding) process.

Glass filler systems are then subject to processing (such as thermal or chemical treatment) and drying processes that produce a filler particle suitable for use. For encapsulated GIC products, the filler system and powder to liquid ratio creates rheological properties that influence the handling of the glass-ionomers. For example, a high viscosity product can obtain higher instrument penetration forces compared to a lower viscosity product. As these materials are multicomponent and their formulations vary significantly, several components of the formulation may influence the handling of the material.

Pre-reacted GIC glass systems have been reported, although these particles are typically transported into resin or adhesive systems to provide "GIC"-like properties (i.e. fluoride release) (Kamijo et al. 2009; Han and Okiji 2011; Shimazu et al. 2012). Glass-ionomer formulations themselves could benefit from this technology, as it allows a certain part of the final matrix to achieve ultimate strength in a controlled and reproducible environment. For example, the setting reaction of these "secondary" particles can be completed prior to the mixing stage, which can potentially give improvements in immediate wear, strength, handling and other properties to the GIC. However, microfiller (0.01–0.1 μm) agglomerated systems, and nanofillers (5–100 nm) have not been widely used as the primary glass filler size range for GIC systems.

7.4 Nanoparticle Technology

Although nano and nano-hybrid filler systems in composites have been available commercially for some time, only one "nano" particle GIC (Ketac^{TM} Nano, 3 M ESPE, St Paul, MN, USA) has become available, although its filler component claims to contain a combination of fluoroaluminosilicate glass, nanoparticles and nanoclusters. The use of smaller nanoparticles is based on the premise that some properties such as gloss retention or wear resistance may be improved. Researchers have found that this type of material has reduced surface roughness values after polishing, although the hardness of the material has not been found to be significantly different from another GIC material (Bala et al. 2012).

However, when transferring nanoparticles or nanocluster technology into encapsulated GIC formulations, difficulties arise in maintaining a usable paste consistency whilst maintaining adequate filler volume content. The evolution of the filler system technologies seen in composite resin material development has potential for translation into future filler types for glass-ionomer systems (Ferracane 2011). As there is a perceived need for GIC materials to possess more aesthetic properties similar to composite resins, it is envisaged that smaller particle types will be introduced.

Various technologies can be employed to achieve nanoparticle systems for use in GICs; these include agglomeration, pre-polymerisation, resin infiltration and the joining of glass systems to nanoparticles. Although other material factors influence optical properties such as gloss, smaller (i.e. nanosize) glass particle composites typically achieve better initial gloss and gloss retention. For GICs, the "nano" phase of research and development is imminent and could provide some exceptional properties particularly in the aesthetic and wear values of GICs. However, it is yet to be shown how a nanoparticle with appropriate chemical properties can adequately replace the current "multicomponent" fluoride-containing glasses commonly employed in commercial GIC formulations.

Although many nanoparticle additions to GIC formulations have been attempted, no nanosized (i.e. <100 nm) universal "multicomponent" reactive glass system has been employed so far. Furthermore, using a combination of two different types of filler or fillers of different compositions could be employed to overcome the problems associated with using nanoparticles as the only filler type. Nano-clays have also been reported to reinforce GIC systems although not yet employed in commercial GICs (Fareed and Stamboulis 2014a, b). Nano-sheets, nano-rods, nano-tubes, nano-films and a diverse range of reported micro-nano structures could be incorporated into GICs to investigate the improvement of various properties.

7.5 Spherical Particles

At present, most GIC materials contain irregularly shaped glass particles. By incorporating spherical particles, it is possible to alter the filler to volume ratio. Some research (Gu et al. 2004) has delved into these spherical glass systems, although they have not been commercially introduced to GICs. Spherical GIC glasses can be produced in different ways, and methods such as sol–gel technology and plasma treatment have been employed. Spheroidisation of glass powders has also been performed by using flame spraying and inductively coupled radio frequency plasma spraying techniques (Gu et al. 2004). Spherical silica additions to RMGICs have also been investigated and have demonstrated improved marginal gap reduction, as well as improvements in compressive, diametral tensile and flexural strength (Irie et al. 2011; Hatanaka et al. 2006).

A potential way of reducing biofilm on glass-ionomers could be by providing a smoother material surface, possibly facilitated by smaller nanosized filler systems, or by different surface chemistries, although this is yet to be introduced (Busscher et al. 2010; Hengtrakool et al. 2006).

7.6 Glass Fibre Reinforcement

Glass fibre composite technology has enabled engineers and chemists to develop advanced composites used in many high technology and demanding situations (Bakis et al. 2002). Reactive glass fibres have been employed in experimental GICs to create fibre-reinforced GICs (FRGIC). They have been found to increase the flexural strength and increases in the work of fracture primarily due to the additional energy required to "pull" the fibres out of the fracture surface (Lohbauer et al. 2003).

Fibres of SiO_2–Al_2O_3–CaF_2–Na_3AlF_6 (430 μm long) have been shown to significantly increase the fracture toughness, as well as providing large increases in the total energy release rate (Lohbauer et al. 2004). However, glass fibres are usually large compared to glass particles, which can be disadvantageous. Short fibres (1000 μm long × 10 μm wide) have also been shown to increase diametral tensile strength, flexural strength, flexural modulus and fracture toughness of GIC (Hammouda 2009). Short fibres from CaO–P_2O_5–Si–O_2–Al_2O_3 glass systems maintain higher flexural strengths after thermo-cycling than unreinforced formulations, as expected from fibre-reinforced materials, although these strengths are inferior to those typically achieved by composites (Kawano et al. 2001).

However, the aesthetic properties of FRGIC materials are compromised, and this together with exposure of fibres due to wear makes the current fibre-reinforced formulations currently non-commercially viable.

Nanofibres with diameters less than 100 nm are now available, although their incorporation into GICs has not become commercially available. Electro-spun inorganic nanofibres based on TiO_2, SiO_2, $Zr0_2$ and Al_2O_3 have been developed (Qizheng et al. 2006; Wessel et al. 2010). This electro-spinning technology developed for the textile industry (Zhou and Gong 2008) could be utilised to produce suitable nanofibres to be incorporated both physically and chemically with GIC systems. Furthermore, as research into nano-tubes and nano-wires continues, the availability of these nano-products will become available for determining their effect on GICs (Zhang et al. 1999). Finally, hybrid organic–inorganic nanofibres are also being investigated in other material science areas and could possibly introduce novel properties to different classes of GICs (Fischer 2003; Wu et al. 2010).

7.7 Incorporation of Polymeric Filler Carriers

Polymer carriers are particles loaded with active molecules or compounds, which are designed to be released or influence the surrounding environment of the restoration/tooth surface interface. These nanosized, monodispersed, spherical particles with functionalities for the immobilisation of chemicals or biomolecules have been used for tissue engineering and controlled-release drug delivery and have been classified as "molecularly imprinted polymer systems". The possibilities for these carrier fillers are endless when applied to GIC systems, and they provide novel systems for releasing future compounds not actively involved in the GIC setting reaction. These particles, loaded with zinc chloride and incorporated into adhesives, have been proposed to inhibit the degradation of collagen by matrix metalloproteinases (MMPs) (Osorio et al. 2014). Their incorporation into GICs could also prove a viable research path for further improving the GIC bond to dentine as it is well known that MMP action can compromise the dentine-adhesive interfaces (Tezvergil-Mutluay et al. 2013).

7.8 Controlled-Release Vehicle Additions to GIC

The controlled release of active ingredients from the GIC matrix could also be facilitated by other technologies. For example, microencapsulated particles have been proposed in order to facilitate tooth mineralisation. Typically these are designed for concentrated release of calcium ($Ca(NO_3)_2$), fluoride (NaF) or phosphate (K_2HPO_4) salts directly to the tooth. Using a semipermeable shell wall, the salt ion permeates through the shell wall at a controlled rate, and these types of particles can provide a diverse delivery platform for different materials (Latta et al. 2014).

New types of interpenetrating polymer networks could also be incorporated in GICs, as they have proven their use in the delivery of a large range of compounds and drugs through different novel carrier systems. These materials are typically based on hydrogels, microspheres, microbeads, microparticles, nanoparticles and other platforms in order to effectively deliver active ingredients (Lohani et al. 2014).

Controlled-release polymer technologies are commonly employed in drug and therapeutic formulations to deliver active ingredients over different time periods. Many of these technologies could be incorporated into GICs to improve the targeted release of future compounds. Typically, nanotechnology delivery systems can be used for improved delivery of poorly soluble drugs, targeted delivery of large molecule actives and the co-delivery of two active compounds (Farokhzad and Langer 2009).

Hydrogel technology, i.e. three-dimensional cross-link networks, can be formulated into micro- or nanoparticles and contain highly porous structures. Their characteristic porosity permits the loading of compounds which can be released at rate-dependent diffusion coefficients through the hydrogel network (Hoare and Kohane 2008). Gelatin hydrogels have also been used for the delivery of bioactive molecules allowing their use in tissue engineering, gene therapy and controlled drug release and could be adapted for use in GICs (Young et al. 2005).

Gold nanoparticles have also been used as controlled-release vehicles, and they are assumed to provide a non-toxic delivery system for active materials coated on their surface (Ghosh et al. 2008). Furthermore, block copolymer micelles have also been utilised as delivery systems for drugs and can provide different mechanisms for delivering micelle-forming polymeric drugs and other compounds (Kazunori et al. 1993). All of these controlled-release technologies could be employed for future use in GIC materials in order to provide the release of specific chemicals beneficial to protecting and repairing the remaining tooth structure.

7.9 Self-Healing Technology

The GIC setting reaction in both the conventional and resin-modified GICs is facilitated by ion-binding and gelation between poly(alkenoic acid) s and metal ions, and the kinetics and reactions have been described in detail previously (Wilson and Nicholson 2005; Wilson 1996; Smith 1998; Nicholson 1998; Walls 1986). A new research topic in polymer science, and one that could be applied to future GIC polymer chemistry and development, involves the study of "self-healing" polymer structures. Self-healing, or autonomously healing polymers and coatings, is a new technology that allows the automatic repair of undetected defects such as cracks, fractures and other damaged areas within a polymer or adhesive interface, which have resulted from chemical, thermal or mechanical fatigue processes. This type of technology could easily be incorporated into GIC materials to provide "smart" multifunctional materials that when subjected to "excess" stress could repair any resultant damage themselves. Glass-ionomers are good candidates for this technology as they already have a significant interaction (i.e. ionic and water transport) with the surrounding oral environment. There are different methods of inducing self-healing technologies, none of which as yet have been applied to GIC chemistry. Several reviews have described the different methods to facilitate self-healing technologies into polymers (Samadzadeh et al. 2010; Yuan et al. 2008; Wu et al. 2008; Wilson et al. 2010).

The incorporation of micro- or nano-capsules releases "repair agents" (Figs. 7.1 and 7.2) specific to the polymer architecture after crack propagation in coatings. In practice, these capsules are presented in the polymer network in sizes ranging from 3 to 800 μm, and they can contain a solid, a liquid or gas components as a "core" material, surrounded by a capsule or shell material (Wu et al. 2008; Samadzadeh et al. 2010).

Interpenetrating polymer networks incorporating linear polymers (e.g. poly(methacrylated phenyl glycidyl ether)) has shown diffusion of the linear polymer phase into the crack interface as a form of self-healing process. SEM images (Fig. 7.2) of damaged areas clearly demonstrate that healing of micro-cracks in the order of 20 μm can be achieved, from mobile chain interdiffusion and entanglement (Peterson et al. 2012).

Polymers incorporating embedded microcapsules of liquid monomers are also used to induce self-healing properties. When the material is damaged, the microcapsules release monomers into the damaged areas and subsequently repair the damage and prevent further fracture. Other approaches include the "mechanochemical" activation of a catalyst in a polymer chain, i.e. when mechanically induced chain scission occurs, a catalytic site is activated, thereby facilitating polymerisation of acrylic monomers. Other approaches are supra-molecular (i.e. non-covalent interactions) and also methods to exploit covalent bond forming repair processes (Colquhoun and Klumperman 2013).

Both intrinsic and extrinsic mechanisms can be used to develop self-healing properties. Polymer architecture such as chain stiffness and cross-link functionality, cross-linking density and content or reversible groups and multiphase polymer structure all have an influence on the self-healing ability of various polymer systems

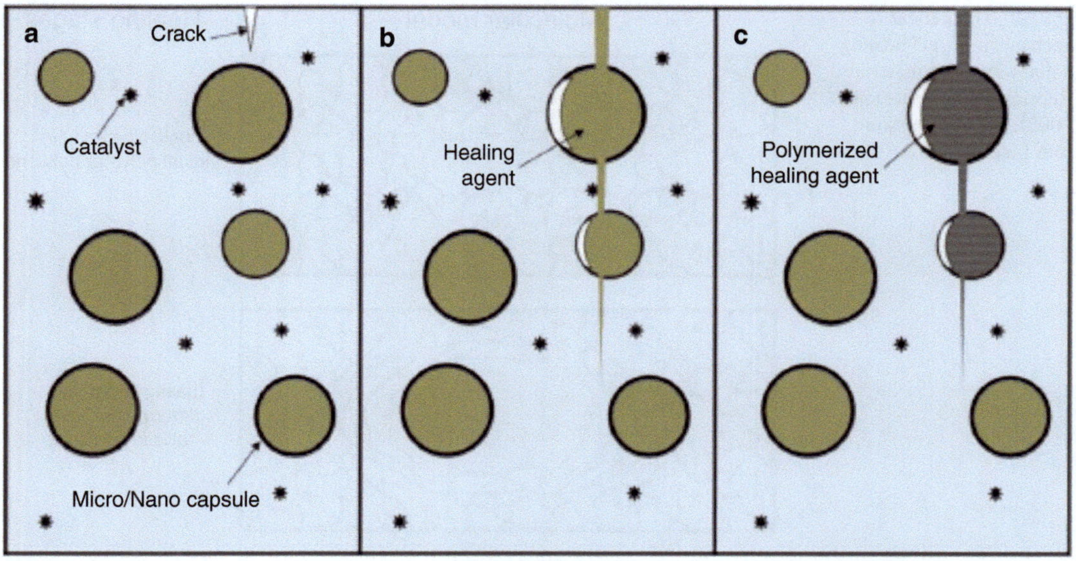

Fig. 7.1 Proposed self-healing concept containing nano-encapsulated healing agent. (**a**) Crack formed due to damage, (**b**) nano-capsule is ruptured releasing healing agent that migrates to crack, and (**c**) healing agent is then polymerised after contacting a catalyst (Reprinted from Samadzadeh et al. (2010). With permission from Elsevier)

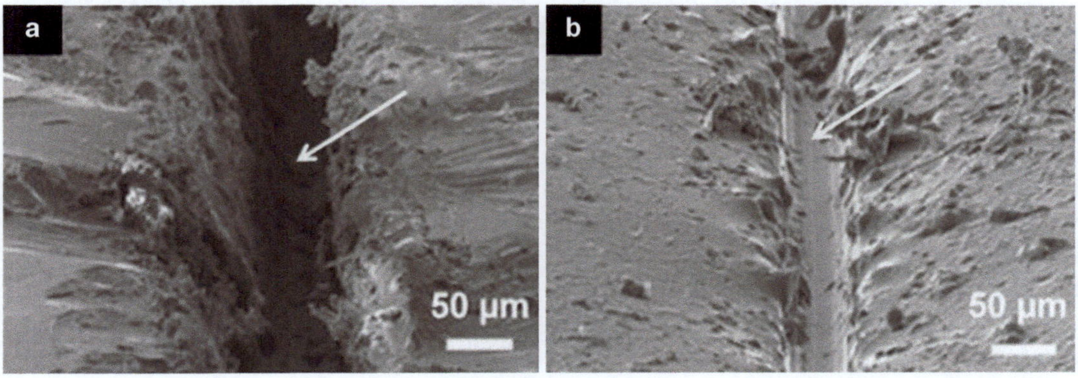

Fig. 7.2 SEM micrographs of micro-crack healing. (**a**) Coating containing scratch defect (*arrowed*) and (**b**) self-healed scratch defect after healing process (Reprinted from Samadzadeh et al. (2010). With permission from Elsevier)

(Garcia 2014). Other approaches incorporating shape memory materials, swollen materials or passivation can also be utilised to impart self-healing properties, and a possible mechanism for GIC repair is shown in Fig. 7.3. The investigation of poly(ethylene-co-methacrylic acid)-based ionomers has also indicated its ability to self-heal (Wu et al. 2008). However, it is yet to be seen how manufacturers will incorporate these new technologies into GICs in an effort to improve their mechanical and adhesive performance.

7.10 Other Novel Polymer Networks for Improvements in Strength and Other Properties

In order to increase the physical properties of GICs, improvements can be achieved by modifying polymer chemistry contained in the liquid component or in the solid form present in the powder component (Guggenberger et al. 1998). Multi-arm poly(acrylic acid-co-itaconic)

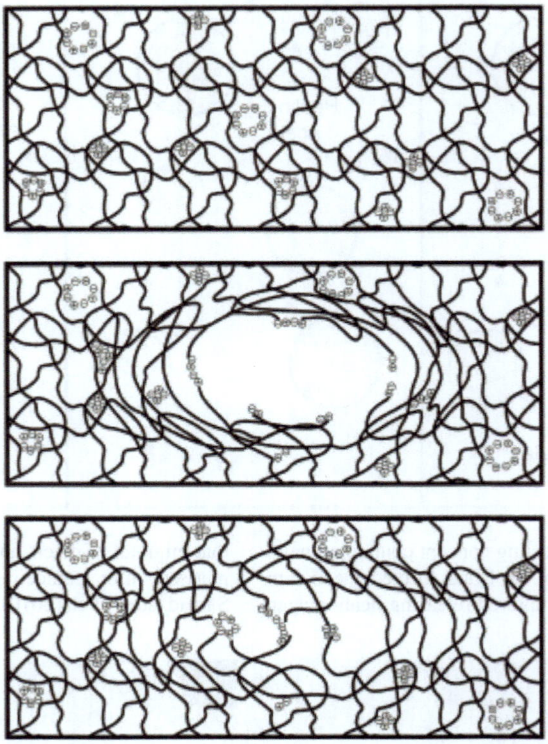

Fig. 7.3 Theoretical mechanism of self-healing in glass-ionomer materials (Reprinted from Wu et al. (2008). With permission from Elsevier)

acids have been prepared and have demonstrated improvements in compressive strength for conventional cured GICs (Xie et al. 2010), and star-shaped poly(carboxylic acid) polymers have been proposed for resin-modified GICs (Weng et al. 2014). Vinyl-containing poly(acrylic acid-co-itaconic acid) copolymers have also shown higher flexural strength leading to a tougher fracture surface and plastic deformation properties (Wu et al. 2003). The polymer chemistry here is complex (Yelamanchili and Darvell 2008), and future improvements in results rely on the interactions between the multicomponent nature of different GIC systems which contain many components, including complex initiating systems.

7.11 Porosity Reduction

As glass-ionomers are mixed together in order for the acid–base reaction to proceed, typically, small voids or air pockets are incorporated into the mix. Although the effects of these voids are not exactly understood, it is assumed that these have a negative effect on the GIC strengths. One method of reducing these voids is to provide both parts of a glass-ionomer in a paste version, which can be hand-mixed by a spatula or through some form of a static mixer (Boehm et al. 2011). However, compared to encapsulated delivery systems, this form of delivery is typically uneconomical and is not widely used. A major advancement for encapsulated versions would be the reduction of voids during the extrusion of the mixed paste, although no such capsule version has yet to be developed.

7.12 Improvements in Fracture Toughness

Fracture toughness is known to be an important material property for successful posterior load-bearing restorations (Lloyd and Adamson 1987). To date, it has been questioned whether the survival of GICs will reach levels achieved by composite resin materials in load-bearing situations (Burke 2013). However, in some studies modern GICs used to restore load-bearing cavities have been demonstrated to perform satisfactorily up to 10 years. This demonstrates that wear properties simulated in a laboratory do not necessarily translate to reduction of anatomical form or surface roughness in real-life situations (Burke 2014).

For primary molar restorations, recent studies have indicated that the survival rate for amalgam restorations is no different from that of atraumatic restorative treatment with a high viscosity (HV) GIC. For both amalgam and HVGIC, the main reason for failure is mechanical, and it has been suggested that for single surfaces of primary teeth, HVGIC is a viable alternative to amalgam (Yamazaki et al. 2006).

Modifications to the polymer component of the GIC have shown to improve the fracture toughness of GICs. Acrylic acid-itaconic acid-N-vinylcaprolactam (NVC) ter-polymers have been synthesised and have shown significantly higher plane-strain fracture toughness (KIc) at 1-day and 1-week storage time periods compared to the control (Fuji IX, GC Corp, Tokyo, Japan) (Moshaverinia et al. 2010). However, issues associated with viscosity increases need to be overcome for the incorporation of any of these new polymers.

Improvements of fracture toughness depend on many variables. It has been shown that modification of the polymer components, such as amino acid-containing GICs, methacryloyl amino acid reactive diluents and a series of other new chemistries are viable paths to improving properties such as fracture toughness of the final cement (Culbertson 2001).

Other novel polymer systems such as 6-arm star-shaped poly(acrylic acid) polymers have also shown significant increases in fracture toughness compared to commercial RMGICs, similar in value to composite material (Zhao et al. 2009). Adjustment of the molecular weight (MW) of polymers has also been investigated for improving properties, although it is unknown how these changes will affect clinical outcomes.

Viscoelastic (i.e. viscous and elastic response of materials to deformation) properties of GICs have also been reported in an effort to understand the mechanical behaviour of these materials. Fracture may involve wear and adhesive debonding modes of failure, as well as the typical bulk fracture of the various GIC materials; both GIC and RMGIC exhibited viscoelastic properties (Yamazaki et al. 2006). Modifications in the powder, for example, particle size reductions and powder to liquid ratios, have also been shown to increase fracture toughness in GIC formulations (Mitsuhashi et al. 2003).

Interfacial fracture toughness has also been studied in order to provide paths for GIC improvements related to failure by fracture. Formulations are investigated at adhesive interfaces, and typically the fracture then continues into the bulk material (Setien et al. 2005; Cheetham et al. 2014b). These studies are extremely relevant for development of improved GIC materials. To improve the longevity of GICs, properties such as fracture toughness of the bulk material and the adhesive properties (interfacial fracture toughness or interfacial work of fracture) need to be improved.

7.13 Improvements in Adhesion to Dentine and Enamel

The critical issue with adhesive dentistry is to place the adhesive material using a method that gives the best chance for long-term stability and the creation of an "effective seal" to the adhesive–tooth interface. In the case of resin-based adhesive systems, there are several strategies that have been proposed in order to optimise the probability of success, and these include application of MMP inhibitors and collagen cross-linkers, additional enamel etching, agitation of the adhesive for deeper penetration, etc. (Manuja et al. 2012). These approaches are also very relevant when trying to improve the bonding reliability of GIC materials. Many original and review articles are available to explain the different concepts involved in adhesion to dentine and enamel (Tyas 2003; Manuja et al. 2012; Atmeh et al. 2012).

Adhesion to dentine and enamel is a complex science and similar to adhesively bonded composite dentistry; successful outcomes depend on many variables (Perdigão 2010; De Munck et al. 2012). Glass-ionomers have also been shown to give a more durable bond compared to other adhesive systems (Van Meerbeek et al. 2010). However, much is unknown about this bond and most importantly the degradation mechanisms of the bond.

The bonding mechanism of new-generation GICs has now demonstrated resin tag formation. Studies investigating the differences between dentine conditioned with phosphoric or polyacrylic acid solutions have shown that both protocols create a surface that allows RMGIC resin tags (Fig. 7.4) to form (Hamama et al. 2014; Korkmaz et al. 2010; El-Askary and Nassif 2011). Other studies demonstrate the intimate chemical interaction with dentine and enamel

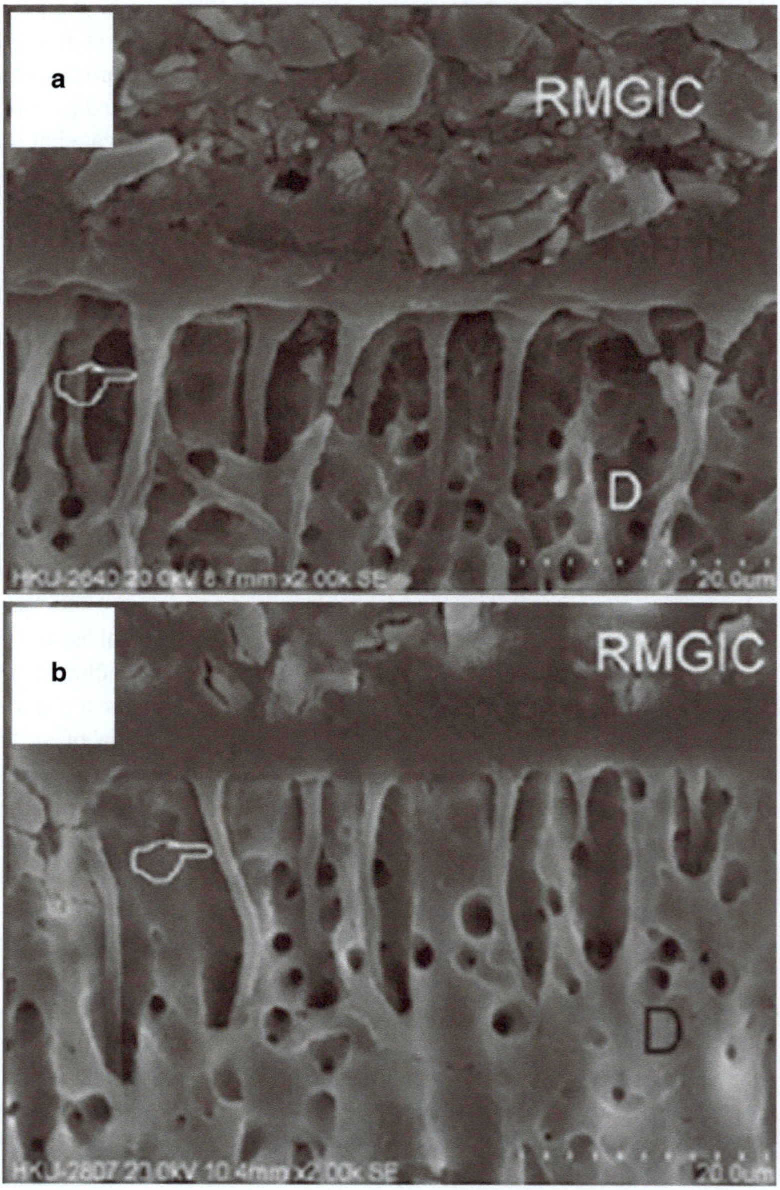

Fig. 7.4 SEM micrographs showing the interface between RMGIC and dentine. The *top image* (**a**) had dentine treated with 37 % phosphoric acid, the *bottom image* (**b**) was treated with a solution of 25–30 % polyacrylic acid conditioner (*D* denotes dentine). The hand pointer indicates the presence of resin tags (Reprinted from Hamama et al. (2014). With permission from John Wiley & Sons)

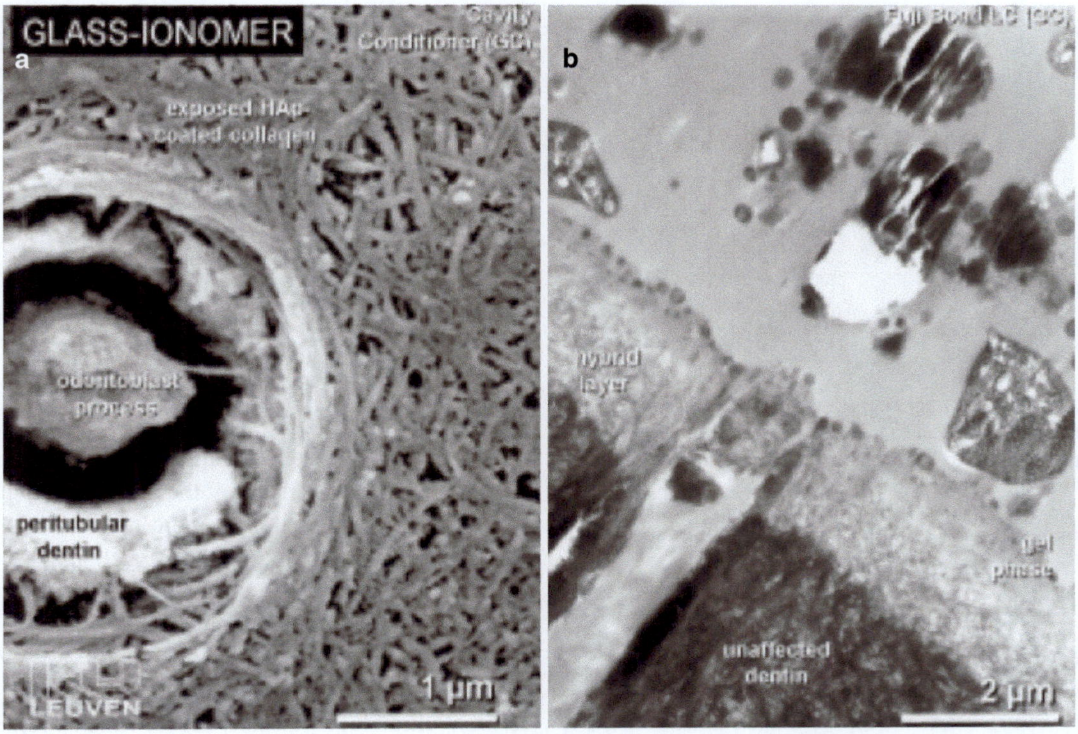

Fig. 7.5 (**a**) SEM image showing the effect of polyacrylic acid conditioner on dentine and (**b**) TEM photomicrograph showing the hybrid layer and gel phase created after RMGIC placement (Reprinted from van Meerbeek et al. (2003). With permission from Operative Dentisitry, Inc.)

surfaces (Fig. 7.5) with exposure of collagen due to dentine pretreatment, with the remaining hydroxyapatite being used as "receptors" for chemical bonding of the GIC. Micropores have also been shown to increase the ability for micromechanical bonding (Van Meerbeek et al. 2003).

The chemical interaction and formation of ionic bonds between carboxylic acid groups with hydroxyapatite have been described previously, and future GICs will use this information to provide materials with stronger, more resilient bonding interfaces (Yoshida et al. 2000).

Further improvements of the bonding to hydroxyapatite, enamel and dentine components will continue to be focused on the incorporation of new polymer chemistries into the GIC formulations. Pioneering work investigating the binding energies of functional groups to these structures as well as the molecular structure of the polyalkenoic acid component has shown that these factors significantly affect the chemical bonding to hydroxyapatite structures (Fukuda et al. 2003; Sennou et al. 1999). This process to gather information on surface interaction will continue to be used to modify resin formulations and optimise chemical adhesion processes for GICs.

Apart from chemically related improvements, other "macro" physical observations of GICs may be utilised to achieve improvements in adhesion. Spherical bodies (Figs. 7.6 and 7.7) have also been shown to be involved in GIC adhesive surfaces which could provide fracture initiation sites for bond failure, although their participation in the adhesive process is not yet fully understood (Yiu et al. 2004a, b). New materials will try to eliminate these porous, randomly incorporated features which disrupt a relatively homogenous and compact solid material. Further understanding of the interfacial properties of GICs with enamel and dentine will inevitably lead to improving the longevity of the GIC bond.

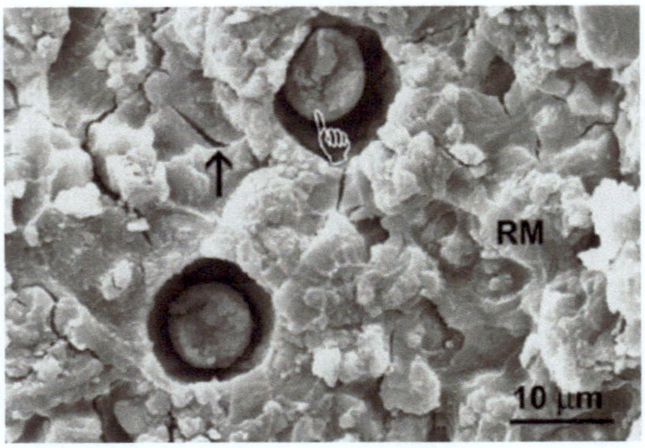

Fig. 7.6 SEM micrograph showing a RMGIC surface fractured adjacent to the GIC–dentine interface, showing the presence of spherical bodies (hand pointer). Dehydration cracks are identified with an *arrow* (Reprinted from Yiu et al. (2004a). With permission from Elsevier)

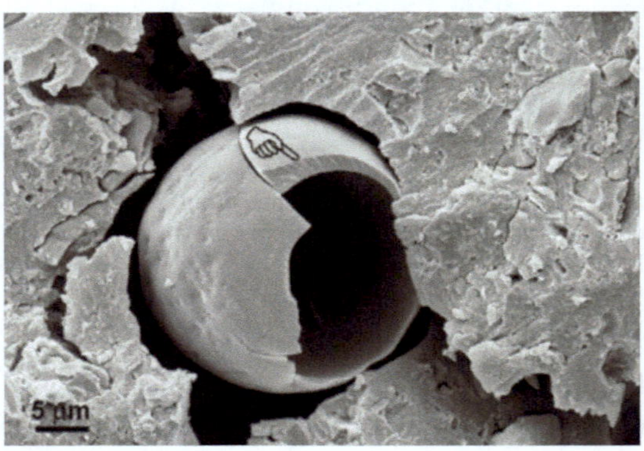

Fig. 7.7 SEM image of a spherical body showing brittle fracture of the spherical structure. The handpointer identifies a fractured eggshell-like structure within the GIC at the GIC–dentine interface [Reprinted from Yiu et al. (2004b). With permission from Sage Publications]

Research on GIC adhesion provides information for understanding the fundamental mechanics and kinetics of the bond formation and subsequent path of bond degradation in order for new adhesive strategies to be devised. Short-term, static bond strengths give limited information when comparing the potential longevity of a GIC bond and understate its adhesive abilities. A fracture mechanics approach, including interfacial fracture toughness and work of fracture testing (Fig. 7.8) showing the "total energy" required to initiate fracture, provides more relevant information on the possible improvements of the bond durability (Cheetham et al. 2014b).

7.14 Future Delivery Systems

The delivery format of glass-ionomers varies from powder–liquid bottle versions and single-use encapsulated systems to dual-barrel syringes (and unit-dose) for paste–paste GICs. Paste–paste systems generally reduce the porosity of the final GIC paste, and single-use formats (Fig. 7.9) have been recently commercialised (Boehm et al. 2011). However, these formats have not been as widely accepted as single-use encapsulated delivery formats for powder–liquid versions of GICs.

Encapsulated systems eliminate the need for measurements to be made by the user, resulting in a dispensed material with more reproducible features such as setting reaction (gel and set time), strength and paste consistency. The other benefits of current GIC capsule systems are the ease of direct delivery and their single use. New-generation GIC capsules (Fig. 7.10) will be able to mix "ultra" high viscosity GICs, which could also allow for a new GIC with very high powder to liquid ratios and strengths not seen in GICs before (Cheetham 2014).

However, a disadvantage of "capsules" is that during the mixing process, they typically introduce some form of subclinical micro-porosity in the paste. Various methods, such as centrifuging the capsule after the mixing process, or vacuum mixers, have been employed to reduce this with limited effect (Suzuki et al. 2004). Theoretically, the reduction of this porosity will increase the physical properties of GICs. The clinician is yet to see the direction of future designs of GIC delivery systems, but it is likely that ease of the use in terms of delivery and reduction of porosity are areas where improvements can be made.

7.15 Wear Improvements

Currently, it is popular to place a coating over the setting GIC in order to protect it during the initial setting stage, which improves the immediate aesthetics of the restoration and acts as a method to fill in any porosity created on the surface (Zoergiebel and Ilie 2013). However, the effect of this coating on GICs placed on occlusal surfaces

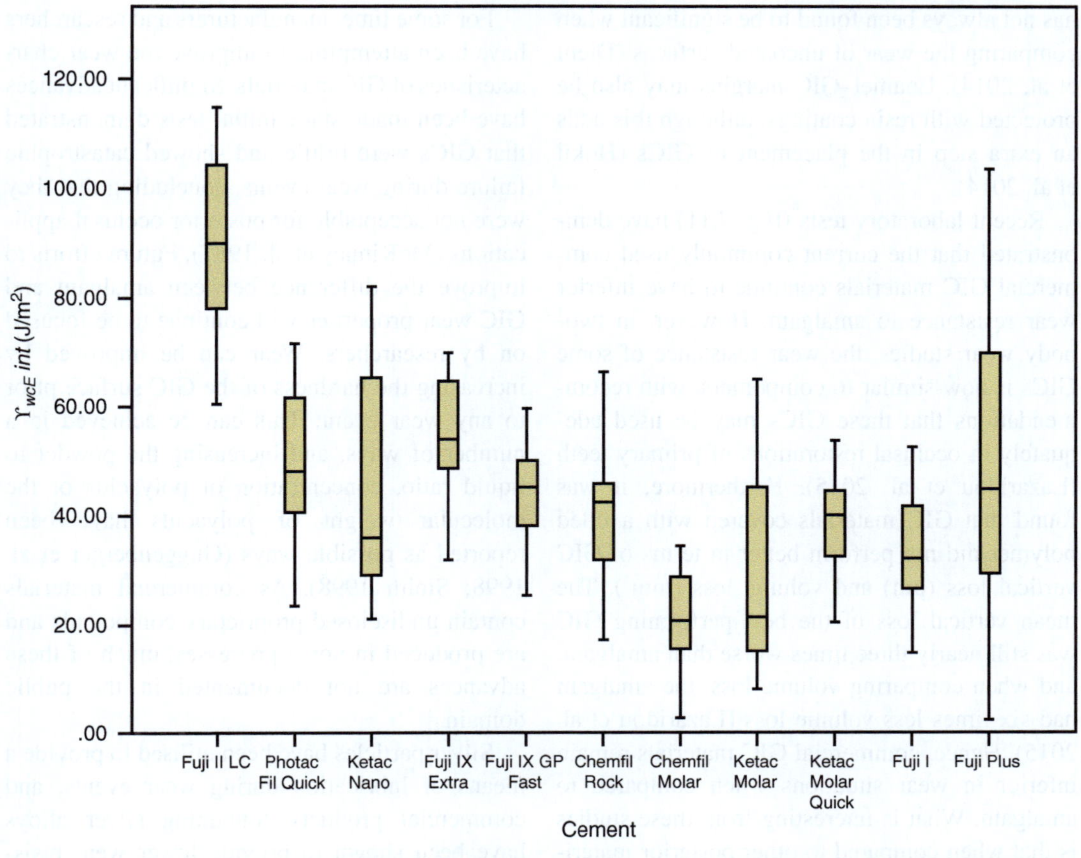

Fig. 7.8 Comparison of the interfacial work of fracture (γ_{wof}int) results (J/m^2) together with standard deviations for glass-ionomer bonded to dentine (Reprinted from Cheetham et al. (2014b). With permission from Elsevier)

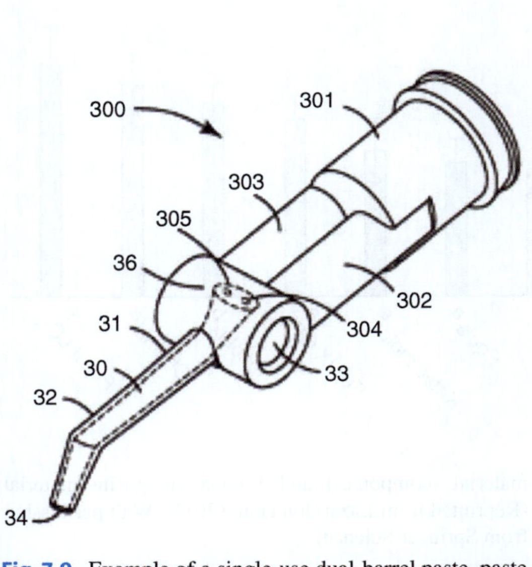

Fig. 7.9 Example of a single-use dual-barrel paste–paste delivery system (Reprinted from Boehm et al. (2011))

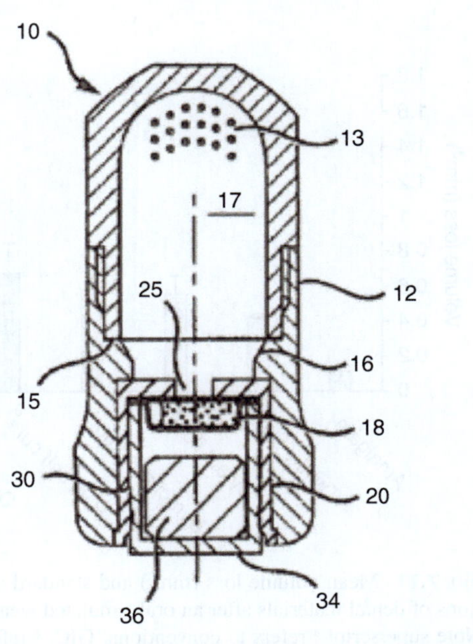

Fig. 7.10 Example of a single-use powder–liquid delivery system (Reprinted from Cheetham (2014))

has not always been found to be significant when comparing the wear of uncoated surfaces (Diem et al. 2014). Enamel–GIC margins may also be protected with resin coatings, although this adds an extra step in the placement of GICs (Hokii et al. 2014).

Recent laboratory tests (Fig. 7.11) have demonstrated that the current commonly used commercial GIC materials continue to have inferior wear resistance to amalgam. However, in two-body wear studies, the wear resistance of some GICs is now similar to compomers, with recommendations that these GICs may be used adequately in occlusal restorations of primary teeth (Lazaridou et al. 2015). Furthermore, it was found that GIC materials covered with a filled polymer did not perform better in terms of GIC vertical loss (μm) and volume loss (mm^3). The mean vertical loss of the best performing GIC was still nearly three times worse than amalgam, and when comparing volume loss, the amalgam had six times less volume loss (Lazaridou et al. 2015). Hence, commercial GIC materials remain inferior in wear situations when compared to amalgam. What is interesting from these studies is that when compared to other posterior materials, some GICs can now be viewed as an alternative option.

For some time, manufacturers and researchers have been attempting to improve the wear characteristics of GIC materials. Significant advances have been made since initial tests demonstrated that GICs were brittle and showed catastrophic failure during wear events, concluding that they were not acceptable for posterior occlusal applications (McKinney et al. 1987). Future efforts to improve the difference between amalgam and GIC wear properties will continue to be focused on by researchers. Wear can be improved by increasing the hardness of the GIC surface prior to any wear event. This can be achieved in a number of ways, and increasing the powder to liquid ratio, concentration of polyacids or the molecular weight of polyacids have been reported as possible ways (Guggenberger et al. 1998; Smith 1998). As commercial materials contain undisclosed proprietary compounds and are produced in novel processes, much of these advances are not documented in the public domain.

Silver particles have been utilised to provide a means of lubrication during wear events, and commercial products containing silver alloys have been shown to provide lower wear resistance (McKinney et al. 1988; Xie et al. 2000). However, from an aesthetic perspective, the

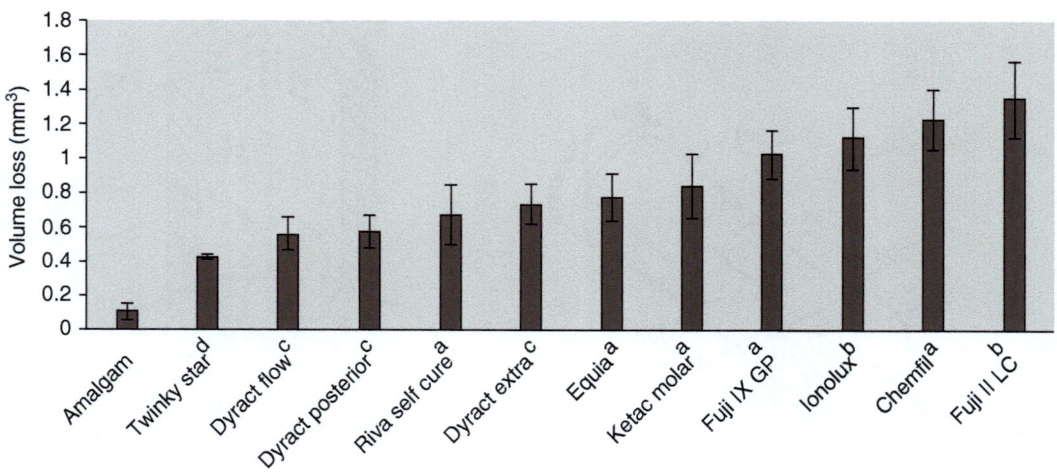

Fig. 7.11 Mean volume loss (mm^3) and standard deviations of dental materials after an oral simulated wear test. Note superscript [a] refers to conventional GIC, [b] refers to RMGIC, and [c] refers to polyacid-modified resin composite material (compomer) and [d] resin composite material (Reprinted from Lazaridou et al. (2015). With permission from Springer Science)

addition of metal particles compromises the clinical outcome, and these materials are not currently widely accepted.

Studies by Xie et al. in 2000 have also shown that the more integrated the GIC microstructure is, the higher the mechanical properties. Furthermore, large glass particle systems have been described as contributing to lower wear properties. The integrity of the interface between the glass filler system and the polymer, the particle sizes of each of the filler systems and the number of voids created during mixing can all influence the wear properties of current GICs (Xie et al. 2000). As GICs age, their wear rate decreases, and differences in wear rates have been described in terms of polyalkenoic acid content, the "overall" chemical composition of the GIC and differences in the filler system and size of fillers used (van Duinen et al. 2005).

Avenues for future improvements in the wear properties of GICs will focus on innovations in these areas described above, in order to provide a harder external surface of GIC restorations, although it is unlikely that the wear properties in the short term will reach those obtained by modern amalgam alternatives.

7.16 Aesthetic Improvements

Compared to modern composite resin materials, the aesthetics of GICs are typically inferior, and much work is being performed in order for GICs to produce aesthetic restorations that blend in with tooth structure. For the future of GICs, the aesthetic properties are an important feature as patients in the "post amalgam age" are demanding that their teeth are restored with more tooth-like materials.

Aesthetics with GICs is likely to continue to evolve. For example, the colour change over time may be reduced with the addition of new polymer and surface chemistries that allow GICs to resist colour change even when subjected to staining media such as beverages or certain foods.

The initial translucency and optical properties (Fig. 7.12) of RMGICs are now similar to leading composite resin materials (Ogledzki et al. 2012). The optical properties, such as translucency and opacity values, together with closer colour matching of shades to Vita™ shades may be improved to follow composite resins. Conventional-cured GICs still lack the translucency properties (Fig. 7.13) of modern-day composites, although improvements are being introduced.

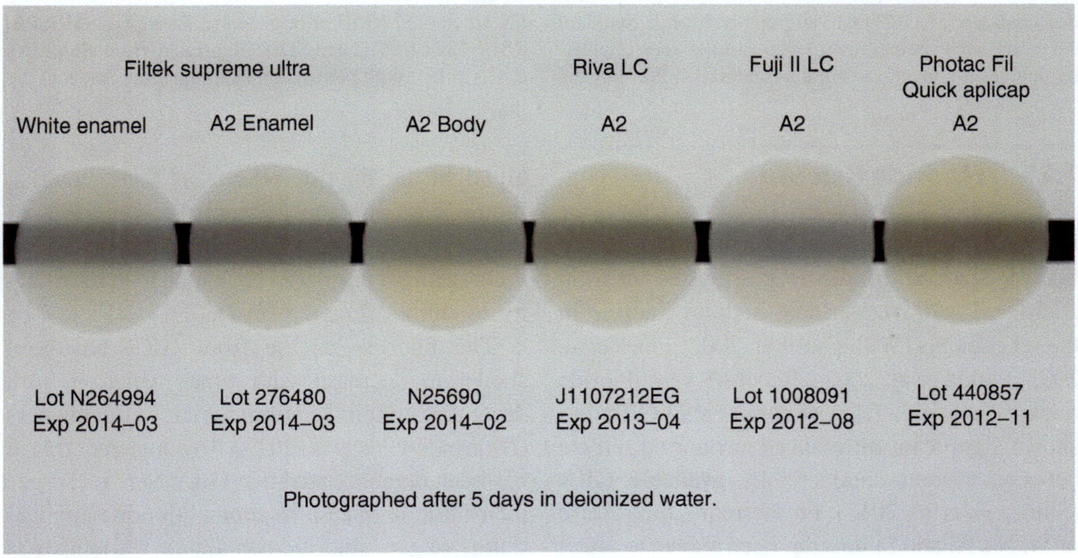

Fig. 7.12 Opacity comparison of a commercial composite resin (Filtek Supreme Ultra) and RMGICs (Riva LC™, Fuji II LC™, Photac Fil Quick Aplicap™) indicating current RMGIC materials can achieve similar opacity levels compared to resin composite (Image courtesy of SDI Limited R&D)

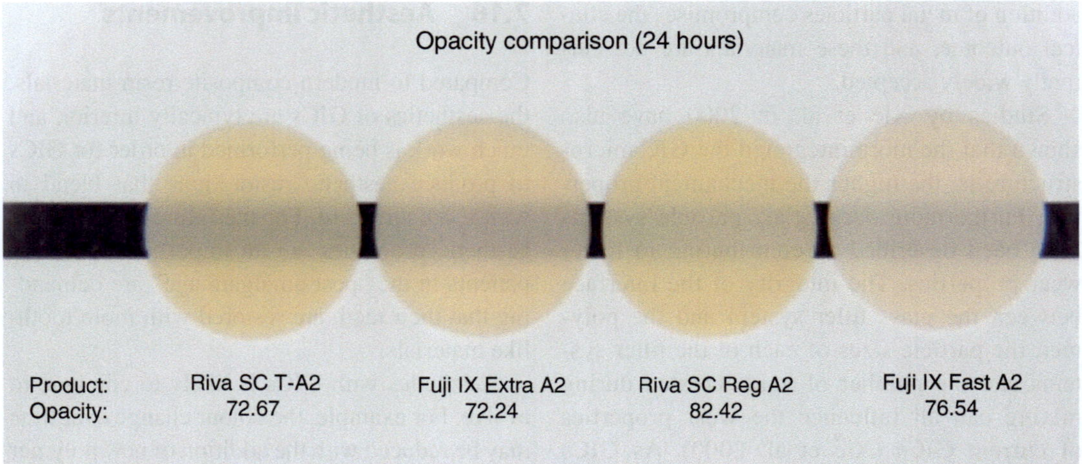

Fig. 7.13 Opacity comparison of commercial GIC demonstrating that they have higher opacities compared to RMGICs shown in Fig. 7.12. All materials are conventional cured type (Image courtesy of SDI Limited R&D)

Time	FEX		FIX		GFX		KME		RSC	
1 day	33.9	(3.9)[a]	19.7	(1.1)[b]	24.5	(3.5)[b]	10.9	(1.3)[c]	30.4	(3.5)[a]
1 week	68.9	(8.5)[d]	35.3	(0.9)[f]	46.2	(6.6)[e]	24.7	(1.2)[g]	70.7	(4.8)[d]
1 month	102.9	(9.5)[i]	54.6	(3.1)[j,k]	66.9	(9.8)[j]	44.8	(1.2)[k]	134.7	(6.4)[h]
3 months	151.5	(11.2)[m]	85.0	(4.6)[n,o]	103.2	(14.3)[n]	72.1	(2.6)[o]	187.1	(11.3)[l]
6 months	184.5	(12.3)[q]	105.9	(5.5)[r,s]	121.1	(19.7)[r]	90.1	(3.7)[s]	231.3	(14.3)[p]
1 year	241.9	(14.1)[u]	137.6	(6.6)[v,w]	153.8	(22.7)[v]	120.1	(5.9)[w]	284.7	(19.0)[t]

Fig. 7.14 Cumulative fluoride release (μg/cm^2) of various commercial GIC materials up to 1 year. Standard deviations are in parentheses, and the same superscript letter denotes homogenous subsets ($p>0.05$) (FEX: Fuji IX GP EXTRA, GC; FIX: Fuji IX GP, GC; GFX: GlasIonomer FX-II, Shofu; KME: Ketac Molar Easymix, 3MESPE; RSC: Riva Self Cure, SDI) (Reprinted from Shiozawa et al. (2013). With permission from Springer Science)

7.17 Fluoride Release

It is well documented that GIC materials release fluoride sourced from their glass system or from additional additives such as sodium fluoride in the set cements (Williams et al. 2002; Jones et al. 2003; Guida et al. 2002). Recent 1-year fluoride release data (Fig. 7.14) of commercial GICs has shown significant differences in fluoride release between current commercially available GICs (Shiozawa et al. 2013). Furthermore, the release of Sr, Na, Al and Si ions has been shown to affect the properties of the glass-ionomers and demonstrate how the GIC can interact with its aqueous environment. This ionic transfer is a unique feature of glass-ionomers not seen in composite resin materials. Although most manufacturers highlight the fluoride release of their material, future glass-ionomers could be designed to release high levels of calcium, phosphate or other ionic species considered beneficial to certain cavity conditions (Forsten 1998).

The fluoride release from GICs has been shown to decrease with time, which in turn decreases their antimicrobial effectiveness (Dionysopoulos et al. 2013). To counteract this, it has been demonstrated that GICs can "recharge" their fluoride release by topical fluoride application (e.g. fluoride-containing toothpaste) (Dionysopoulos et al. 2013; Arbabzadeh-Zavareh et al. 2012). Studies have shown that covering aged GIC with 0.1 % fluoride toothpaste or 1.25 % fluoride gel significantly increases the fluoride release (Seppa et al. 1993).

Glass-ionomer cements based on strontium glass systems have also been shown to release strontium ions originating from the glass structure to the adjacent tooth structure. Although these ions do not have any antibacterial effect, it is envisaged that they are rapidly exchanged for calcium ions, and a synergistic relationship with fluoride could facilitate antimicrobial properties (Dabsie et al. 2009). New-generation GICs will aim to maintain a constant relevant supply of fluoride ions over their life, without degradation of the cement, and any improvement in the release of fluoride should be incorporated into future GICs.

Addition of potassium and fluoride has also been previously made to the liquid components of GICs, and this has demonstrated ion release up to 500 days (Williams et al. 1999). Glass-ionomers immersed into potassium fluoride exhibited ion release twenty times greater than specimens that had additions to their liquid component, and this process could be adapted for pre-reacted GIC filler systems that act as reservoirs for specific ions (Williams et al. 1999).

7.18 Bioremineralisation/ Biopromoting Improvements

Although most manufacturers highlight the fluoride release of their GIC material/s, future GICs could be designed to release high levels of calcium, phosphate or other ionic species considered beneficial to certain cavity conditions. This release could originate from (a) glass systems involved in the main setting reaction, (b) glass systems not involved in the setting reaction or (c) other additives (e.g. amorphous calcium phosphate).

Calcium phosphate has also been added to two low viscosity GICs in the form of nano-amorphous calcium phosphate and ACP-CPP. Although the benefits of these additives have not yet been clinically proven, it shows attempts at using the GIC matrix as a vehicle for delivering specific agents to the tooth. Spray-dried amorphous calcium phosphate (ACP) nanoparticles incorporated in composite materials have been shown to release calcium ions when subjected to acidic conditions and decreasing the pH resulted in greater ion release (Xu et al. 2011).

Although ACP has been used in GICs for some time, a newly developed GIC contains casein phosphopeptide-amorphous calcium phosphate (CPP-ACP) incorporated in the powder component. This has been shown to release fluoride, calcium and phosphate ions under acidic conditions, potentially minimising the effects of demineralisation resulting from caries attacks (Zalizniak et al. 2013).

Micro- or nano-hydroxyapatite nanoparticles have also been proposed as additives to further promote bioremineralisation in GICs and have been found to increase GIC properties (Moshaverinia et al. 2008). Biomimetic fluorhydroxyapatite/polyacrylic acid nanostructures have also been proposed as additive structures, which have structures very similar to human enamel (Roche and Stanton 2015). However, these promising compounds have not yet been incorporated into commercial GICs.

7.19 Biofilm Alteration

Biofilms are formed over tooth and GIC surfaces due to the diverse range of microbial species and communities present in the oral cavity. There are various stages of film formation, including the formation of a pellicle, colonisation, propagation and finally steady-state existence on the surface (Steinberg 2000; Teughels et al. 2006). GICs have been shown to have rougher surfaces than composite resin materials (Carlén et al. 2001). Their surface chemistry is complex, and the surface free energy components of these surfaces (i.e. total surface free energy, nonpolar, acid–base components as well as acid and basic contribution) changes when comparing polished and unpolished materials. Unpolished GIC surfaces have also been shown to contain more positively charged components, which collect more proteins and increase bacterial adhesion compared to composite resin (Carlén et al. 2001). This colonisation causes a deterioration of the GIC surface and eventually the development of caries around the interface of the material and the tooth (Busscher et al. 2010). In vitro studies have shown that the release of fluoride from GIC is not adequate to prevent biofilm formation, possibly due to the low levels of fluoride release (Al-Naimi et al. 2008). It would be advantageous for GICs to improve their protective mechanisms from biofilm attack, and a number of strategies could be employed including increased fluoride release, antimicrobial properties and the incorporation of other additives.

7.20 Self-Cleaning Glass Technology

A technology known as "self-cleaning" glass has been developed, but has not been previously adapted to biomaterials in order to reduce biofilm accumulation or to at least favourably alter the biofilm. Generally, these glass surfaces are coated with a thin layer of material that facilitates photo-oxidative self-cleaning or some other cleaning process. For example, titanium dioxide (TiO_2) has been used to coat commercial glasses in layers less than 10 nm, and with photo-activation, it has been shown to be capable of killing gram-positive and gram-negative bacteria, although it is unknown how much energy is required to produce this effect (Foster et al. 2011; Guan 2005). Other self-cleaning surfaces have been described, but the hydrophobicity resulting from their properties may not allow them to be incorporated into GICs. However, it could be assumed that investigations into incorporating some form of "self-cleaning" mechanisms or technologies into GICs could be introduced and may potentially reduce biofilm accumulation in critical areas such as the enamel-restoration margin whilst maintaining biocompatible properties (Blossey 2003).

7.21 Antimicrobial Properties/Bio-protection of GICs

Topical antimicrobial therapy has been used as a technique to reduce and manage caries. For early childhood caries, these materials are used to reduce caries progression, as well as actively reduce the pathogenic oral microorganism levels. Antimicrobials employed and reported are fluoride, silver diamine fluoride, chlorhexidene, povidone iodine and xylitol (Jayabal and Mahesh 2014; Mei et al. 2013). Some in situ anti-cariogenic potential properties of glass-ionomers have been documented (Benelli et al. 1993), and the cariostatic effect of GICs has been demonstrated clinically, with reduced rates of secondary caries and marginal staining compared to composite. However, it is questionable whether this "inhibiting" effect can completely arrest the carious process (Van Amerongen 1996).

Incorporating additional antimicrobial compounds into the GIC formulation could be beneficial in maximising the protection of an already vulnerable tooth interface damaged by a cariogenic attack (Tyas 1991). Incorporating antimicrobial compounds into GICs and using GICs as a "carrier" has been suggested, although these highly antimicrobial materials face a difficult task of passing biocompatibility tests and material registration issues required for dental materials (Dimkov et al. 2009; Yli-Urpo et al. 2003). It has also been shown that placing antimicrobials such as benzalkonium chloride into GICs releases chloride ions as well as fluoride ions, further increasing the antimicrobial efficacy of GICs (Dimkov et al. 2009).

Other strategies have employed bioactive glasses, known to exhibit antimicrobial properties in GIC formulations. GICs incorporating these glasses at levels up to 30 % have demonstrated antimicrobial effects on *Candida albicans* and *Streptococcus mutans* and generally reducing bacterial growth levels (Yli-Urpo et al. 2003).

Macromolecules containing quaternary ammonium salts have also been investigated by incorporating poly(acrylic acid-co-itaconic acid) with pendant ammonium salts. Studies have shown that the antimicrobial effect of these polymers can be longer lasting than compounds that leach out of GICs over time (Weng 2011).

Other synthesised poly(quaternary ammonium salt)-containing polyacids have also demonstrated antimicrobial properties of GICs, although other considerations such as strength need to be taken into account when incorporating such polymers (Xie et al. 2011).

Loading GICs with nanoparticle antimicrobial release agents has also been proposed. Nanoparticles of chlorhexidine hexametaphosphate have been added to filler systems in 1–20 wt% range to provide a "broad spectrum antimicrobial agent", which would theoretically release chlorhexidine in a controlled manner (Hook

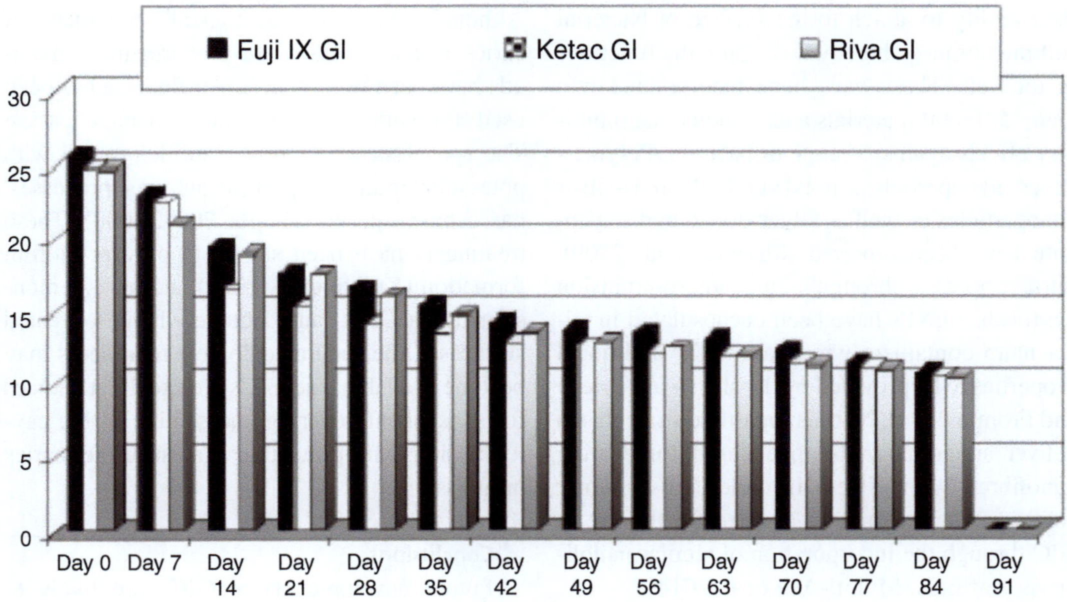

Fig. 7.15 Means of free *Streptococcus mutans* areas (mm) in GIC materials containing 1 % chlorhexidine treatment; circular inhibition zones (*y* axis) produced around the GIC samples are demonstrated up to 84 days. The three materials are convention cured GICs (Reprinted from El-Baky and Hussien (2013). With permission from Synergy Publishers)

et al. 2014). Chlorhexidine is reported to provide antimicrobial action against oral bacteria. However, due to the fact that GIC restorations still fail from secondary caries, it could be concluded that fluoride release alone is not adequate to inhibit bacterial ingress into cavities.

Current data suggests that the antimicrobial effect of GICs diminishes after 1 month (El-Baky and Hussien 2013). With the addition of 1 % chlorhexidine diacetate powder (Fig. 7.15), the antibacterial effect of the GICs is significantly increased up to 84 days (El-Baky and Hussien 2013). Although these tests are laboratory based, they demonstrate the effectiveness of GIC matrices as carriers for antimicrobial additives and offer many avenues for future material improvements, particularly in high caries prevalence situations.

7.22 Antibiotic Additions

Glass-ionomers generally possess some form of antimicrobial properties compared to other inert dental materials. Considering a carious lesion is formed primarily from the acidic by-product attack of microbial species, antimicrobial properties can be viewed as a positive feature of glass-ionomers. As GIC materials are required to pass biocompatibility tests defined in standards such as ISO 7405 (ISO 2008) and ISO 10993 (ISO 2009), there will be limits to the level of antimicrobial action a GIC can possess. Antibiotics (ciprofloxacin and metronidazole) have been previously added to GICs and have been shown to increase the inhibitory effect of *Streptococcus mutans* and *Lactobacillus casei*. Furthermore, the addition of antibiotics increased the fluoride release of the GIC, possibly by the creation of voids that allow water ingress into the material (Prabhakar et al. 2013). Initial clinical trials have also shown the benefits of using GIC loaded with metronidazole, ciprofloxacin and cefaclor antibiotics in the sealing of infected dentine in atraumatic restoration in primary molars. However, to date, no commercial GIC is available that contains an antibiotic, and other additives considered safer could be the preferred path for future developments (Ferreira et al. 2013).

Silver nanoparticles (Ag NPs) have been known to possess antimicrobial properties by their ability to attach to the surface of bacterial cell membranes, thereby disturbing the functions of the cell. These have been incorporated into many different materials and demonstrate inhibitory effects against a range of bacteria. Polymer-silver nanoparticles, poly(vinyl alcohol)-silver nanoparticles as well as silver-doped hydroxyapatite have been reported (Sharma et al. 2009). Furthermore, through a micro-emulsion approach, AgNPs have been encapsulated in silica nano containers which allow for additional properties to be provided by the shell wall (Priebe and Fromm 2014). Non-nanoparticle strategies to deliver silver have also been used for coating nanofibres with silver ion releasing polymer coatings, which could be adapted for the use in GIC through the incorporation of similar nanofibrous scaffolds (Mohiti-Asli et al. 2014).

7.23 Future Pit and Fissure Sealing

Pit and fissure sealing of occlusal surfaces has principally been performed by resin sealants. Future GICs may possess "ideal" rheological and wetting properties to replace resin sealants, as well as all of the other properties that GICs possess, including the option of visible light-curing (VLC). The progressive stages of occlusal lesion formation have been described since well over a century ago (Bate 1864). Sealing fossae with an anti-cariogenic material is a logical protocol. Although low viscosity GICs lack the wear resistance of resin sealants, their dynamic interaction with the tooth together with excellent adhesive properties and bond longevity could make VLC and self-cured low viscosity GIC sealants for pit and fissure sealing a standard protocol in the future.

7.24 Participation in Future Pharmacological Approaches to Caries Reduction

The treatment of carious lesions can follow a number of protocols that generally involve the removal of the infected and affected carious regions. Although the "pharmacological" treatment of caries is not common, several treatment methods have been proposed. Silver fluoride has been used for some time to safely manage caries. The use of silver diamine fluoride, coated with potassium iodide to prevent staining processes, has been proposed (Knight 2007, 2008). These treatments have been shown to prevent biofilm formation (Knight et al. 2009) and have demonstrated that GICs can adequately bond to treated surfaces. Other pharmacological treatments may become available, and GICs are excellent choices for subsequent covering and sealing of the cavity, adding extra protection against further caries progression.

Conclusions

Future developments in GICs are likely to deliver improvements in strength, wear resistance and aesthetic properties. These improvements will allow the material to increase its longevity in load-bearing situations, thus allowing the material to become a viable alternative to amalgam restorations. Other new features likely to be focused on include optimising biomimetic, biomineralising or antimicrobial properties to provide new-generation GICs. Glass-ionomer cements will continue to be considered as "smart" materials due to their dynamic interaction with tooth structure and the surrounding environment.

References

Al-Naimi O, Itota T, Hobson R, Mccabe J. Fluoride release for restorative materials and its effect on biofilm formation in natural saliva. J Mater Sci Mater Med. 2008;19:1243–8.

Altunsoy M, Botsali MS, Korkut E, Kucukyilmaz E, Sener Y. Effect of different surface treatments on the shear and microtensile bond strength of resin-modified glass ionomer cement to dentin. Acta Odontol Scand. 2014;72:1–6.

Arbabzadeh-Zavareh F, Gibbs T, Meyers IA, Bouzari M, Mortazavi S, Walsh LJ. Recharge pattern of contemporary glass ionomer restoratives. Cord Conf Proc. 2012;9:139–45.

Atmeh AR, Chong EZ, Richard G, Festy F, Watson TF. Dentin-cement interfacial interaction: calcium silicates and polyalkenoates. J Dent Res. 2012;91:454–9.

Bakis C, Bank LC, Brown V, Cosenza E, Davalos J, Lesko J, Machida A, Rizkalla S, Triantafillou T. Fiber-reinforced polymer composites for construction-state-of-the-art review. J Compos Constr. 2002;6:73–87.

Bala O, Arisu HD, Yikilgan I, Arslan S, Gullu A. Evaluation of surface roughness and hardness of different glass ionomer cements. Eur J Dent. 2012;6:79–86.

Bate CS. The pathology of dental caries. Odontological Society of Great Britain London: Cox & Wyman; 1864.

Benelli EM, Serra MC, Rodrigues Jr AL, Cury JA. In situ anticariogenic potential of glass ionomer cement. Caries Res. 1993;27:280–4.

Blossey R. Self-cleaning surfaces – virtual realities. Nat Mater. 2003;2:301–6.

Boehm AJR, Peuker M, Walter A, Broyles BR, Oxman JD, Dubbe JW, Hartung MG, Guggenmos S. Mixer for mixing a dental composition. United States Patent Application 20110189059. 2011.

Burke FJ. Dental materials – what goes where? The current status of glass ionomer as a material for load-bearing restorations in posterior teeth. Dent Update. 2013;40:840–4.

Burke FJ. Reinforced glass-ionomer restorations. Dent Abstr. 2014;59, E79.

Busscher HJ, Rinastiti M, Siswomihardjo W, Van Der Mei HC. Biofilm formation on dental restorative and implant materials. J Dent Res. 2010;89:657–65.

Carlén A, Nikdel K, Wennerberg A, Holmberg K, Olsson J. Surface characteristics and in vitro biofilm formation on glass ionomer and composite resin. Biomaterials. 2001;22:481–7.

Cheetham JJW. Dental capsule. United States Patent Application 20140305816. 2014.

Cheetham JJ, Palamara JE, Tyas MJ, Burrow MF. A comparison of resin-modified glass-ionomer and resin composite polymerisation shrinkage stress in a wet environment. J Mech Behav Biomed Mater. 2014a;29:33–41.

Cheetham JJ, Palamara JEA, Tyas MJ, Burrow MF. Evaluation of the interfacial work of fracture of glass-ionomer cements bonded to dentin. J Mech Behav Biomed Mater. 2014b;29:427–37.

Colquhoun H, Klumperman B. Self-healing polymers. Polym Chem. 2013;4:4832–3.

Culbertson BM. Glass-ionomer dental restoratives. Prog Polym Sci. 2001;26:577–604.

Dabsie F, Gregoire G, Sixou M, Sharrock P. Does strontium play a role in the cariostatic activity of glass ionomer? Strontium diffusion and antibacterial activity. J Dent. 2009;37:554–9.

De Munck J, Mine A, Poitevin A, Van Ende A, Cardoso MV, Van Landuyt KL, Peumans M, Van Meerbeek B. Meta-analytical review of parameters involved in dentin bonding. J Dent Res. 2012;91:351–7.

Diem VT, Tyas MJ, Ngo HC, Phuong LH, Khanh ND. The effect of a nano-filled resin coating on the 3-year clinical performance of a conventional high-viscosity glass-ionomer cement. Clin Oral Investig. 2014;18:753–9.

Dimkov A, Nicholson JW, Gjorgievska E. On the possibility of incorporating antimicrobial components into glass-ionomer cements. Prilozi. 2009;30:219–37.

Dionysopoulos D, Koliniotou-Koumpia E, Helvatzoglou-Antoniades M, Kotsanos N. Fluoride release and recharge abilities of contemporary fluoride-containing restorative materials and dental adhesives. Dent Mater J. 2013;32:296–304.

El-Askary FS, Nassif MS. The effect of the pre-conditioning step on the shear bond strength of nano-filled resin-modified glass-ionomer to dentin. Eur J Dent. 2011;5:150–6.

El-Baky RMA, Hussien SM. Comparative antimicrobial activity and durability of different glass ionomer restorative materials with and without chlorohexidine. J Adv Biotech Bioeng. 2013;1:14–21.

Fareed MA, Stamboulis A. Effect of nanoclay dispersion on the properties of a commercial glass ionomer cement. Int J Biomater. 2014a.

Fareed MA, Stamboulis A. Nanoclays reinforced glass ionomer cements: dispersion and interaction of polymer grade (Pg) montmorillonite with poly(acrylic acid). J Mater Sci Mater Med. 2014;25:91–9.

Farokhzad OC, Langer R. Impact of nanotechnology on drug delivery. ACS Nano. 2009;3:16–20.

Ferracane JL. Resin composite—state of the art. Dent Mater. 2011;27:29–38.

Ferreira JM, Pinheiro SL, Sampaio FC, Menezes VA. Use of glass ionomer cement containing antibiotics to seal off infected dentin: a randomized clinical trial. Braz Dent J. 2013;24:68–73.

Fischer H. Polymer nanocomposites: from fundamental research to specific applications. Mater Sci Eng C. 2003;23:763–72.

Forsten L. Fluoride release and uptake by glass-ionomers and related materials and its clinical effect. Biomaterials. 1998;19:503–8.

Foster HA, Ditta IB, Varghese S, Steele A. Photocatalytic disinfection using titanium dioxide: spectrum and mechanism of antimicrobial activity. Appl Microbiol Biotechnol. 2011;90:1847–68.

Fukuda R, Yoshida Y, Nakayama Y, Okazaki M, Inoue S, Sano H, Suzuki K, Shintani H, Van Meerbeek B. Bonding efficacy of polyalkenoic acids to hydroxyapatite, enamel and dentin. Biomaterials. 2003;24:1861–7.

Garcia SJ. Effect of polymer architecture on the intrinsic self-healing character of polymers. Eur Polym J. 2014;53:118–25.

Gerdolle DA, Mortier E, Droz D. Microleakage and polymerization shrinkage of various polymer restorative materials. J Dent Child. 2008;75:125–33.

Ghosh P, Han G, De M, Kim CK, Rotello VM. Gold nanoparticles in delivery applications. Adv Drug Deliv Rev. 2008;60:1307–15.

Giray F, Peker S, Durmus B, Kargül B. Microleakage of new glass ionomer restorative materials in permanent teeth. Eur J Paediatr Dent. 2014;15:122–6.

Gu YW, Yap AU, Cheang P, Kumar R. Spheroidization of glass powders for glass ionomer cements. Biomaterials. 2004;25:4029–35.

Guan K. Relationship between photocatalytic activity, hydrophilicity and self-cleaning effect of Tio2/Sio2 films. Surf Coat Technol. 2005;191:155–60.

Guggenberger R, May R, Stefan K. New trends in glass-ionomer chemistry. Biomaterials. 1998;19:479–83.

Guida A, Hill RG, Towler MR, Eramo S. Fluoride release from model glass ionomer cements. J Mater Sci Mater Med. 2002;13:645–9.

Hamama HH, Burrow MF, Yiu C. Effect of dentine conditioning on adhesion of resin-modified glass ionomer adhesives. Aust Dent J. 2014;59:193–200.

Hammouda IM. Reinforcement of conventional glass-ionomer restorative material with short glass fibers. J Mech Behav Biomed Mater. 2009;2:73–81.

Han L, Okiji T. Evaluation of the ions release / incorporation of the prototype S-Prg filler-containing endodontic sealer. Dent Mater J. 2011.

Hatanaka K, Irie M, Tjandrawinata R, Suzuki K. Effect of spherical silica filler addition on immediate interfacial Gap-formation in class V cavity and mechanical properties of resin-modified glass-ionomer cement. Dent Mater J. 2006;25:415–22.

Hengtrakool C, Pearson GJ, Wilson M. Interaction between GIC and S. sanguis biofilms: antibacterial properties and changes of surface hardness. J Dent. 2006;34:588–97.

Hoare TR, Kohane DS. Hydrogels in drug delivery: progress and challenges. Polymer. 2008;49:1993–2007.

Hokii Y, Yoshimitsu R, Yamamoto K, Fukushima S, Fusejima F, Kumagai T. Protection of enamel-glass ionomer restorative margins by resin-coatings. Dent Mater. 2014;30 Suppl 1:E107.

Hook ER, Owen OJ, Bellis CA, Holder JA, O'sullivan DJ, Barbour ME. Development of a novel antimicrobial-releasing glass ionomer cement functionalized with chlorhexidine hexametaphosphate nanoparticles. J Nanobiotechnol. 2014;12:3.

Huo X, Torres V, Elsner O, Pfefferkorn F. Texture analysis of glass ionomers. IADR 89th General Session San Diego, USA, 2011.

Irie M, Nagaoka N, Tamada Y, Maruo Y, Nishigawa G, Minagi S, Finger WJ. Effect of spherical silica additions on marginal gaps and compressive strength of experimental glass-ionomer cements. Am J Dent. 2011;24:310–4.

ISO 2008. ISO 7405:2008 Dentistry-evaluation of biocompatibility of medical devices used in dentistry.

ISO 2009. International Standards Organisation 10993 – biological evaluation of medical devices part 1: evaluation and testing.

Jayabal J, Mahesh R. Current state of topical antimicrobial therapy in management of early childhood caries. ISRN Dent. 2014;2014:5.

Jones FH, Hutton BM, Hadley PC, Eccles AJ, Steele TA, Billington RW, Pearson GJ. Fluoride uptake by glass ionomer cements: – a surface analysis approach. Biomaterials. 2003;24:107–19.

Kamijo K, Mukai Y, Tominaga T, Iwaya I, Fujino F, Hirata Y, Teranaka T. Fluoride release and recharge characteristics of denture base resins containing surface pre-reacted glass-ionomer filler. Dent Mater J. 2009;28:227–33.

Kawano F, Kon M, Kobayashi M, Miyai K. Reinforcement effect of short glass fibers with Cao–P2o5–Sio2–Al2o3 glass on strength of glass-ionomer cement. J Dent. 2001;29:377–80.

Kazunori K, Glenn SK, Masayuki Y, Teruo O, Yasuhisa S. Block copolymer micelles as vehicles for drug delivery. J Control Release. 1993;24:119–32.

Knight GM. The pharmacological management of caries. Dental Asia, September/October 2007.

Knight GM. The pharmacological management of dentine to protect against plaque microorganism degradation. PhD thesis, University of Adelaide; 2008.

Knight GM, Mcintyre JM, Craig G, Zilm PS, Gully N. Inability to form a biofilm of Streptococcus mutans on silver fluoride-and potassium iodide-treated demineralized dentin. Quin Int. 2009;40:155.

Korkmaz Y, Ozel E, Attar N, Ozge Bicer C. Influence of different conditioning methods on the shear bond strength of novel light-curing nano-ionomer restorative to enamel and dentin. Lasers Med Sci. 2010;25:861–6.

Latta M, Gross SM, Mchale WA. Microencapsulated compositions and methods for tissue mineralization. United States Patent Application 8889161. 2014.

Lazaridou D, Belli R, Kramer N, Petschelt A, Lohbauer U. Dental materials for primary dentition: are they suitable for occlusal restorations? A two-body wear study. Eur Arch Paediatr Dent. 2015;16(2):165–72.

Lloyd CH, Adamson M. The development of fracture toughness and fracture strength in posterior restorative materials. Dent Mater. 1987;3:225–31.

Lohani A, Singh G, Bhattacharya SS, Verma A. Interpenetrating polymer networks as innovative drug delivery systems. J Drug Deliv. 2014;2014:583612.

Lohbauer U. Dental glass ionomer cements as permanent filling materials?–Properties, limitations and future trends. Materials. 2009;3:76–96.

Lohbauer U, Walker J, Nikolaenko S, Werner J, Clare A, Petschelt A, Greil P. Reactive fibre reinforced glass ionomer cements. Biomaterials. 2003;24:2901–7.

Lohbauer U, Frankenberger R, Clare A, Petschelt A, Greil P. Toughening of dental glass ionomer cements with reactive glass fibres. Biomaterials. 2004;25:5217–25.

Mackey TK, Contreras JT, Liang BA. The Minamata convention on mercury: attempting to address the global controversy of dental amalgam use and mercury waste disposal. Sci Total Environ. 2014;472:125–9.

Manuja N, Nagpal R, Pandit IK. Dental adhesion: mechanism, techniques and durability. J Clin Pediatr Dent. 2012;36:223–34.

Mckinney JE, Antonucci JM, Rupp NW. Wear and microhardness of glass-ionomer cements. J Dent Res. 1987;66:1134–9.

Mckinney JE, Antonucci JM, Rupp NW. Wear and microhardness of a silver-sintered glass-ionomer cement. J Dent Res. 1988;67:831–5.

Mei ML, Li Q-L, Chu C-H, Lo EC-M, Samaranayake LP. Antibacterial effects of silver diamine fluoride on multi-species cariogenic biofilm on caries. Ann Clin Microbiol Antimicrob. 2013;12:4.

Mitsuhashi A, Hanaoka K, Teranaka T. Fracture toughness of resin-modified glass ionomer restorative materials: effect of powder/liquid ratio and powder particle size reduction on fracture toughness. Dent Mater. 2003;19:747–57.

Mohiti-Asli M, Pourdeyhimi B, Loboa EG. Novel, silver-ion-releasing nanofibrous scaffolds exhibit excellent antibacterial efficacy without the use of silver nanoparticles. Acta Biomater. 2014;10: 2096–104.

Moshaverinia A, Ansari S, Moshaverinia M, Roohpour N, Darr JA, Rehman I. Effects of incorporation of hydroxyapatite and fluoroapatite nanobioceramics into conventional glass ionomer cements (GIC). Acta Biomater. 2008;4:432–40.

Moshaverinia A, Brantley WA, Chee WWL, Rohpour N, Ansari S, Zheng F, Heshmati RH, Darr JA, Schricker SR, Rehman IU. Measure of microhardness, fracture toughness and flexural strength of N-vinylcaprolactam (NVC)-containing glass-ionomer dental cements. Dent Mater. 2010;26:1137–43.

Moshaverinia A, Roohpour N, Chee WW, Schricker SR. A review of powder modifications in conventional glass-ionomer dental cements. J Mater Chem. 2011;21:1319–28.

Nicholson JW. Chemistry of glass-ionomer cements: a review. Biomaterials. 1998;19:485–94.

Ogledzki M, Perry RD, Kugel G. Translucency of resin modified glass ionomer restoratives. AADR annual meeting, Tampa; 21–24 Mar 2012.

Osorio R, Osorio E, Medina-Castillo AL, Toledano M. Polymer nanocarriers for dentin adhesion. J Dent Res. 2014;93(12):1258–63.

Perdigão J. Dentin bonding – variables related to the clinical situation and the substrate treatment. Dent Mater. 2010;26:E24–37.

Peterson AM, Kotthapalli H, Rahmathullah MAM, Palmese GR. Investigation of interpenetrating polymer networks for self-healing applications. Compos Sci Technol. 2012;72:330–6.

Peumans M, Kanumilli P, De Munck J, Van Landuyt K, Lambrechts P, Van Meerbeek B. Clinical effectiveness of contemporary adhesives: a systematic review of current clinical trials. Dent Mater. 2005;21: 864–81.

Powis D, Folleràs T, Merson S, Wilson A. Materials science improved adhesion of a glass ionomer cement to dentin and enamel. J Dent Res. 1982;61:1416–22.

Prabhakar AR, Prahlad D, Kumar SR. Antibacterial activity, fluoride release, and physical properties of an antibiotic-modified glass ionomer cement. Pediatr Dent. 2013;35:411–5.

Priebe M, Fromm KM. One-pot synthesis and catalytic properties of encapsulated silver nanoparticles in silica nanocontainers. Part Part Syst Char. 2014;31(6):645–51.

Qizheng C, Xiangting D, Weili Y, Jinxian W, Huiru W, Xiaofeng Y, Xiaohui Y. New developments of inorganic nanofibers fabricated by electrospinning. Rare Met Mater Eng. 2006;35:1167.

Roche KJ, Stanton KT. Precipitation of biomimetic fluorhydroxyapatite/polyacrylic acid nanostructures. J Cryst Growth. 2015;409:80–8.

Samadzadeh M, Boura SH, Peikari M, Kasiriha S, Ashrafi A. A review on self-healing coatings based on micro/nanocapsules. Prog Org Coat. 2010;68:159–64.

Seemann R, Flury S, Pfefferkorn F, Lussi A, Noack MJ. Restorative dentistry and restorative materials over the next 20 years: a Delphi survey. Dent Mater. 2014;30(4):442–8.

Sennou HE, Lebugle AA, Gregoire GL. X-Ray photoelectron spectroscopy study of the dentin-glass ionomer cement interface. Dent Mater. 1999;15:229–37.

Seppa L, Forss H, Øgaard B. The effect of fluoride application on fluoride release and the antibacterial action of glass lonomers. J Dent Res. 1993;72:1310–4.

Setien VJ, Armstrong SR, Wefel JS. Interfacial fracture toughness between resin-modified glass ionomer and dentin using three different surface treatments. Dent Mater. 2005;21:498–504.

Sharma VK, Yngard RA, Lin Y. Silver nanoparticles: green synthesis and their antimicrobial activities. Adv Colloid Interface Sci. 2009;145:83–96.

Shimazu K, Ogata K, Karibe H. Caries-preventive effect of fissure sealant containing surface reaction-type pre-reacted glass ionomer filler and bonded by self-etching primer. J Clin Pediatr Dent. 2012;36: 343–7.

Shiozawa M, Takahashi H, Iwasaki N. Fluoride release and mechanical properties after 1-year water storage of recent restorative glass ionomer cements. Clin Oral Investig. 2013;18:1–8.

Smith DC. Development of glass-ionomer cement systems. Biomaterials. 1998;19:467–78.

Steinberg D. Studying plaque biofilms on various dental surfaces. In: An Y, Friedman R, editors. Handbook of bacterial adhesion. Totowa, NJ: Humana Press; 2000.

Suzuki YI-K, Aoyagi S, Kaneko M, Mukasa Y. Vacuum assisted mixer for capsule of dental restoration material. United States Patent Application 6776516. 2004.

Teughels W, Van Assche N, Sliepen I, Quirynen M. Effect of material characteristics and/or surface topography on biofilm development. Clin Oral Implants Res. 2006;17:68–81.

Tezvergil-Mutluay A, Mutluay M, Seseogullari-Dirihan R, Agee KA, Key WO, Scheffel DL, Breschi L, Mazzoni A, Tjaderhane L, Nishitani Y, Tay FR, Pashley DH. Effect of phosphoric acid on the degradation of human dentin matrix. J Dent Res. 2013;92:87–91.

Tyas MJ. Cariostatic effect of glass ionomer cement: a five-year clinical study. Aust Dent J. 1991;36:236–9.

Tyas MJ. Milestones in adhesion: glass-ionomer cements. J Adhes Dent. 2003;5:259–66.

Van Amerongen WE. Dental caries under glass ionomer restorations. J Public Health Dent. 1996;56:150–4; discussion 161–3.

Van Duinen RNB, Kleverlaan CJ, De Gee AJ, Werner A, Feilzer AJ. Early and long-term wear of 'fast-Set' conventional glass–ionomer cements. Dent Mater. 2005;21:716–20.

Van Meerbeek B, De Munck J, Yoshida Y, Inoue S, Vargas M, Vijay P, Van Landuyt K, Lambrechts P, Vanherle G. Adhesion to enamel and dentin: current status and future challenges. Oper Dent. 2003;28:215–35.

Van Meerbeek B, Peumans M, Poitevin A, Mine A, Van Ende A, Neves A, De Munck J. Relationship between bond-strength tests and clinical outcomes. Dent Mater. 2010;26:E100–21.

Walls A. Glass polyalkenoate (glass-ionomer) cements: a review. J Dent. 1986;14:231–46.

Weng Y. Advanced antibacterial glass ionomer cements for improved dental restoratives. PhD 3481168, Purdue University; 2011.

Weng Y, Howard L, Xie D. A novel star-shaped poly (carboxylic acid) for resin-modified glass-ionomer restoratives. J Biomater Sci Polym Ed. 2014;18:1–15.

Wessel C, Ostermann R, Dersch R, Smarsly BM. Formation of inorganic nanofibers from preformed TiO2 nanoparticles via electrospinning. J Phys Chem C. 2010;115:362–72.

Williams JA, Billington RW, Pearson GJ. Comparison of Ion release from a glass ionomer cement as a function of the method of incorporation of added ions. Biomaterials. 1999;20:589–94.

Williams JA, Billington RW, Pearson GJ. The glass ionomer cement: the sources of soluble fluoride. Biomaterials. 2002;23:2191–200.

Wilson AD. Acidobasicity of oxide glasses used in glass ionomer cements. Dent Mater. 1996;12:25–9.

Wilson AD, Nicholson JW. Acid–base cements: their biomedical and industrial applications. New York, NY, USA: Cambridge University Press; 2005.

Wilson GO, Andersson HM, White SR, Sottos NR, Moore JS, Braun PV. Self-healing polymers. In: Encyclopedia of polymer science and technology. Hoboken, NJ: Wiley-Interscience. 2010.

Wu N, Xia X, Wei Q, Huang F. Preparation and properties of organic/inorganic hybrid nanofibres. Fibres and Textiles in Eastern Europe. 2010;18(78):21–3.

Wu W, Xie D, Puckett A, Mays JW. Synthesis and formulation of vinyl-containing polyacids for improved light-cured glass-ionomer cements. Eur Polym J. 2003;39:663–70.

Wu DY, Meure S, Solomon D. Self-healing polymeric materials: a review of recent developments. Prog Polym Sci. 2008;33:479–522.

Xie D, Brantley WA, Culbertson BM, Wang G. Mechanical properties and microstructures of glass-ionomer cements. Dent Mater. 2000;16:129–38.

Xie D, Zhao J, Weng Y. Synthesis and application of novel multi-arm poly(carboxylic acid)s for glass-ionomer restoratives. J Biomater Appl. 2010;24:419–36.

Xie D, Weng Y, Guo X, Zhao J, Gregory RL, Zheng C. Preparation and evaluation of a novel glass-ionomer cement with antibacterial functions. Dent Mater. 2011;27:487–96.

Xu HH, Moreau JL, Sun L, Chow LC. Nanocomposite containing amorphous calcium phosphate nanoparticles for caries inhibition. Dent Mater. 2011;27:762–9.

Yamazaki T, Schricker SR, Brantley WA, Culbertson BM, Johnston W. Viscoelastic behavior and fracture toughness of six glass-ionomer cements. J Prosthet Dent. 2006;96:266–72.

Yelamanchili A, Darvell BW. Network competition in a resin-modified glass-ionomer cement. Dent Mater. 2008;24:1065–9.

Yiu CK, Tay FR, King NM, Pashley DH, Carvalho RM, Carrilho MR. Interaction of resin-modified glass-ionomer cements with moist dentine. J Dent. 2004a;32:521–30.

Yiu CK, Tay FR, King NM, Pashley DH, Sidhu SK, Neo JC, Toledano M, Wong SL. Interaction of glass-ionomer cements with moist dentin. J Dent Res. 2004b;83:283–9.

Yli-Urpo H, Narhi T, Soderling E. Antimicrobial effects of glass ionomer cements containing bioactive glass (S53p4) on oral micro-organisms in vitro. Acta Odontol Scand. 2003;61:241–6.

Yoshida Y, Van Meerbeek B, Nakayama Y, Snauwaert J, Hellemans L, Lambrechts P, Vanherle G, Wakasa K. Evidence of chemical bonding at biomaterial-hard tissue interfaces. J Dent Res. 2000;79:709–14.

Young S, Wong M, Tabata Y, Mikos AG. Gelatin as a delivery vehicle for the controlled release of bioactive molecules. J Control Release. 2005;109:256–74.

Yuan Y, Yin T, Rong M, Zhang M. Self healing in polymers and polymer composites. Concepts, realization and outlook: a review. Exp Polym Lett. 2008;2:238–50.

Zalizniak I, Palamara JE, Wong RH, Cochrane NJ, Burrow MF, Reynolds EC. Ion release and physical properties of CPP-ACP modified GIC in acid solutions. J Dent. 2013;41:449–54.

Zhang M, Bando Y, Wada K, Kurashima K. Synthesis of nanotubes and nanowires of silicon oxide. J Mater Sci Lett. 1999;18:1911–3.

Zhang L, Tang T, Zhang ZL, Liang B, Wang XM, Fu BP. Improvement of enamel bond strengths for conventional and resin-modified glass ionomers: acid-etching vs. conditioning. J Zhejiang Univ Sci B. 2013;14:1013–24.

Zhao J, Weng Y, Xie D. In vitro wear and fracture toughness of an experimental light-cured glass–ionomer cement. Dent Mater. 2009;25:526–34.

Zhou F-L, Gong R-H. Manufacturing technologies of polymeric nanofibres and nanofibre yarns. Polym Int. 2008;57:837–45.

Zoergiebel J, Ilie N. Evaluation of a conventional glass ionomer cement with new zinc formulation: effect of coating, aging and storage agents. Clin Oral Investig. 2013;17:619–26.

Index

S.K. Sidhu (ed.), *Glass-Ionomers in Dentistry*, DOI 10.1007/978-3-319-22626-2

MIX
Papier aus verantwortungsvollen Quellen
Paper from responsible sources
FSC® C105338

If you have any concerns about our products,
you can contact us on
ProductSafety@springernature.com

In case Publisher is established outside the EU,
the EU authorized representative is:
Springer Nature Customer Service Center GmbH
Europaplatz 3, 69115 Heidelberg, Germany

Printed by Libri Plureos GmbH
in Hamburg, Germany